Radiotherapy for Head and Neck Cancers

Indications and Techniques

THIRD EDITION

■■ **K. KIAN ANG, MD, PHD**

Professor of Radiation Oncology
Gilbert H. Fletcher Distinguished Chair
Department of Radiation Oncology
The University of Texas M.D. Anderson Cancer Center
Houston, Texas

■■ **ADAM S. GARDEN, MD**

Professor of Radiation Oncology
Section Chief, Head and Neck Radiation Oncology
Department of Radiation Oncology
The University of Texas M.D. Anderson Cancer Center
Houston, Texas

◆ LIPPINCOTT WILLIAMS & WILKINS
A **Wolters Kluwer** Company

Philadelphia • Baltimore • New York • London
Buenos Aires • Hong Kong • Sydney • Tokyo

Acquisitions Editor: Jonathan W. Pine, Jr.
Managing Editor: Anne E. Jacobs
Project Manager: Alicia Jackson
Senior Manufacturing Manager: Benjamin Rivera
Associate Director of Marketing: Adam Glazer
Creative Director: Doug Smock
Production Services: Laserwords Private Limited
Printer: Quebecor World-Kingsport

© 2006 by Lippincott Williams & Wilkins
530 Walnut Street
Philadelphia, PA 19106

1st Edition: 1993 by Lea & Febiger
2nd Edition: 2002 by Lippincott Williams & Wilkins

Library of Congress Cataloging-in-Publication Data

Ang, K. K. (K. Kian)
    Radiotherapy for head and neck cancers : indications and techniques / K. Kian Ang, Adam S. Garden.
    -- 3rd ed.
        p. ; cm.
    Includes bibliographical references and index.
    ISBN 0-7817-6093-3
    1. Head--Cancer--Radiotherapy. 2. Neck--Cancer--Radiotherapy. I. Garden, Adam S. II. Title.
    [DNLM: 1. Head and Neck Neoplasms--radiotherapy. 2. Radiotherapy--methods. WE 707 A581r 2006]
RC280.H4A54 2006
616.99'4910642--dc22

                            2005021780

Care has been taken to confirm the accuracy of the information presented and to describe generally accepted practices. However, the authors, editors, and publisher are not responsible for errors or omissions or for any consequences from application of the information in this book and make no warranty, expressed or implied, with respect to the currency, completeness, or accuracy of the contents of the publication. Application of this information in a particular situation remains the professional responsibility of the practitioner.

The authors, editors, and publisher have exerted every effort to ensure that drug selection and dosage set forth in this text are in accordance with current recommendations and practice at the time of publication. However, in view of ongoing research, changes in government regulations, and the constant flow of information relating to drug therapy and drug reactions, the reader is urged to check the package insert for each drug for any change in indications and dosage and for added warnings and precautions. This is particularly important when the recommended agent is a new or infrequently employed drug.

Some drugs and medical devices presented in this publication have Food and Drug Administration (FDA) clearance for limited use in restricted research settings. It is the responsibility of health care providers to ascertain the FDA status of each drug or device planned for use in their clinical practice.

The publishers have made every effort to trace copyright holders for borrowed material. If they have inadvertently overlooked any, they will be pleased to make the necessary arrangements at the first opportunity.

To purchase additional copies of this book, call our customer service department at (800) 638-3030 or fax orders to (301) 824-7390. Lippincott Williams & Wilkins customer service representatives are available from 8:30 am to 6:30 pm, EST, Monday through Friday, for telephone access. Visit Lippincott Williams & Wilkins on the Internet: http://www.lww.com.

10 9 8 7 6 5 4 3 2 1

Contents

iii

Preface

The first two editions of this book summarized the treatment philosophy and the radiotherapy techniques for the management of patients with head and neck cancer as practiced at The University of Texas M.D. Anderson Cancer Center up to 2001. Although the compilation of resident teaching materials began in the mid-1980s, it was the encouragement by many visitors who found this type of practical handbook useful for day-to-day reference that stimulated us to publish the first edition of this book in 1993. We received many constructive comments and suggestions and benefited from exchange of ideas that resulted from the publication of this work.

Many randomized clinical trials testing the value of radiobiologically sound-altered regimens and combinations of radiation with cytotoxic agents were designed and completed in the 1990s. The emergence of results of critical clinical trials gradually changed the treatment methodologies during the late 1990s. Therefore, it was necessary to update the manual. So, the second edition was completed in the latter part of 2001.

Innovations in computerized radiotherapy planning and delivery technology have picked up momentum in changing the philosophy and practice training of head and neck radiation oncology. The ability to deliver high doses of radiation to target volumes of irregular shapes while minimizing exposure to close but uninvolved normal tissues by intensity-modulated radiation therapy (IMRT) offers the prospect to reduce rather taxing morbidity such as xerostomia. This development opens the possibility of defining different regions with various densities and the probability of tumor infestation instead of outlining a broad initial target volume and a cone-down to boost volume usually on the basis of surface and bony landmarks. Therefore, a new terminology has been introduced to describe such approach. In terms of actual radiation treatment, there is a general move from delivering a homogenous dose at each fraction and reducing the size of target volume after a defined number of fractions of therapy to delivering the radiation in a fixed number of fractions but varying the dose per fraction, and therefore the total dose, to distinct target volumes that are judged to have different densities of infestation. Expertise in defining the target volumes is, however, essential to safely implement and benefit from this elegant mode of treatment delivery. Knowledge about head and neck anatomy, proficiency in performing clinical head and neck examination (including endoscopy), understanding the pattern of disease extension, and familiarity with head and neck imaging are critical elements for making a successful transition.

Encouraged by the promising results of single institutional trials, the use of IMRT in the treatment of head and neck carcinoma is increasing at a rapid pace, although the concept of target delineation and the technical aspects are still evolving. This third edition provides a more systematic description of general principles, nomenclature, and examples of IMRT as we practice in our center.

Preface to the Second Edition

The first edition of this book summarized the treatment philosophy and radiotherapy techniques for management of patients with head and neck cancer as practiced at The University of Texas M.D. Anderson Cancer Center up to 1992. Many residents and radiation oncologists have found this handbook practical and useful for training and day-to-day reference. We received many constructive comments and suggestions and benefited from exchange of ideas resulting from the publication of this work.

The last decade has witnessed many exciting accomplishments in head and neck cancer research. Design and completion of key randomized clinical trials testing the value of radiobiologically sound new radiation regimens and combination of radiation with cytotoxic agents have changed the standard of care for a number of head and neck cancers. Astonishing advancements of molecular biology methodology and concepts and emergence of new data have improved our understanding of the carcinogenesis and behavior of a number of head and neck cancers; these serve as the basis for the development of novel multidisciplinary therapy strategies. Many new therapy approaches are undergoing preclinical studies and a few have moved on to phase I–II clinical trials.

Innovations in physics, dosimetry, and radiation delivery technology have generated enthusiasm for thorough testing of the value of conformal, precision radiotherapy in increasing the efficacy and/or reducing the morbidity of radiotherapy, leading to improvement of quality of life.

As a result, the treatment philosophy and techniques for a number of tumor sites and stages have been continuously refined since the publication of the first edition. We realized the need for updating the handbook a few years ago but competing commitments have delayed such undertaking until now. Upon request of many colleagues and trainees, we also incorporate common prescriptions, frequently used supportive care guidelines, and dosimetry principles and examples.

Preface to the First Edition

Primary cancers of the head and neck region are relatively rare. The estimated yearly number of new cases, excluding skin cancers located in the head and neck area, is about 42,000, which represents 4% to 5% of the total number of cancers diagnosed per annum in the United States. Although the vast majority of head and neck cancers arise from epithelial elements, their natural history differs considerably according to the disease location. This is related to regional anatomical peculiarities that dictate patterns of contiguous and lymphatic spread. The extent of the lesion and the presence of numerous critical normal tissues in the head and neck area, injury to which could result in serious functional impairment, are obstacles to local-regional disease eradication. Therefore, failure to achieve local-regional control is the leading cause of cancer-related death in patients with head and neck neoplasms.

Radiotherapy plays a very important role in the management of patients with head and neck cancers. In early-stage lesions, radiotherapy is frequently preferred because it is as effective as surgery in controlling the disease and is generally better in preserving cosmetic and organ functions. In advanced tumors, radiation treatment is complementary to surgery in obtaining maximal local-regional control. Sound knowledge of the behavior of various head and neck cancers is essential for selecting proper indications for radiotherapy for different subsets of patients. Thorough command of the regional anatomy, technical bases of radiotherapy, and awareness of available data on radiation effects on critical normal tissues are necessary for optimizing the treatment outcome. The choice of radiation target volume and dose is based on the best trade-off between control probability and likelihood of severe treatment-induced complication.

The natural history of head and neck cancers, general treatment strategies and therapy results obtained at different institutions are summarized in a number of textbooks and chapters. However, so far there is no handbook on the technical detail of radiotherapy for head and neck cancers. This manual serves as a practical reference to head and neck radiotherapy. We chose to present the basic concepts and specific indications and techniques for various common types of head and neck cancers, i.e., carcinoma and melanoma, as practiced at The University of Texas M.D. Anderson Cancer Center rather than compiling all available techniques in an encyclopedic fashion. The treatment policies described in this manual evolved during the past one-half century through gradual refinements based on results of systematic analysis of causes of failure and complications in cohorts of patients treated in a disciplined and consistent way. This philosophy introduced by the late Dr. Gilbert H. Fletcher has continued to the present day.

Acknowledgments

We wish to thank our family members for their support for the completion of this task, our mentors for training and for guiding us to pursue an academic career, and our trainees for the stimulating discussions.

We appreciate the contribution of members of the Head and Neck Radiation Oncology Service for continuously refining the treatment strategy, technique, and delivery procedure and for providing valuable feedback in shaping the third edition. The contribution of Dr. Mark Chambers in updating the guidelines for dental care is acknowledged. We are also grateful to our patients for participating in many clinical studies and thereby contributing to continuous refinement of therapy.

Many of the treatment policies described in this manual have been developed through a long track record of program project grant funding, PO1 CA06294, awarded by the National Institutes of Health. The Gilbert H. Fletcher Distinguished Chair provided supplemental support for the revision of this manual. We would also like to thank Ms. Cathy Ramirez for administrative assistance.

PART 1

General Principles of Head and Neck Radiotherapy

The head and neck region contains numerous delicate, intricately organized organs essential for basic physiologic functions and critical for appearance, expression, and social interactions. Although representing approximately 4% of cancers, a variety of neoplasms with diverging natural histories arise in this relatively small body region. Depending on the site, size, and pattern of spread, head and neck cancers can cause varying degrees of structural deformations and functional handicaps compromising well-being, self-esteem, and social integration. In addition, treatments of head and neck tumors can induce additional mutilations, worsening quality of life. These features make head and neck cancers very challenging to manage. Knowledge of the basic principles of oncology and expertise in patient assessment and in individual specialty are essential for staging workup of patients and for treatment selection. Integrated interdisciplinary collaborations among surgical, radiation, medical, and dental oncologists and oncologist interaction with pathologists, radiologists, plastic surgeons, nurses, speech pathologists, and other health care personnel are essential ingredients for optimal management and rehabilitation of head and neck cancer patients. Well-functioning, coordinated care is essential to yield the highest complication-free cure rate with maximal cosmetic and functional outcome.

Close collaborations between radiation oncologists, dosimetrists, medical physicists, radiation radiotherapists (technologists), and oncology nurses are important to deliver high-quality radiation treatment. The first part of this manual describes the basic principles of radiation oncology relevant for head and neck radiotherapy along with guidelines and examples of general supportive care during and after radiation treatment.

Overview

Head and neck cancers have been the subject of intensive laboratory research and clinical investigations. Recent advances in molecular biology techniques have facilitated research addressing molecular epidemiology, genetic predisposition, genetic tumor progression models, and so on. Because of the ease of clinical assessment and a relatively low incidence of systemic spread, head and neck cancers are good models for testing the efficacy of new therapy concepts that are aimed primarily at improving local-regional disease control. Most of the clinical radiobiology research on altered fractionations, for example, has been conducted on patients with locally advanced head and neck cancers. Such long-term investment in cancer research has come to fruition for certain cancers. After increasing for decades, the mortality rate of most cancers in the United States has decreased since 1975 (1). Many advances have been achieved in the understanding of the biology, natural history, and treatment of head and neck cancers. A detailed depiction of recent progress is beyond the scope of this handbook—this brief introductory summary highlights a few interesting evolving concepts and recent findings of clinical interest in the carcinogenesis, biology, and treatment of head and neck cancers.

MOLECULAR BIOLOGY AND ECOGENETICS

The molecular tumor progression model was initially proposed by Fearon and Vogelstein (2). This model states that tumors progress by activating oncogenes and by inactivating tumor suppressor genes (TSGs), each producing a growth advantage for a clonal population of cells, and that specific genetic events usually occur in a distinct order (multistep carcinogenesis) that is not necessarily the same for each tumor. For head and neck carcinomas, Califano and associates (3) described a preliminary tumor progression model using allelic loss or imbalance as a molecular marker for oncogene amplification or TSG inactivation. They identified *p16* (9p21), *p53* (17p), and *Rb* (13q) as candidate TSGs, and cyclin D1 (11q13) as a candidate proto-oncogene. The results of this work support the initial observations of the colorectal molecular progression model, in that clonal genetic changes occur early in the histopathologic continuum of tumor progression. About one third of histopathologically benign squamous hyperplasias already consist of a clonal population of cells with shared genetic anomalies characterizing head and neck cancer. Identification of such early events facilitates discovery of genetic alterations associated with further transformation and aggressive clinical behavior. With further validation, this knowledge will contribute a great deal to the development of screening strategies focusing on the earlier steps of the estimated ten or more genetic alterations required to generate an invasive tumor phenotype and to the conception of early pharmacologic or genetic therapy approaches.

Tobacco and alcohol exposure have long been recognized as the dominant risk factors in head and neck carcinogenesis. Although their consumption was estimated to account for approximately three fourths of oral and pharyngeal carcinomas in the United States (4), neoplasms develop in only a small fraction of exposed individuals. This intriguing information raised the notion of the contribution of genetic susceptibility or predisposition and other cofactors (for examples of cofactors, see "Virus Etiology" section) to carcinogenesis. The potential pathways are thought to include genetic polymorphism influencing environmental carcinogen absorption and detoxification, individual sensitivity to carcinogen-induced genotypic alterations, and so on. These ideas can now be tested more comprehensively because of recent progress in molecular biology concepts and assay methodology. For example, the ability to identify smokers with a high risk of development of cancer will have important practical clinical implications in selecting individuals for more aggressive screening programs or for enrollment into intensive chemoprevention trials (see subsequent text).

VIRAL ETIOLOGY

Nasopharyngeal carcinoma (NPC) has been an excellent model for studying viral etiology in human cancer. Although the association between *Epstein-Barr virus* (EBV) and NPC was recognized for about four decades, major progress has been made in this field only recently. For example, the EBV genome was characterized (reviewed by Liebowitz [5]) to consist of a linear, 172-kb, double-stranded DNA having five unique sequences separated by four internal repeats and two terminal repeats. The DNA circularizes by homologous recombination at random locations within terminal repeats in the nucleus of infected cells. The length of terminal repeat is therefore specific for each infected cell, and this is the basis for clonality assay, which may be useful in determining the putative primary tumor in patients presenting with nodal metastasis from an unknown source. The genome encodes several families of proteins, such as early antigens (EAs), Epstein-Barr nuclear antigens (EBNAs), and latency membrane proteins (LMPs). Many of these proteins control viral behavior and affect cell proliferation regulatory mechanisms, and are thought to play a role in transformation and carcinogenesis and to influence tumor response to therapy. EBNA-1 regulates viral genome replication during cell division and was found to induce growth and dedifferentiation of an NPC cell line not infected by EBV (6). LMP-1 seems to alter growth of epithelial cells and induce well-differentiated squamous carcinomas from human epithelial cell-line transfectants, and is associated with bcl-2 expression in tumors (7,8).

More work has been done on the molecular genetics of NPC. Many NPCs were found to have deletions of the short arm, or some regions of the short arm, of chromosomes 3 and 9, suggesting the possibility of the existence of TSGs in these regions (9,10). For example, more recent studies (11,12) revealed that the combined frequency for chromosome 3p/9p (bearing *p16* and *RASSF1A*) losses in the normal nasopharyngeal epithelium among southern Chinese in Hong Kong (a population at high risk for NPC) was 82.6% as opposed to 20% in the low-risk populations. In contrast, latent EBV infection was detected only in high-grade nasopharyngeal dysplasia or in NPC. Consequently, it was postulated that the abnormal genetic changes in chromosomes 3p and 9 predispose nasopharyngeal cells to sustain latent EBV infection, and this combination promotes a cascade of events leading to malignancy.

The causal relation between *human papillomaviruses* (HPV) and some human neoplasms has been established, particularly for carcinoma of the uterine cervix. Nearly all cervical cancers contain integrated HPV-DNA, most commonly of high-risk types HPV-16 and HPV-18n (13). Cell culture studies clearly demonstrated that the high-risk HPVs can transform and immortalize epithelial cells from cervix, foreskin, and oral cavity (14–16). In contrast, HPV-6 and HPV-11, associated more often with benign lesions, do not possess this capability (17,18). Expression of *E6* and *E7* open reading frames of HPV-16 or HPV-18 genome is sufficient for immortalization (19,20).

The potential role of HPV in head and neck carcinogenesis has attracted more attention recently (reviewed by Herrero [21]). Carcinomas of the tonsil, oral tongue, and floor of mouth were found to have a relatively high prevalence of HPV-DNA (22–24). A high proportion of verrucous carcinomas—rare, locally invasive carcinomas with papillomatous morphology—are also associated with HPV (25,26). Verrucous carcinomas of the larynx predominantly contain HPV-6, HPV-11, or HPV-16, or related DNA (25,27). The evidence for the role of HPVs in carcinogenesis of tonsillar carcinomas is increasing because these tumors not only contain HPV-DNA in most of the cells but also express readily detectable levels of HPV-RNA (28). In a series of 253 patients, Gillison and associates (29) detected HPV in 25% of tumors, with HPV-16 present in 90% of the positive neoplasms. The presence of HPV was most frequent in oropharyngeal carcinoma occurring in individuals with no history of smoking and alcohol consumption, having basaloid subtype without TP53 mutation. Laboratory data showing that transcriptionally active, integrated HPV-16 DNA persisting in an oral carcinoma cell line having features indistinguishable from those of the primary tumor (30) provide strong evidence of an active role of HPV in carcinogenesis.

Knowledge of HPV etiology and mechanisms of HPV-induced malignant conversion are essential for developing strategies for preventing HPV infection and viral-associated carcinogenesis such as blocking expression of *E6* and *E7* proteins.

TREATMENT OF RELATIVELY ADVANCED CANCERS

Refinement in surgical resection–reconstructive techniques and advances in radiotherapy planning and delivery technology yield good outcome in most patients with early head and neck cancers. Unfortunately, therapy consisting of surgical resection and preoperative or postoperative radiotherapy still achieves rather poor results in terms of disease control, preservation of organ function, or both in patients with locally advanced cancer. Consequently, there has been a continuous search for better treatment approaches. This quest, along with the simplicity of clinical evaluation and well-characterized pattern of relapse, makes head and neck carcinomas ideal models for testing the relative efficacy of novel therapy concepts and modalities. For example, most clinical radiobiologic investigations have been conducted in patients with head and neck cancers.

Clinical Radiobiology

Radiobiologic concepts derived from more than two decades of integrated laboratory and clinical investigations led to the conception of two classes of new fractionation schedules for the treatment of head and neck cancers. These altered fractionation regimens are referred to as *hyperfractionation* and *accelerated fractionation schedules*. Hyperfractionation exploits the difference in fractionation sensitivity between tumors and normal tissues manifesting late morbidity. In contrast, accelerated fractionations attempt to reduce tumor proliferation as a major cause of radiotherapy failure. Although there are many permutations in accelerating radiation treatment, the existing schedules can be conceptually grouped into two categories, namely, pure and hybrid accelerated fractionation regimens, depicting the absence and presence of concurrent changes in other fractionation parameters, respectively. These radiobiologically sound fractionation regimens have been extensively tested in patients with intermediate and advanced head and neck carcinomas, mainly of the oropharynx. This line of clinical research is nearing conclusion. The results of the completed Phase III clinical trials have been reviewed recently (31,32). A brief overview of overall results and conclusions is presented in subsequent text.

Hyperfractionation
The clinical trial results, most notably that of the European Organization for Research on Treatment of Cancer (EORTC), show a moderate (10% to 15%) but consistent improvement in the local control of T2–T3 N0–1 oropharyngeal carcinomas (33). The incidence of late toxicity of a 10% to 15% total dose increment delivered in smaller than the standard fraction sizes, twice a day, was within the toxicity range observed with conventional fractionation schedules, although none of the studies were designed to test equivalency of late morbidity.

Accelerated Fractionation
The trial results indicate that mucosal toxicity limits the magnitude of overall time reduction to at most 2 weeks, without decreasing the total dose. With *pure accelerated* fractionations (no change or minimal change in the total dose and in the fraction size relative to conventional schedule), delivery of ten fractions per week (Vancouver trial [34]) induced very severe acute mucositis. Administration of continuous daily irradiations without a weekend break (Gliwice trial [35]), on the other hand, caused severe late effects, which were thought to be of the "consequential" type. With *hybrid accelerated* fractionations, delivery of three fractions of 1.6 Gy per day, separated by an approximate 6-hour interval, without reduction of the total dose (EORTC trial [36]), increased late complications such as soft tissue fibrosis, peripheral neuropathy, and myelopathy. On the basis of the repair kinetic data obtained from experimental spinal cord and skin models and from human

skin, these late morbidities can, at least in part, be ascribed to the occurrence of compounding incomplete cellular repair of sublethal injury. A 12-Gy total dose reduction (as in continuous hyperfractionated accelerated radiotherapy [CHART] [37]) seems more than sufficient to offset the compounding incomplete repair associated with the delivery of three fractions per day and, thereby, results in reduced severity in a number of late complications. These were skin telangiectasia, mucosal ulceration, and laryngeal edema. However, CHART did not improve tumor control in patients with a variety of advanced head and neck carcinomas. This study shows that it is possible to substitute radiation dose by overall time reduction and, thereby, provides indirect evidence for the importance of tumor clonogenic proliferation in determining local cure by radiation. Theoretically, this regimen should benefit a subset of patients with very rapidly proliferating tumors. The results of subset analyses reveal that this subgroup may well be those with T3 to T4, well-differentiated carcinomas of the larynx. It would be interesting to study this analysis further.

A pure accelerated fractionation regimen, by delivering six fractions per week in a trial of the Danish Head and Neck Cancer Study Group (DAHANCA 7) (38) and a hybrid variant by concomitant boost (Radiation Therapy Oncology Group [RTOG] trial [39]), yielded improved local control rate of advanced head and neck cancers without increasing the morbidity. The Danish trial randomized a total of 1,485 patients eligible for primary radiotherapy alone to receive 66 to 68 Gy in 33 to 34 fractions given in either five or six fractions per week. The compliance rate of therapy regimens was high. The incidence of acute severe mucositis and dysphagia was higher in patients receiving six fractions per week, but there was no difference in the incidence of late edema or fibrosis. The 5-year actuarial local-regional control (LRC) rates in 1,476 evaluable patients were 70% and 60% for accelerated and conventional regimens, respectively ($P = 0.0005$). The whole benefit for acceleration resulted from improvement in primary tumor control.

The RTOG 9003 randomized trial (39) compared the relative efficacy of three altered fractionation regimens with the standard 70-Gy regimen in 35 fractions over 7 weeks (39). The test radiation schedules were hyperfractionation (81.6 Gy in 68 fractions over 7 weeks, 1.2 Gy twice daily), split-course accelerated fractionation (67.2 Gy in 42 fractions over 6 weeks, including a 2-week break, 1.6 Gy twice daily), and concomitant boost regimen (72 Gy in 42 fractions over 6 weeks, 1.8 Gy daily for 3.6 weeks, and 1.8 Gy + 1.5 Gy, 6 hours apart, for 2.4 weeks). Recent analysis of 1,073 enrolled patients showed that concomitant boost and hyperfractionation regimens yielded significantly higher LRC rates than those of standard fractionation. The split-course accelerated regimen, however, did not improve LRC rate over that of the standard fractionation. The acute mucosal reactions were more severe in patients receiving altered fractionation regimens, but there was no difference in the complication rates at 6, 12, 18, and 24 months after therapy.

Conclusion

More than two decades of intensive clinical investigations on altered fractionations have finally settled and produced conceptually interesting and clinically important findings. Trials addressing hyperfractionation show that this biologically sound regimen yields a moderate but consistent improvement in LRC of moderate-to-advanced head and neck squamous cell carcinoma (HNSCC). The late toxicity of a 10% to 15% increment in total dose, delivered in smaller than the standard fraction sizes twice a day, was within the range of toxicity observed with conventional schedules, although no study was designed to test the equivalency of late morbidity.

The results of accelerated fractionation indicate that acute mucosal toxicity limits the magnitude of overall time reduction to at most 2 weeks, and that late complications resulting from compounding incomplete repair compromise delivery of three fractions of 1.6 Gy per day without total dose reduction. However, acceleration of radiotherapy by delivering six fractions per week and by concomitant boost yielded significantly improved local tumor control rates, relative to standard fractionation, without increasing the morbidity in the treatment of predominantly advanced carcinomas. These two types of regimens are conceptually similar in that radiotherapy duration is shortened by 1 week without reducing the total radiation dose or introducing an interruption in the regimen.

All in all, well-organized clinical trials enrolling more than 6,000 patients to test the relative efficacy of various altered fractionation regimens have generated important data. Radiobiologically, the trial results demonstrated the existence of differential fractionation sensitivity between head and neck carcinomas and late-responding normal tissues, and provided firm evidence that tumor clonogenic proliferation is a major obstacle to curing advanced head and neck cancers with fractionated radiotherapy. Clinically, the results of these trials call for changing radiotherapy practice for the treatment of moderate-to-locally advanced head and neck carcinomas. Because the magnitudes of therapeutic gain achieved with hyperfractionation, six-fraction-per-week schedule, and concomitant boost regimen are similar, the economic and logistic considerations determine the choice of the new standard treatment. For considerations of cost, resource utilization, and patient convenience, many centers have adopted the relatively simple concomitant boost regimen as the standard radiotherapy for patients with intermediate-stage head and neck carcinomas and for those with advanced cancers who are not eligible for protocol studies or for those choosing to receive radiotherapy alone. Finally, the data open the challenge for conceiving creative approaches to integrate the altered fractionation regimen with cytotoxic and/or biologic agents to further improve the therapy outcome. Several concepts have been or are being subjected to preclinical and clinical testing.

Combination of Radiation with Chemotherapy

Sequential versus Concurrent Radiation Chemotherapy Combination

Most combined radiation–chemotherapy regimens that have been tested have evolved empirically by administering drugs found to have some activity against tumors of interest in a dose and time sequence known to be tolerated in a single modality therapy setting. Meta-analyses of available data of randomized trials in head and neck cancer undertaken a few years ago showed that in spite of a high initial response rate, multiagent chemotherapy given before radiation treatment (neoadjuvant setting) has a small impact on the LRC and survival rates (40). Concurrent radiation and chemotherapy, on the other hand, yielded a higher survival rate close to the 10-percentage point compared to radiation alone (41). Unfortunately, the complication rates of combined regimens are also higher than those of radiotherapy alone (41).

The Meta-analysis of Chemotherapy on Head and Neck Cancer (MACH–NC) Collaborative Group undertook a very extensive meta-analysis. The project investigators obtained updated patient data of 63 randomized trials enrolling a total of 10,741 patients. This study revealed tremendous heterogeneity in eligibility criteria and in results between studies exploring chemotherapy for patients with nonmetastatic head and neck carcinoma, which made a simple conclusion on the role of chemotherapy difficult. Nonetheless, the analysis revealed a small, statistically significant benefit with the addition of chemotherapy to local-regional therapy, which consists of a 4% improvement in survival at 2 and 5 years. The benefit was due primarily to the favorable effect of concurrent and alternating radiation and chemotherapy, resulting in an 8% overall improvement in survival. However, the greatest heterogeneity was also seen in these groups. The authors conclude that concurrent chemoradiation should remain experimental, particularly when toxicity and cost–benefit ratios are taken into account, in addition to survival (42).

Results of many recently published Phase III trials (43–49) confirm the finding of meta-analyses that chemotherapy given concurrently with radiation yield better LRC and survival rates than radiation alone in patients with locally advanced HNSCC. Two trials also have shown the benefit of a concurrent radiation–chemotherapy given in a postoperative adjuvant setting (50,51). The combined radiation–chemotherapy regimen most extensively tested is the combination of conventionally fractionated radiotherapy (70 Gy in 35 fractions over 7 weeks) with cisplatin. In earlier trials, cisplatin was given in a dose of 100 mg per m^2 administered during weeks 1, 4, and 7 of radiotherapy (approximately one third of patients were not able to tolerate the last dose). The systemic and mucosal toxicities of such a high-dose, intermittent cisplatin regimen are rather severe. There are now four trials showing LRC and/or survival benefit of alternative cisplatin regimens—that is, five dosages of 20 mg per m^2 over 5 consecutive days or four dosages of 25 mg per m^2 over 4 sequential days during weeks 1, 4, and 7 (52,53); weekly fixed doses of 50 mg during the 7- to-9-week course of postoperative radiotherapy (54); or 6 mg/m^2/day, 5 days a week during the 7-week course of radiotherapy (49).

Unfortunately, recording and reporting of the late morbidity of combined radiation–chemotherapy have not been sufficiently consistent and systematic (55). A thorough report of the long-term results of a French Groupe d'Oncologie Radiotherapie Tete et Cou (GORTEC) trial reveals that the late complication rate of the combination of radiation with concurrent carboplatin and fluorouracil was significantly higher than that of radiation alone (46). Because of lack of adequate reporting, controversy still exists as to whether the late toxicity of the combination of standard radiation with 100 mg per m² of cisplatin administered every 3 weeks might also be higher than that of radiation alone. Hopefully, longer and more complete follow-up data on late morbidities will be reported in the future. Despite this uncertainty, many oncologists consider 100 mg per m² of cisplatin administered during weeks 1, 4, and 7 of conventionally fractionated radiotherapy as the current standard of care for patients with locally advanced head and neck carcinomas who are found to be medically fit to receive chemotherapy.

Principles for Optimizing Combination of Radiation with Systemic Therapy

Clear understanding of the therapy objective is essential for designing a logical combined therapy regimen. The purpose for combining radiation and systemic therapy in the treatment of neoplastic diseases can be to eliminate hematogenous micrometastases that have occurred before initiation of local-regional therapy, to improve the probability of eradicating primary tumors and involved regional nodes, or both. Depending on the pattern of failure, one or both objectives may be desirable in given clinical settings. It is obvious that the primary objective determines the choice of the agent(s) and the timing of drug administration relative to radiation. If the main aim is to reduce the probability of metastatic relapse, then it is logical to select least-toxic agents with proven antitumor activity and to administer radiation and systemic therapy sequentially, rather than concurrently, to minimize direct drug–radiation interactions that may increase normal tissue toxicity within the radiation portals. On the other hand, if the major purpose is to increase local tumor control, then it is more logical to select drugs on the basis of mechanisms of action and to administer systemic therapy concurrently with radiation to maximize drug–radiation interactions. In the latter scenario, therapeutic benefit only occurs when the combined therapy enhances tumor response more than it increases normal tissue toxicity.

Analysis of the data of randomized trial RTOG 9003 on altered fractionations for advanced head and neck carcinomas, which enrolled more than 1,000 patients, 60% of whom had stage IV disease, revealed that local-regional relapse is the predominant pattern of failure. Overall, the actuarial local-regional tumor recurrence rate was close to 50%, as opposed to less than 20% for distant metastasis (39). Consequently, for the time being, the effort should preferentially focus on developing combined therapy aimed at improving LRC for patients with advanced HNSCC. The finding that concurrent radiation and systemic therapy, but not sequential combined therapy, improved outcome is consistent with this first principle. Such confirmation should be taken into account in the design of future trials.

Despite three decades of clinical research, many scientific questions related to combination of radiation and chemotherapy remain unanswered. These include whether cisplatin is beneficial when added to altered fractionation, whether newer cytotoxic agents have higher efficacy, and whether neoadjuvant chemotherapy can further improve the outcome of concurrent radiation and chemotherapy. Factors to be taken into account in selecting agents for combination with radiation include mechanisms of drug–radiation interaction, pharmacodynamic characteristics, and clinical activity in inducing tumor response in a single modality therapy setting. A large number of laboratory studies have been undertaken to optimize combination of radiation with chemotherapy, particularly using newer cytotoxic and biologic agents such as taxanes and inhibitors of growth factor receptor signaling pathways.

HIGH-PRECISION RADIOTHERAPY

Advances in computerized radiotherapy planning and delivery technology open the possibility to conform irradiation to an irregular tumor target volume (conformal radiation therapy [CRT]) (56). Consequently, it is feasible to reduce the radiation dose to more of the crucial normal tissues surrounding the tumor without compromising dose delivery to the intended target volume, resulting in a reduction in morbidity. Reduced toxicity would, in turn, permit escalation of the radiation dose or combining radiotherapy with intensive chemotherapy, each of which has the prospect of improving HNSCC control. Basic expertise in anatomy, imaging, and pattern of tumor spread are, however, vital for clinical application of precision radiotherapy.

Such precision radiotherapy can be accomplished by the use of an array of x-ray beams individually shaped to conform to the projection of the target, which is referred to as *three-dimensional conformal radiation therapy* (3-D CRT). In addition, technology is also available to modify the intensity of the beams across the irradiation field as an added degree of freedom to enhance the capability of conforming dose distributions in three dimensions. This radiotherapy technique is called *intensity-modulated radiation therapy* (IMRT). Proton beams offer even a higher magnitude of normal tissue sparing, which is more desirable for the treatment of, for example, skull base neoplasms and pediatric cancers.

The role of 3-D CRT and, particularly, IMRT in reducing morbidity and, perhaps, in improving control of squamous cell carcinoma through radiation dose escalation is being tested in a number of centers. Results already reveal that it is effective in sparing parotid glands from receiving high radiation dose, thereby diminishing radiation-induced permanent xerostomia in select patients (57).

Single institutional studies testing the role of IMRT in the management of NPC and oropharyngeal cancers yielded exciting results. In patients with NPC, IMRT was given alone or, for locally advanced stage, in combination with chemotherapy consisting of concurrent cisplatin and adjuvant cisplatin plus 5-fluorouracil (58). In a series of 67 patients with a median follow-up of 31 months, the 4-year estimates of local progression-free, local-regional progression-free, distant metastasis-free, and overall survival rates were 98%, 97%, 66%, and 88%, respectively. The worst acute toxicity was grade 1 to 2 in 51 patients (76%), grade 3 in 15 patients (22%), and grade 4 in one patient (2%). The worst late morbidity was grade 1 in 20 patients (30%), grade 2 in 15 (22%), grade 3 in seven patients (10%), and grade 4 in one (2%) patient. Xerostomia was less pronounced than after 3-D CRT and its intensity decreased with time. At 3 months after IMRT, 8% of patients had no dry mouth, 28% had grade 1 xerostomia, and 64% had grade 2 xerostomia. Of the 41 patients evaluated at 2 years, 66% had no dry mouth, 32% had grade 1 xerostomia, and 2% had grade 2 xerostomia.

In a series of 74 patients with oropharyngeal carcinoma reported by Chao and associates (59), 14 received IMRT alone, 17 had IMRT combined with cisplatin-based chemotherapy, and 43 underwent surgery followed by postoperative IMRT. With a median follow-up of 33 months, the 4-year estimates of LRC, distant metastasis-free survival, disease-free survival, and overall survival rates were 87%, 90%, 81%, and 87%, respectively. Grade 1 and 2 late xerostomia were reported in 32 and nine patients, respectively. Late skin toxicity occurred in three patients (two grade 1 and one grade 2), mucositis in three (all grade 1), and trismus in three patients.

Inspired by the encouraging single institutional data, a number of multi-institutional trials addressing the role of IMRT in the treatment of head and neck carcinomas (e.g., RTOG trial 0022 for early stage oropharyngeal carcinoma and trial 0225 for NPC) have been launched. The results will be available in the next 2 to 3 years.

Of note is that more developments are needed to fully benefit from this sophisticated technology. Areas needing improvement to refine margins of coverage include topographic and biologic tumor imaging to better define target volumes, quantification of day-to-day anatomic variations occurring during the course of radiotherapy due to motion and changes in tumor and normal tissue volume, and so on.

Although results of IMRT and particle therapy are encouraging, the observation that most recurrences originated from the high-dose region indicates that radiation dose escalation alone will only improve outcome in a subset of patients. Further advances in the treatment of solid tumors would likely come through the application of new knowledge on tumor biology, as exemplified by translational research addressing the role of epidermal growth factor receptor (EGFR) in tumor progression and as a target for therapeutic intervention.

BIOMARKERS AND MOLECULAR TARGETING

Progress in searching for useful markers for early detection of tumor, estimation of tumor burden, prediction of response to therapy, and monitoring disease progression has been slow. A prototypical marker is prostate-specific antigen (PSA), which proved to be quite useful for prostatic cancer screening and for the prognostic grouping and monitoring of the therapeutic response of prostate carcinoma. Unfortunately, equivalent markers have yet to be identified for most other solid tumors. However, recent studies in head and neck carcinomas have generated optimism.

Review of literature data up to a few years ago identified p53; EGFR and one of its ligands, transforming growth factor-α (TGF-α); and cyclin D1 as promising prognostic biomarkers for HNSCC (60–62). A few recent studies (63–65) corroborated the prognostic value of EGFR. Our own study using HNSCC specimens of patients enrolled into a Phase III trial of the RTOG (39) and randomized to receive standard radiotherapy (SFX) (65), for example, revealed no correlation between EGFR expression and T-stage, N-stage, American Joint Committee (AJC) stage grouping, and recursive partitioning analysis classes (66) (r: –0.07 to +0.17). However, patients with greater than median EGFR-expressing tumors, as measured using an image-analysis–based immunohistochemical (IA-IHC) assay, were found to have significantly lower overall and disease-free survival rates secondary to significantly higher local-regional relapse rate. Multivariate analysis showed that EGFR expression was a strong, independent predictor of survival and of local-regional relapse.

A recently completed follow-up study using a validation set of patients enrolled into the same trial revealed high reproducibility of the IA-IHC assay and confirmed the absence of correlation between EGFR expression and tumor stage and other clinical prognostic variables (r: –0.20 to +0.18). The results validated our previous finding that higher tumor EGFR expression predicted for worse survival, disease-free survival, and local-regional relapse, with hazard ratios of 1.97, 2.15, and 3.12, respectively. However, whether EGFR predicts for the risk for metastasis and whether EGFR is a marker for tumor clonogen proliferation have not been resolved.

The recognition of the importance of erbB family tyrosine kinase receptors in coregulating cell proliferation, death, and angiogenesis led to the development of several strategies targeting the EGFR signaling pathway for cancer treatment. Two of these strategies—monoclonal antibody (e.g., cetuximab) and small molecule kinase inhibitors (e.g., gefitinib and erlotinib)—have gone through various stages of preclinical and clinical development in various types of cancers. A number of recently published reviews summarize the current status of clinical investigations (65,67–69). Randomized trials in colorectal adenocarcinoma (70) and in HNSCC (71) showed that cetuximab given in combination with irinotecan or cisplatin yielded higher objective response rates (23% and 26%, respectively) than chemotherapy alone. However, the higher response rates to combined therapies have not translated into improved overall survival relative to monotherapy. On the other hand, two Phase III trials in patients with non–small cell lung cancer show that gefitinib did not improve response rate or survival when added to cisplatin–gemcitabin or carboplatin–paclitaxel doublets (72,73).

In contrast to the results of combinations of EGFR antagonists with chemotherapy, data of the combination of cetuximab with radiotherapy in patients with locally advanced HNSCC are very impressive. A recently completed international Phase III trial (ImClone Systems Incorporated CP02-9815) revealed that, compared with radiotherapy alone, adding cetuximab to radiation therapy resulted in a significant improvement both in overall survival and LRC rates without increasing mucositis or dysphagia (74). These findings validate the notion that selective enhancement of tumor response leading to durable LRC can be achieved by "designer drugs" targeting a specific molecular pathway.

Progress has also been made in identifying a prognostic marker in patients with NPC. The study of Chan and associates (75) showed in a series of 170 patients that the post-treatment plasma level of EBV DNA was strongly correlated with progression-free and overall survival, more so than the pretreatment titer. For example, the relative risk for NPC recurrence was 11.9 (95% confidence interval: 5.53 to 25.43) for patients with higher post-therapy EBV DNA titer, as opposed to 2.5 (1.14 to 5.70) for patients with higher pretreatment EBV DNA. The positive and negative predictive values for recurrence for higher post-therapy EBV DNA were 83% (58% to 98%) and 98% (76% to 89%), respectively. When validated in larger series, this marker would be useful in identifying the high-risk patient for testing more aggressive therapy and monitoring response to treatment.

PREVENTION OF HEAD AND NECK CANCERS

The concept of "field cancerization" was first described by Slaughter and associates in 1953 (76) and has long been validated by clinical data. This evolving notion describes diffuse subcellular injury to epithelium, resulting from interactions between prolonged carcinogen exposure and individuals' genetic profiles, rendering the whole anatomic field at risk for developing invasive cancers through stepwise progressive accumulation of genetic alterations. It follows that an individual who develops and survives an upper aerodigestive cancer is at a higher risk (susceptible) for forming a second primary tumor (SPT) in the same anatomic field during the ensuing years. The field cancerization and multistep carcinogenesis concepts form the basis for research on cancer chemoprevention.

Results of relatively large series revealed that patients cured of their first head and neck cancer had more than 20% projected lifetime risk of development of SPT. The estimated annual SPT development rate ranged from 4% to 6% for at least 8 years after the diagnosis of the first cancer (77,78). In fact, SPT is the leading cause of death in patients with early head and neck cancers (79). This patient population has served as a model for addressing the efficacy of *adjuvant chemoprevention* regimens. Initial trial testing the role of *cis*-retinoic acid in preventing SPT had yielded encouraging results (80). Unfortunately, a recently completed large, multi-institutional, randomized trial did not confirm its benefit (unpublished data).

Leukoplakia and erythroplakia carry increased risk for transformation into squamous carcinomas. Therefore, this patient subset has been used as a model to test *chemoprevention of malignant transformation*. The weaknesses of this model are that the natural history of leukoplakia is rather variable, with spontaneous improvement occurring in many cases, and that the malignant transformation rate at 8 years may vary from 18% to 36%, depending on the degree of dysplasia observed histologically (81). Consequently, large series and prolonged follow-up studies are required to properly test the efficacy of a given primary chemoprevention strategy.

Identification of key genetic changes resulting in development of malignant clones and markers of multistep carcinogenesis will aid in selecting patients with highest risk for enrollment into chemoprevention trials, thereby reducing the required sample size. Markers can also serve as intermediate surrogate end points for assessing the efficacy of chemoprevention regimens and thereby shortening the length of the required follow-up.

SUMMARY

It has been exciting and gratifying to participate in laboratory research and/or clinical trials on head and neck cancer during the past two decades. Advances in molecular biology techniques opened new research avenues yielding new concepts or knowledge, such as multistep tumor progression model, genetic susceptibility to environmental carcinogen-induced tumorigenesis, and processes of viral-induced changes in cellular behavior, factors, and mechanisms governing cellular and tissular radiation response. Some of the new wisdom has already found applications in developing novel therapy strategies that have completed or are undergoing preclinical and clinical testing. Examples include altered fractionation regimens, mechanism- or molecular-oriented combined therapy modalities, and conformal radiotherapy. All in all, the basic and translational research efforts have finally paid off in that the head and neck cancer mortality rate in the United States has declined since the inception of record keeping. For example, the annual death rate for men due to oral cavity and pharyngeal cancers in the United States decreased by an average of 1.9% and 3% between 1975–1993 and 1993–2001, respectively (1).

It is very likely that the pace of discovery will even increase in the coming years. For example, it is reasonable to envisage that, before long, sensitive methods for detecting occult tumor foci for screening and staging purposes would be developed and new approaches in characterizing the genetic profile of cancers would accurately depict their individual virulence, predict therapy response, and guide treatment selection. Optimism in developing rational novel therapeutic strategies aimed at specific molecular targets to prevent malignant transformation or to reverse malignant phenotype is also increasing. Hopefully, the new insights and technologies gained from further research will have an additional sizable impact in reducing the mortality rate caused by head and neck cancers.

The high pace of new discoveries and the large number of research directions make it increasingly complex to determine what constitutes the standard therapy for a variety of patient subsets. In situations where several treatment options can yield approximately the same local-regional tumor control rate, other determinants to be taken into account in selecting the treatment of choice include cosmetic and functional outcome, acute and long-term morbidity (quality of life), resource utilization (cost), physician expertise, and patient convenience.

REFERENCES

1. Jemal A, Clegg LX, Ward E, et al. Annual report to the nation on the status of cancer, 1975–2001, with a special feature regarding survival. Cancer 2004;101:3–27.
2. Fearon ER, Vogelstein BA. A genetic model for colorectal tumorigenesis. Cell 1990;61:759–767.
3. Califano J, van der Riet P, Westra W, et al. Genetic progression model for head and neck cancer: implications for field cancerization. *Cancer Res* 1996;56:2488–2492.
4. Blot WJ, McLaughlin JK, Winn DM, et al. Smoking and drinking in relation to oral and pharyngeal cancer. *Cancer Res* 1988;48:3282–3287.
5. Liebowitz D. Nasopharyngeal carcinoma: the Epstein-Barr virus association. *Semin Oncol* 1994;21:376–381.
6. Sheu LF, Chen A, Meng CL, et al. Enhanced malignant progression of nasopharyngeal carcinoma cells mediated by the expression of Epstein-Barr nuclear antigen 1 in vivo. *J Pathol* 1996;180:243–248.
7. Nicholson LJ, Hopwood P, Johannessen I, et al. Epstein-Barr virus latent membrane protein does not inhibit differentiation and induces tumorigenicity of human epithelial cells. *Oncogene* 1997;15:275–283.
8. Murray PG, Swinnen LJ, Constandinou CM, et al. BCL-2 but not its Epstein-Barr virus-encoded homologue, BHRF1, is commonly expressed in posttransplantation lymphoproliferative disorders. *Blood* 1996;8287:706–711.
9. Choi PHK, Suen MWM, Path MRC, et al. Nasopharyngeal carcinoma: genetic changes, Epstein-Barr virus infection, or both. *Cancer* 1993;72:2873–2878.
10. Huang DP, Lo KW, van Hasselt CA, et al. A region of homozygous deletion on chromosome 9p21-22 in primary nasopharyngeal carcinoma. *Cancer Res* 1994;54:4003–4006.
11. Chan ASC, To KF, Lo KW, et al. High frequency of chromosome 3p deletion in histologically normal nasopharyngeal epithelia from Southern Chinese. *Cancer Res* 2000;60:5365–5370.
12. Chan ASC, To KF, Lo KW, et al. Frequent chromosome 9P losses in histologically normal nasopharyngeal epithelia from Southern Chinese. *Int J Cancer* 2002;102:300–303.
13. zur Hausen H, Schneider A. The role of papillomaviruses in human anogenital cancer. In: Salzman NP, Howley PM, eds. *The popovaviridae*, Vol 2. New York: Plenum Publishing; 1987.
14. Woodworth CD, Bowden PE, Doniger J, et al. Characterization of normal human exocervical epithelial cells immortalized in vitro by papillomavirus types 16 and 18 DNA. *Cancer Res* 1988;48:4620–4628.
15. Kaur P, McDougall JK. Characterizaton of primary human keratinocytes transformed by human papillomavirus type 18. *J Virol* 1988;62:1917–1924.
16. Park NH, Min BM, Li SL, et al. Immortalization of normal human oral keratinocytes with type 16 human papillomavirus. *Carcinogenesis* 1991;12:1627–1631.
17. Schlegel R, Phelps WC, Zhang YL. Quantitative keratinocyte assay detects two biological activities of human papillomavirus DNA and identifies viral types associated with cervical carcinoma. *EMBO J* 1988;7:3181–3187.
18. Pecoraro G, Morgan D, Defendi V. Differential effects of human papillomavirus type 6, 16, and 18 DNAs on immortalization and transformation. *Proc Natl Acad Sci U S A* 1989;86:563–567.
19. Barbosa MS, Schlegel R. The E6 and E7 genes of HPV-18 are sufficient for inducing two-stage in vitro transformation of human keratinocytes. *Oncogene* 1989;4:1529–1532.
20. Munger K, Phelps WC, Bubb V, et al. The E6 and E7 genes of the human papillomavirus type 16 together are necessary and sufficient for transformation of primary human keratinocytes. *J Virol* 1989;63:4417–4421.
21. Herrero R. Human papillonmavirus and cancer of the upper aerodigestive tract. *J Natl Cancer Inst Monogr* 2003;31:47–51.
22. Brachman DG, Graves D, Vokes E, et al. Occurrence of p53 gene deletions and human papilloma virus infection in human head and neck cancer. *Cancer Res* 1992;52:4832–4836.
23. Ogura H, Watanabe S, Fukushima K, et al. Human papillomavirus DNA in squamous cell carcinoma of the respiratory and upper digestive tracts. *Jpn J Clin Oncol* 1993;23:221–225.
24. Brandwein M, Zeitlin J, Nuovo GJ, et al. HPV detection using "hot start" polymerase chain reaction in patients with oral cancer: a clinicopathological study of 64 patients. *Mod Pathol* 1994;7:720–727.
25. Brandsma JL, Steinberg BM, Abramson AL, et al. Presence of human papillomavirus type 16 related sequences in verrucous carcinoma of the larynx. *Cancer Res* 1986;46:2185–2188.
26. Noble-Topham SE, Fliss DM, Hartwick WJ. Detection and typing of human papillomavirus in verrucous carcinoma of the oral cavity using the polymerase chain reaction. *Arch Otolaryngol Head Neck Surg* 1993;119:1299–304.
27. Fliss DM, Noble-Topham SE, McLachlin M, et al. Laryngeal verrucous carcinoma: a clinicopathologic study and detection of human papillomavirus using polymerase chain reaction. *Laryngoscope* 1994;104:146–152.
28. Snijders PJ, Cromme FV, van den Brule AJ, et al. Prevalence and expression of human papillomavirus in tonsillar carcinomas, indicating a possible viral etiology. *Int J Cancer* 1992;51:845–850.
29. Gillison ML, Koch WM, Capone RB, et al. Evidence for a causal association between human papillomavirus and a subset of head and neck cancers. *J Natl Cancer Inst* 2000;92:709–720.
30. Steenbergen R, Hermsen M, Walboomers J, et al. Integrated human papillomavirus type 16 and loss of heterozygosity at 11q22 and 18q21 in an oral carcinoma and its derivative cell line. *Cancer Res* 1995;55:5465–5471.
31. Nguyen LN, Ang KK. Radiotherapy for cancer of the head and neck: altered fractionation regimens. *Lancet Oncol* 2002;3:693–701.
32. Bernier J, Bentzen SM. Altered fractionation and combined radio-chemotherapy approaches: pioneering new opportunities in head and neck oncology. *Eur J Cancer* 2003;39:560–571.
33. Horiot JC, LeFur RN, Guyen T, et al. Hyperfractionation versus conventional fractionation in oropharyngeal carcinoma: final analysis of a randomized trial of the EORTC cooperative group of radiotherapy. *Radiother Oncol* 1992;25:231–241.
34. Jackson SM, Weir LM, Hay JH, et al. A randomised trial of accelerated versus conventional radiotherapy in head and neck cancer. *Radiother Oncol* 1997;43:39–46.
35. Skladowski K, Maciejewski J, Golen M, et al. Randomized clinical trial on 7-day continuous accelerated irradiation (CAIR) of head and neck cancer—report on 3-year tumor control and normal tissue toxicity. *Radiother Oncol* 2000;55:93–102.
36. Horiot JC, Bontemps P, van den Bogaert V, et al. Accelerated fractionation (AF) compared to conventional fractionation (CF) improved head and neck cancers: results of the EROTC 22851 randomized trial. *Radiother Oncol* 1997;44:111–121.
37. Dische S, Saunders M, Barrett A, et al. A randomised multicentre trial of CHART versus conventional radiotherapy in head and neck cancer. *Radiother Oncol* 1997;44:123–136.
38. Overgaard J, Hansen HS, Specht L, et al. Five compared with six fractions per week of conventional radiotherapy of squamous-cell carcinoma of head and neck: DAHANCA 6 and 7 randomised controlled trial. *Lancet* 2003;362:933–940.
39. Fu KK, Pajak TF, Trotti A, et al. A radiation therapy oncology group (RTOG) phase III randomized study to compare hyperfractionation and two variants of accelerated fractionation to standard fractionation radiotherapy for head and neck squamous cell carcinomas: first report of RTOG 9003. *Int J Radiat Oncol Biol Phys* 2000;48:7–16.
40. Munro AJ. An overview of randomised controlled trials of adjuvant chemotherapy in head and neck cancer. *Br J Cancer* 1995;71:83–91.
41. El-Sayed S, Nelson N. Adjuvant and adjunctive chemotherapy in the management of squamous cell carcinoma of the head and neck region. A meta-analysis of prospective and randomised trials. *J Clin Oncol* 1996;14:838–847.
42. Pignon JP, Bourhis J, Domenge C, et al. Chemotherapy added to locoregional treatment for head and neck squamous-cell carcinoma: three meta-analyses of updated individual data. *Lancet* 2000;355:949–955.

43. Adelstein DJ, Li Y, Adams GL, et al. An intergroup phase III comparison of standard radiation therapy and two schedules of concurrent chemoradiotherapy in patients with unresectable squamous cell head and neck cancer. *J Clin Oncol* 2003;21:92–98.
44. Al-Sarraf M, LeBlance M, Shanker PG, et al. Chemoradiotherapy versus radiotherapy in patients with advanced nasopharyngeal cancer: phase III randomized intergroup study 0099. *J Clin Oncol* 1998;16:1310–1317.
45. Forastiere AA, Goepfert H, Maor M, et al. Concurrent chemotherapy and radiotherapy for organ preservation in advanced laryngeal cancer. *NEJM* 2003;349:2091–2098.
46. Denis F, Garaud P, Bardet E, et al. Late toxicity results of the GORTEC 94-01 randomized trial comparing radiotherapy with concomitant radiochemotherapy for advanced-stage oropharynx carcinoma: comparison of LENT/SOMA, RTOG/EORTC, and NCI-CTC scoring systems. *Int J Radiat Oncol Biol Phys* 2003;55:93–98.
47. Wendt TG, Grabenbauer GG, Rodel CM, et al. Simultaneous radiochemotherapy versus radiotherapy alone in advanced head and neck cancer: a randomized multicenter study. *J Clin Oncol* 1998;16:1318–1324.
48. Brizel DM, Albers ME, Fisher SR, et al. Hyperfractionated irradiation with or without concurrent chemotherapy for locally advanced head and neck cancer. *NEJM* 1998;338:1798–1804.
49. Jeremic B, Shibamoto Y, Milicic B, et al. Hyperfractionated radiation therapy with or without concurrent low-dose daily cisplatin in locally advanced squamous cell carcinoma of the head and neck: a prospective randomized trial. *J Clin Oncol* 2000;18:1458–1464.
50. Bernier J, Domenge C, Ozsahin M, et al. Postoperative irradiation with or without concurrent chemotherapy for locally advanced head and neck cancer. *NEJM* 2004;350:1945–1952.
51. Cooper JS, Pajak TF, Forastiere AA, et al. Postoperative concurrent radiotherapy and chemotherapy for high-risk squamous-cell carcinoma of the head and neck. *NEJM* 2004;350:1937–1944.
52. Huguenin P, Beer KT, Allal A, et al. Concomitant cisplatin significantly improves loco-regional control in advanced head and neck cancers treated with hyperfactionated radiotherapy. *J Clin Oncol* 2004;22:4665-4673.
53. Wee J, Tan EH, Tai BC, et al. Phase III randomized trial of radiotherapy versus concurrent chemoradiotherapy followed by adjuvant chemotherapy in patients with AJCC/UICC (1997) stage 3 and 4 nasopharyngeal cancer of the endemic variety. *Ann Mtg Proc Am Soc Clin Oncol* 2004;23:487.
54. Bachaud J-M, Cohen-Jonathan E, Alzieu C, et al. Combined postoperative radiotherapy and weekly cisplatin infusion for locally advanced head and neck carcinoma: final report of a randomized trial. *Int J Radiat Oncol Biol Phys* 1996;36:999–1004.
55. Trotti A, Bentzen SM. The need for adverse effects reporting standards in oncology clinical trials. *J Clin Oncol* 2004;22:19–22.
56. Verhey LJ. Comparison of three-dimensional conformal radiation therapy and intensity-modulated radiation therapy systems. *Semin Radiat Oncol* 1999;9:78–98.
57. Eisbruch A, Ten Haken RK, Kim HM, et al. Dose, volume, and function relationships in parotid salivary glands following conformal and intensity-modulated irradiation of head and neck cancer. *Int J Radiat Oncol Biol Phys* 1999;45:577–587.
58. Lee N, Xia P, Quivey JM, et al. Intensity-modulated radiotherapy in the treatment of nasopharyngeal carcinoma: an update of the UCSF experience. *Int J Radiat Oncol Biol Phys* 2002;53:12–22.
59. Chao KSC, Ozyigit G, Blanco AI, et al. Intensity-modulated radiation therapy for oropharyngeal carcinoma: impact of tumor volume. *Int J Radiat Oncol Biol Phys* 2004;59:43–50.
60. Smith BD, Haffty BG. Molecular markers as prognostic factors for local recurrence and radioresistance in head and neck squamous cell carcinoma. *Radiat Oncol Investig* 1999;7:125–144.
61. Salesiotis AN, Cullen KJ. Molecular markers predictive of response and prognosis in the patient with advanced squamous cell carcinoma of the head and neck: evolution of a model beyond TNM staging. *Curr Opin Oncol* 2000;12:229–239.
62. Quon H, Liu FF, Cummings BJ. Potential molecular prognostic markers in head and neck squamous cell carcinomas. *Head Neck* 2001;23:147–159.
63. Maurizi M, Almadori G, Ferrandina G, et al. Prognostic significance of epidermal growth factor receptor in laryngeal squamous cell carcinoma. *Br J Cancer* 1996;74:1253–1257.
64. Grandis J, Melhem M, Gooding W, et al. Levels of TGF-a and EGFR protein in head and neck squamous cell carcinoma and patient survival. *J Natl Cancer Inst* 1998;90:824–832.
65. Ang KK, Berkey BA, Tu X, et al. Impact of epidermal growth factor receptor expression on survival and pattern of relapse in patients with advanced head and neck carcinoma. *Cancer Res* 2002;62:7350–7356.
66. Cooper J, Farnum N, Asbell S, et al. Recursive partitioning analysis of 2,105 patients treated in RTOG studies of head and neck cancer. *Cancer* 1996;77:1905–1911.
67. Ang KK, Andratschke NH, Milas L. Epidermal growth factor receptor and response of head-and-neck carcinoma to therapy. *Int J Radiat Oncol Biol Phys* 2004;58:959–965.
68. Mendelsohn J, Baselga J. Status of epidermal growth factor receptor antagonists in the biology and treatment of cancer. *J Clin Oncol* 2003;21:2787–2799.
69. Harari PM, Huang S-M, Combining EGFR inhibitors with radiation or chemotherapy: will preclinical studies predict clinical results? *Int J Radiat Oncol Biol Phys* 2004;58:976–983.
70. Cunningham D, Humblet Y, Siena S, et al. Cetuximab monotherapy and cetuximab plus irionotecan in irinotecan-refractory metastic colorectal cancer. *NEJM* 2004;351:337–345.
71. Burtness B, Li Y, Flood W, et al. Phase III trial of cisplatin+placebo versus cisplatin+C225 a monoclonal antibody directed to the epidermal growth factor-receptor: an Eastern Cooperative Group trial. AACR-NCI-EORTC International Conference on Molecular Targets and Cancer Therapeutics, Boston, MA, 2003.
72. Giaccone G, Herbst RS, Manegold C, et al. Gefitinib in combination with gemcitabine and cisplatin in advanced non–small-cell lung cancer: a phase III trial—INTACT 1. *J Clin Oncol* 2004;22:777–784.
73. Herbst RS, Giaccone G, Schiller JH, et al. Gefitinib in combination with paclitaxel and carboplatin in advanced non–small-cell lung cancer: a phase III trial—INTACT 2. *J Clin Oncol* 2004;22:785–794.
74. Bonner JA, Giralt J, Harari PM, et al. Cetuximab prolongs survival in patients with locoregionally advanced squamous cell carcinoma of head and neck: a phase III study of high dose radiation therapy with or without cetuximab. *Proc Am Soc Clin Oncol* 2004;23:488.
75. Chan ATC, Lo YMD, Zee B, et al. Plasma Epstein-Barr virus DNA and residual disease after radiotherapy for undifferentiated nasopharyngeal carcinoma. *J Natl Cancer Inst* 2002;94:1614–1619.
76. Slaughter DP, Southwick HW, Smejkal W. "Field cancerization" in oral stratified squamous epithelium: clinical implications of multicentric orgin. *Cancer* 1953;6:963–968.
77. Cooper JS, Pajak TF, Rubin P, et al. Second malignancies in patients who have head and neck cancer: incidence, effect on survival and implications based on the RTOG experience. *Int J Radiat Oncol Biol Phys* 1989;17:449–456.
78. Vokes EE, Weichselbaum RR, Lippman SM, et al. Head and neck cancer. *N Engl J Med* 1993;328:184–193.
79. Lippman SM, Hong WK. Second malignant tumors in head and neck squamous cell carcinoma: the overshadowing threat for patients with early stage disease. *Int J Radiat Oncol Biol Phys* 1989;17:691–694.
80. Hong WK, Lippman SM, Jtri LM, et al. Prevention of second primary tumors with isotretinoin in squamous-cell carcinoma of the head and neck. *NEJM* 1990;323:795–801.
81. Silverman SJ, Gorsky M, Lozada F. Oral leukoplakia and malignant transformation: a follow-up study of 257 patients. *Cancer* 1984;53:563–568.

Modes of Therapy

2

External Beam Irradiation (Teletherapy)

Most primary radiotherapy is delivered through external beam irradiation with 6- or 18-MV x-rays, less frequently with ^{60}Co γ-rays (when available), and 6- to 20-MeV electron beams. The choice of the beam type and energy is based on the location and geometric parameters of the target volumes. Occasionally, orthovoltage x-rays are used, for example, for treatment of skin cancers or for intraoral cone therapy for accessible, well-circumscribed tumors of the oral cavity or anterior oropharynx.

The initial target volume for external beam therapy includes both the gross tumor, as determined by clinical examinations and diagnostic imaging, and the potential routes of subclinical (microscopic) disease spread. A shrinking field technique is generally used, whereby the target volume is reduced after a dose sufficient to sterilize subclinical disease is reached to deliver additional boost dose to the demonstrable gross tumor. The boost dose may be given after or concomitantly with the initial large-field target volume irradiations. In the latter scenario, the boost irradiations are administered as second daily fractions.

The common practice in the United States up to the late 1990s was to administer primary radiotherapy in 2-Gy fractions, once a day, 5 days a week, to total doses ranging from 66 to 70 Gy depending on the tumor stage and site. As summarized in Chapter 1, intensive clinical investigations conducted during the past two decades revealed the superiority of hyperfractionation (e.g., 81.6 Gy given in 1.2 Gy per fractions, twice a day with 6-hour intervals, over 7 weeks) and two types of accelerated fractionation—concomitant boost (54 Gy given in 30 fractions over 6 weeks plus 18 Gy boost dose given in 1.5 Gy fractions, as second daily fractions during the last 2.5 weeks) and 6 fractions of 2 Gy per week regimens—in yielding local-regional control (1). Consequently, many centers have adopted one of these regimens as the current standard for the treatment of patients with intermediate-stage head and neck carcinomas or those with locally advanced cancers who are not medically fit to receive chemotherapy.

Intensity-Modulated Radiation Therapy

As presented in Chapter 1, advances in computing and engineering technologies have greatly improved the flexibility and precision of aiming the radiation beam at irregular volumes. Such precision radiotherapy can be achieved with intensity-modulated photon beams in intensity-modulated radiation therapy (IMRT) or with proton beams. With IMRT, all target volumes are irradiated during every radiation session, but a lower dose is delivered to the subclinical disease volume at each fraction. In addition, the overall treatment time for subclinical disease is prolonged from the conventional 5 weeks (50 Gy in 25 fractions) up to 6.5 to 7 weeks (33 to 35 fractions). Therefore, it is prudent to adjust the dose to the electively irradiated regions to correct for these changes. Consequently, when IMRT is given in 6 weeks to deliver a total dose of 66 Gy in 30 fractions to the gross tumor volume (GTV), such as in the treatment of T1-2 oropharyngeal carcinoma, we currently prescribe 54 Gy (1.8 Gy per fractions) to the elective volume. When a total dose of 70 Gy is given in 32 to 35 fractions over 6.5 to 7 weeks (2.12 to 2.0 Gy per fraction, respectively) to the GTV for treatment of larger tumors, we prescribe 56 to 59.5 Gy (1.75 to 1.70 Gy per fraction) to the elective clinical target volume (CTV).

Brachytherapy

Brachytherapy is usually combined with external beam therapy. The rationale for this combination is that areas at risk of harboring subclinical disease are irradiated with external beams to a dose sufficient to sterilize microscopic deposits and that gross lesion is boosted with a brachytherapy system to higher doses. This results in exposing a smaller volume of normal tissues to high-radiation doses. Therefore, if applied appropriately, tumor control can be obtained with low treatment morbidity.

Brachytherapy is used in the form of interstitial implants (e.g., primary cancer of the base of tongue or tonsillar fossa extending into the base of tongue), molds (e.g., lesion of the hard palate), or intracavitary applicators (e.g., recurrent nasopharyngeal cancer).

In selected situations, brachytherapy is used alone. Examples of such applications include treatment of superficial lip cancers, small nasal vestibule neoplasms, and alveolar ridge carcinomas.

POSTOPERATIVE RADIOTHERAPY

Advanced head and neck cancers (e.g., those invading the mandible or neck soft tissues) are often treated with a combination of surgery and radiation. The general indications for postoperative radiotherapy include close or positive surgical margins, perineural spread, lymph–vascular invasion, contiguous tumor extension into bone or neck soft tissue, multiple nodes, and extracapsular extension (ECE) of nodal disease.

In the postoperative setting, especially when a neck dissection has been performed, it is important to choose beam energies that do not provide excessive skin sparing, because part of the target volume is immediately subjacent to the skin. Therefore, in most patients, ^{60}Co γ-rays, when available, may be preferred for most postoperative treatments; that is, the initial large-field irradiations to a dose of 44 to 45 Gy. When using 6-MV x-rays, a 3-mm scar bolus is often considered. The remaining part of the treatment, off–spinal cord and boost irradiations, can be delivered with 6-MV x-rays without bolus and electrons (for administering supplemental dose to the posterior cervical nodal areas) to avoid the need to set up patients on two therapy units.

As a general principle, the entire operative bed is included in the postoperative target volume. The donor sites of skin grafts or flaps may not be considered part of the operative bed in this context.

The dose prescribed to sterilize subclinical disease in the postoperative setting is somewhat higher than in the surgically undisturbed state. Target volume to receive boost dose and the total doses prescribed are based on surgical pathologic findings. Several field reductions may be necessary to deliver desired doses to the undissected nodal basins, surgical bed, and region at higher risk of recurrence, such as sites of extensive ECE or positive margins.

In the presence of perineural invasion of major or named nerves, our general policy is to treat the course of involved major nerves at least to the skull base. However, if only minor unnamed nerves are histologically involved, slightly larger portals (e.g., with margins of an additional 2 to 3 cm) are generally selected and no attempt is made to trace the course of major nerves to the skull base.

The general rule is to start radiotherapy as soon as the surgical wound has healed, usually 3 to 4 weeks after surgery. With good communication between surgical, radiation, and dental oncologists, simulation generally can take place 3 to 4 weeks after surgery, and radiotherapy can start a few days later in most patients. This requires that dental assessment occur before surgery to determine the need for extractions when postoperative radiotherapy is contemplated. When recommended, dental care can be provided at the time of cancer surgery to avoid the need for a second anesthesia for full mouth dental extraction and unnecessary delay in initiating radiotherapy.

Our series revealed that completion of combined therapy within 11 weeks yielded a better local-regional control and better survival rates than in 11 to 13 weeks, and finishing combined therapy in more than 13 weeks resulted in a worse outcome (2). When delayed wound healing postpones postoperative radiation beyond 5 to 6 weeks, we prescribe accelerated fractionation by delivering twice-a-day irradiations for 1 week, usually to take place at the end of the radiation course, to reduce the potential deleterious effects of prolonged cumulative treatment time. Using this strategy, a dose of 60 Gy is given in 5 weeks, which was found to induce a more severe mucositis but without increasing the late complication rate.

PREOPERATIVE RADIOTHERAPY

Preoperative radiotherapy is rarely used in our practice because of the surgeons' preference to operate in an unirradiated field where frozen section control of surgical margins can be obtained. In certain circumstances, however, planned preoperative radiotherapy may be given.

These include situations where the cancer is marginally resectable or has a very rapid growth history. Patients with small radiocurable primary tumors and large adenopathy may be treated with definitive radiation to the primary tumor and preoperative radiation to the neck with a planned neck dissection to follow radiation. This strategy is particularly appealing in patients with bulky disease in level IV nodal region, to eliminate the need to administer a total dose of 70 Gy to the brachial plexus. Neck dissection is performed approximately 6 weeks following radiotherapy.

For most preoperative treatments, the dose is limited to that required for sterilization of subclinical disease; that is, 50 Gy in 25 fractions over 5 weeks. In very advanced tumors, a dose of 60 Gy in 30 fractions over 6 weeks may be administered. Surgery may also be performed, however, after full dose primary radiotherapy if residual disease persists 6 or more weeks after completion of treatment. This situation occurs mostly in the presence of a large nodal mass. The timing for surgery is generally about 6 weeks after completion of radiation.

RADIOTHERAPY FOLLOWING CHEMOTHERAPY

Neoadjuvant chemotherapy yielding complete or partial response of the tumor occurs in approximately 20% and 60% of patients, respectively. In spite of these occasional impressive responses, overall control rates in randomized trials have been at most a few percentage points better than those achievable with radiotherapy alone. For this reason, we do not generally recommend neoadjuvant chemotherapy outside the protocol study setting. For occasional patients referred after chemotherapy, we irradiate the entire original tumor volume with adequate margins to equivalent doses as primary radiotherapy alone. A small dose reduction is sometimes made when acute reactions are excessive.

CONCURRENT RADIATION AND CHEMOTHERAPY

Data from a number of recently completed clinical trials demonstrate that concurrent radiation–chemotherapy regimens improve the local-regional control rate of locally advanced head and neck cancers, and some regimens also improve the survival rate over that of radiation alone. However, some of the combined regimens studied so far appear to induce higher normal tissue toxicity, as well. The challenge is to develop mechanism-driven combined regimens to yield more pronounced effects on tumors than normal tissues or to conceive creative approaches to integrate altered fractionation regimen with cytotoxic and/or biologic agents to further improve the effects on tumors. Therefore, most patients with T3 to T4, N2 to N3 head and neck carcinomas are being enrolled into clinical trials addressing new radiation–chemotherapy regimens, combination of altered fractionation with chemotherapy, or combination of radiotherapy with biologics with or without chemotherapy.

Outside of the protocol study setting, however, the combination of conventional fractionation (70 Gy in 35 fractions over 7 weeks) with cisplatin (100 mg per m^2, given during weeks 1, 4, and 7) is currently preferred because this regimen has the longest and most solid track record. Results of

Phase III trial showed that as primary therapy, this regimen improves local-regional control and survival as compared with radiation alone in patients with locally advanced nasopharyngeal carcinoma (3) and other head and neck carcinomas (4). It also increases the larynx preservation rate (5). The combination of conventionally fractionated radiotherapy with cisplatin given as postoperative adjunctive therapy also improves local-regional control and disease-free survival (6,7) and survival (6) in patients with high-risk surgical pathologic features, particularly in the presence of ECE and positive section margins.

REFERENCES

1. Nguyen LN, Ang KK. Radiotherapy for cancer of the head and neck: altered fractionation regimens. *Lancet Oncol* 2002;3:693–701.
2. Ang KK, Trotti A, Brown BW, et al. Randomized trial addressing risk features and time factors of surgery plus radiotherapy in advanced head and neck cancer. *Int J Radiat Oncol Biol Phys* 2001;51:571–578.
3. Al-Sarraf M, LeBlance M, Shanker PG, et al. Chemoradiotherapy versus radiotherapy in patients with advanced nasopharyngeal cancer: phase III randomized intergroup study 0099. *J Clin Oncol* 1998;16:1310–1317.
4. Adelstein DJ, Li Y, Adams GL, et al. An intergroup phase III comparison of standard radiation therapy and two schedules of concurrent chemoradiotherapy in patients with unresectable squamous cell head and neck cancer. *J Clin Oncol* 2003;21:92–98.
5. Forastiere AA, Goepfert H, Maor M, et al. Concurrent chemotherapy and radiotherapy for organ preservation in advanced laryngeal cancer. *N Engl J Med* 2003;349:2091–2098.
6. Bernier J, Domenge C, Ozsahin M, et al. Postoperative irradiation with or without concomitant chemotherapy for locally advanced head and neck cancer. *N Engl J Med* 2004;350:1945–1952.
7. Cooper JS, Pajak TF, Forastiere AA, et al. Postoperative concurrent radiotherapy and chemotherapy for high-risk squamous-cell carcinoma of the head and neck. *N Engl J Med* 2004;350:1937–1944.

Practical Aspects of External Beam Therapy

3

PATIENT POSITIONING

The supine position is most frequently used to deliver radiation through isocentric opposed–lateral fields matched to a lower-neck portal, three-field techniques with or without matching neck portal (e.g., paranasal sinuses), or opposed anterior and posterior (AP–PA) fields.

The "open neck" position, in which the head is rotated on the trunk, resulting in flattening of the contours of the neck, is used for irradiating lateralized tumors and the ipsilateral neck. This position is suitable for irradiations with adjoining appositional electron fields or with a wedge-pair photon portal matched to an appositional electron field for lower neck.

The true lateral position is used in select cases, for example, postoperative situations in which patients are unable to control secretions in the supine position but nonetheless need to be treated with opposed–lateral fields.

The seated position is used for certain patients, primarily those who have difficulty managing their secretions or those who have difficulty breathing in the supine position. Treatment is accomplished using a specially designed chair mounted to the treatment couch. This chair enables the same immobilization and allows the same treatment accessories to be used as in the supine position. The chair is generally used only if other options are not feasible because complex treatment planning and dosimetry are difficult and because most computed tomographic scanners cannot accommodate patients in this position.

PATIENT IMMOBILIZATION

Virtually all patients nowadays are immobilized with thermoplastic masks that are individually made in the desired treatment position. A variety of commercial neck pads and head holders are now available for the purpose of immobilization in different positions. When making a mask, care should be taken to stretch the thermoplastic sufficiently thin to avoid unwanted bolus effect. For treatments limited to the neck region, the mask can be constructed so as to avoid the portals altogether. Figures 3.1 and 3.2 outline briefly the general procedure of constructing immobilization devices.

Introduction of conformal radiotherapy to reduce radiation morbidity or to escalate radiation dose to improve tumor control demands more precise and reproducible immobilization technology. Several methods have been introduced, which can be grouped into invasive and noninvasive techniques. Invasive techniques use head immobilization frames similar to those used for stereotactic radiosurgery. The frame is affixed to the patient's skull by several screws, usually placed by the neurosurgeon.

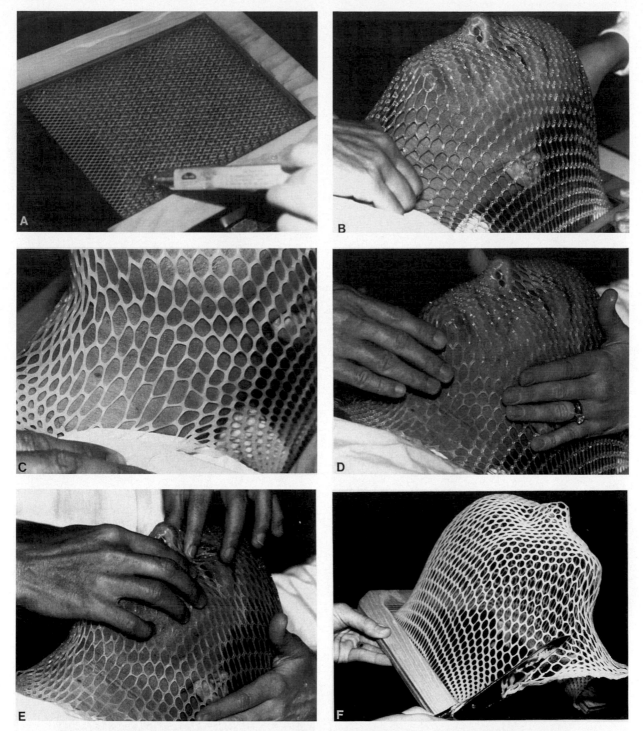

Figure 3.1 Procedure for making a thermoplastic mask in a supine position. **A:** Thermoplastic sheet attached to a wood or plastic frame is submerged in a warm water bath (72°C) until it becomes flexible. **B:** The thermoplastic sheet is stretched over the head of the patient, aligned in the desired position, and the frame is then fixed to a Perspex head holder by clamps. **C:** Care is taken to stretch the thermoplastic sheet sufficiently thin to avoid unwanted bolus effect. **D,E:** Gentle pressure is applied to make the thermoplastic sheet conform to the contour of the face. Portals can be simulated when the mask becomes more rigid. **F:** The mask can be trimmed, if desired, after completion of simulation.

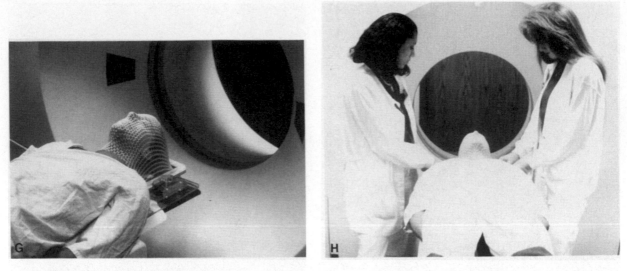

Figure 3.1 (*continued*) **G,H:** The immobilization system is also used to obtain a computed tomography scan for dosimetric planning.

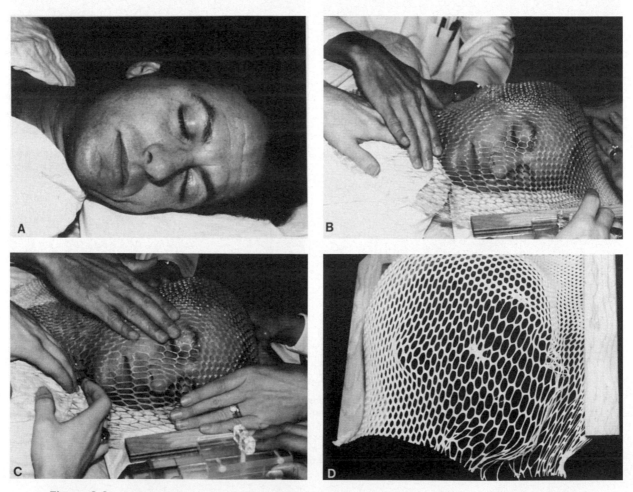

Figure 3.2 Procedure for making a thermoplastic mask for treatment in an open-neck position. **A:** The patient is positioned with the head rotated on the trunk to flatten the contours of the neck. **B:** The thermoplastic sheet is stretched over the head of the patient and the frame is then fixed to a special Perspex head holder by clamps. **C:** Gentle pressure is applied to make the thermoplastic sheet conform to the contour of the patient. Portals can be simulated when the mask becomes more rigid. **D:** The mask can be trimmed, if desired, after completion of simulation.

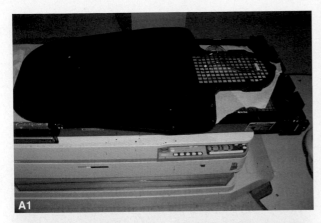
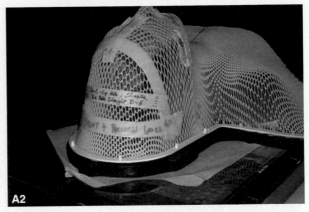
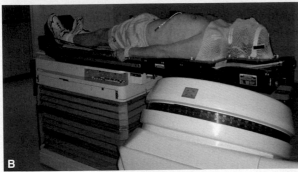

Figure 3.3 Thermoplastic immobilization mask for conformal therapy. **A:** Headboard (*1*) and mask (*2*) used for conformal therapy. **B:** Patient setup with mask and shoulder straps.

Numerous noninvasive immobilization techniques have been described. They are based on thermoplastic mask immobilization or customized polyurethane cradles. Thermoplastic masks can be reinforced with additional straps to increase rigidity. Some systems add individualized cradles for support of the occiput. We currently use a longer headboard for attachment of a mask that extends from the vertex of the scalp to the upper chest, giving additional support for the lower neck and shoulder (see Fig. 3.3).

RADIOPAQUE MARKERS AND STENTS

Although computed tomography (CT) scan–based simulation and dosimetry are increasingly used, radiopaque markers are still useful for delineating the primary lesion and scars in select cases. It is important to realize that it is often difficult to visualize superficial tumors in the planning CT scan. This simple procedure helps in designing treatment portals to minimize the risk of a geographic miss and to avoid unnecessary inclusion of normal tissues. Several types of custom-made stents are useful in reducing the volume of normal tissues irradiated.

Wires and seeds placed on the skin or on the thermoplastic mask or inserted into the tissue are helpful in marking the boundaries of the primary tumor, nodal biopsy sites, or surgical scar, and to indicate relevant structures (e.g., orbital canthi, lacrimal gland, external auditory canals, and oral commissures).

Stents can be custom-made, such as those used to depress or shield the tongue or to protrude the lip. In general, these devices can be categorized into two basic types: shielding stents and positional stents. A shielding device serves to reduce the radiation dose administered to normal tissues by incorporating shielding material, whereas a positional device serves to displace normal tissues out of the treatment fields (see Figs. 3.4–3.8).

An ancillary function of positional stents is to facilitate the use of internal bolus to fill surgical cavities; for example, to fill the cavity after maxillectomy or orbital exenteration (see Fig. 3.9).

Fortunately, progress in reconstructive techniques allows the surgeon to fill such tissue defects, even the palate, using a vascular flap. In addition to improving functional and cosmetic outcome, such a flap eliminates the need to use internal bolus.

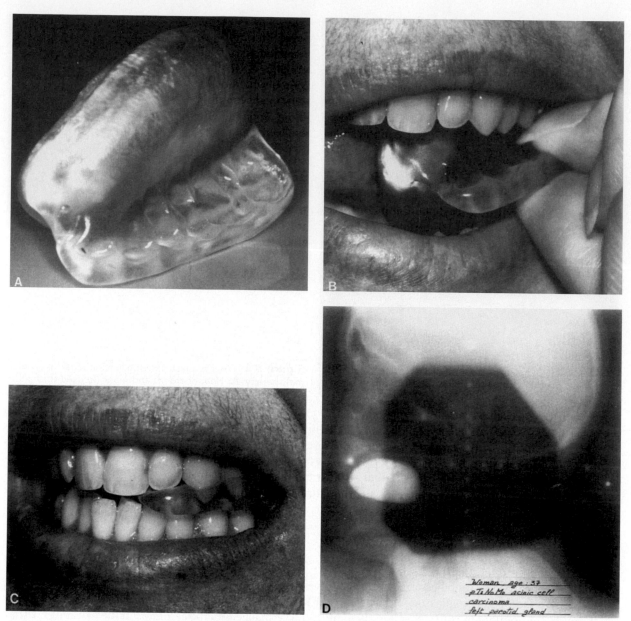

Figure 3.4   A 37-year-old woman presented with a 1.5 cm mass at the left angle of the mandible. The head and neck examination was otherwise unremarkable and the facial nerve function was intact. Material for cytologic study was obtained by fine needle aspiration and was interpreted as pleomorphic adenoma. At surgery, the tumor was found to be mainly located in the deep lobe of the parotid gland. It was well encapsulated and was dissected out along with the surrounding normal parotid tissue. The facial nerve was preserved. Pathologic examination revealed an acinic cell carcinoma measuring 2.4 cm in maximum diameter. All gross tumor was resected, but tumor cells extended to the surgical margin. For this reason, postoperative radiotherapy was recommended. The left parotid bed was treated with an ipsilateral appositional field using a combination of 20-MeV electrons and 18-MV photons, weighted 4:1 respectively. A dose of 56 Gy was delivered in 2-Gy fractions, specified at the 90% isodose line. To reduce the dose to the underlying brain during the electron treatments, 2 cm of beveled bolus was placed over the superior part of the field. After a dose of 44 Gy, the field was reduced off the spinal cord, and treatment to the postauricular and posterior cervical area was completed with 12-MeV electrons. A custom-made intraoral stent containing cerrobend (Lipowitz's metal, Cerro Metal Product, Bellefonte, PA, or Belmont Metal Inc, Brooklyn, NY) was used to shield the tongue and contralateral oral mucosa from the electron beam treatments by positioning between the alveolar processes and the tongue, displacing the tongue toward the contralateral side. The stent was held in place by the teeth fitting in the ridge on the lateral side (**A–C**). Although the cerrobend was sufficiently thick to reduce the transmitted dose to approximately 10% when treating with electrons, it would have increased the dose directly behind the stent when treating with high-energy photons because of the forward scatter of secondary electrons. For this reason, when the patient was treated with photons, a duplicate stent without the lead alloy was used to maintain the treatment field geometry. Because 80% of the dose was delivered by electrons, there was still a significant protection of the tongue and contralateral oral mucosa so that mucositis could be prevented in these areas. **A–D:** The intraoral stent used for shielding the tongue and contralateral oral mucosa during ipsilateral radiation treatment of a parotid gland tumor. **A:** Lateral view—the flange on the lateral side of the stent containing occlusal registration. **B:** Stent insertion. **C:** Device in treatment position. **D:** Port film showing the position of the stent in relation to the radiation field. (From Kaanders JH, Fleming TJ, Ang KK, et al. Devices valuable in head and neck radiotherapy. *Int J Radiat Oncol Bio Phys* 1992;23:639–645, with permission.)

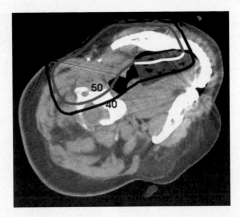

Figure 3.5 Axial computed tomographic (CT) scan images of patient with parotid carcinoma treated with an appositional 16-MeV electron field. A dose of 50 Gy was prescribed to the 90% line. To avoid artifact, a wax pattern of the stent was used for obtaining CT scan images. The stent captures the 50-Gy line at the edge of where the lateral tongue would normally be positioned. Without the stent, the 40-Gy line would have penetrated to the midline of the oral tongue.

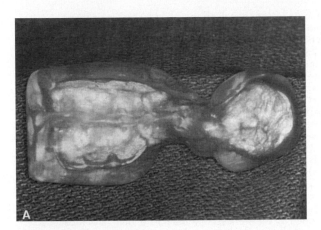

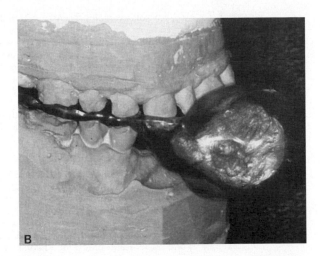

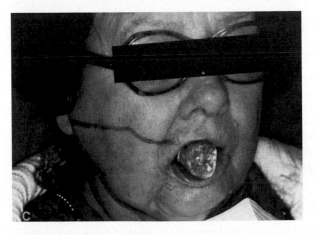

Figure 3.6 A 66-year-old woman presented with a right buccal mucosa lesion. On physical examination, she was found to have an infiltrative tumor measuring approximately 3.5 cm in largest diameter, extending anteriorly almost to the oral commissure. The tumor was 1.0 to 1.5 cm thick, without apparent skin involvement. There were two right submandibular nodes palpable, the largest measuring 2 cm in diameter. Biopsy revealed squamous cell carcinoma. The patient underwent resection of the tumor and a right modified neck dissection. Pathologic examination revealed a well-differentiated squamous cell carcinoma of the buccal mucosa with microscopic extension into the skeletal muscle and skin of the cheek. Nine lymph nodes were recovered in the surgical specimen, four of which contained metastatic squamous cell carcinoma with extension beyond the capsule. The patient received postoperative radiotherapy. The tumor bed and right upper neck were subjected to an ipsilateral appositional 13-MeV electron field to a given dose of 60 Gy in 30 fractions. The ipsilateral mid and lower jugular nodes and the posterior cervical chain were encompassed by a 9-MeV electron field. These areas were treated to a given dose of 50 Gy in 25 fractions. The scar extending into the mid-neck was given a 4-Gy boost with 6-MeV electrons. A variation of the stent as described in Figure 3.3 was used for this patient. As in the previous case, the stent-containing cerrobend was placed between the alveolar processes and the tongue, serving to displace the tongue and to shield the tongue and contralateral oral mucosa. In this case, the right oral commissure needed to be included in the field and, therefore, fall off was required anteriorly. The stent protruded anteriorly to shield the contralateral part of both lips and the left oral commissure. **A–C:** The stent used for protection of the tongue and contralateral oral mucosa and commissure during ipsilateral radiation treatment of a tumor of the buccal mucosa. **A:** Lateral view. **B:** Stent mounted on an articulator. **C:** Anterior end of the stent protrudes through the mouth for shielding part of the lips and the left oral commissure. (From Kaanders JH, Fleming TJ, Ang KK, et al. Devices valuable in head and neck radiotherapy. *Int J Radiat Oncol Bio Phys* 1992;23:639–645, with permission.)

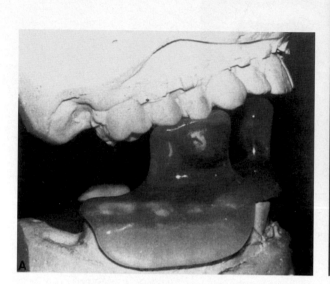
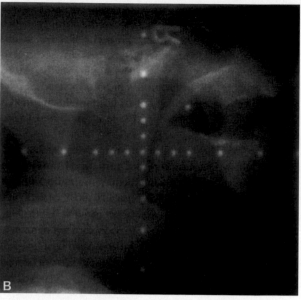

Figure 3.7   A 49-year-old woman presented with a 3-month history of enlarging neck masses. On examination she was found to have a 3-cm exophytic lesion on the left side of the tongue base, extending laterally to the glossopharyngeal sulcus. Mobility of the tongue was normal. There were three palpable nodes in the neck (a 3.5×3 cm right upper jugular node, a 2.5×2 cm left jugulodigastric node, and a 2×2 cm left mid-jugular node). Biopsy of the primary lesion revealed squamous cell carcinoma. The patient received radiotherapy followed by neck dissection. The primary tumor and upper neck nodes were treated with lateral parallel-opposed portals using ^{60}Co photons to a dose of 45 Gy, in 25 fractions, delivered to the isocenter. Reduction of the spinal cord was made and therapy was continued with 6-MV photons to a tumor dose of 54 Gy in 30 fractions. The posterior cervical strips were supplemented with electron beams. The mid and lower jugular nodes were treated through an anterior appositional ^{60}Co field and were supplemented with a smaller posterior field to a tumor dose of 54 Gy in 30 fractions. During the last 2.5 weeks of this basic treatment, the primary tumor and palpable nodes were boosted to a total tumor dose of 72 Gy. The boost was delivered in 1.5 Gy per fraction, given as second daily treatments using the concomitant boost technique. The stent for this patient consisted of a horizontal tongue positioner with protrusions fitting the occlusal surfaces of the mandibular and maxillary teeth, which served to separate the upper and lower jaws. The horizontal portion depressed the tongue so that it could be treated with adequate margins without encompassing the palate, upper gums, and most of the buccal mucosa. **A:** Stent mounted on maxillary and mandibular casts. **B:** Portal film showing the position of the tongue held down by the depressor and the mouth kept open by the stent so that the palate, gum, and most of the buccal mucosa were excluded from the field. (From Kaanders JH, Fleming TJ, Ang KK, et al. Devices valuable in head and neck radiotherapy. *Int J Radiat Oncol Bio Phys* 1992;23:639–645, with permission.)

SIMULATION

Simulation is a crucial procedure in planning the technical aspects of radiotherapy. The general treatment strategy (target volumes, field arrangement, treatment unit, etc.) should be determined before the onset of simulation. During simulation, attention is paid to mark relevant structures, to set up and immobilize patients in the desired position, and to obtain simulation films or CT scan images for portal design. The following sequence is usually applied.

Marking Anatomic Structures and Patient Positioning

When indicated, wires are used to mark the boundaries of the nodes or surgical scars and to indicate relevant structures (e.g., orbital canthi, lacrimal gland, external auditory canals, and oral commissures). For accessible tumors, seeds can be implanted to indicate the borders. The next step, before making an immobilization mask, is to set up the patient in a suitable position and to verify, with fluoroscopy or CT scan simulator, the appropriate orientation of the patient's anatomy (e.g., no axial rotation and the desired degree of neck extension) and stent position when applicable (e.g., tongue depressor). Subsequently, the thermoplastic mask is made and the patient's position is preserved. Care must be taken to ensure that the marking wires are not displaced when

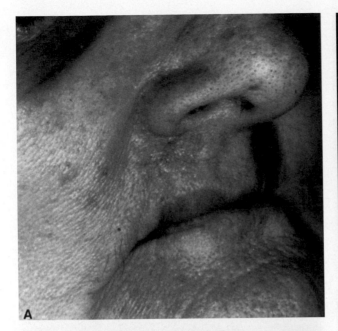

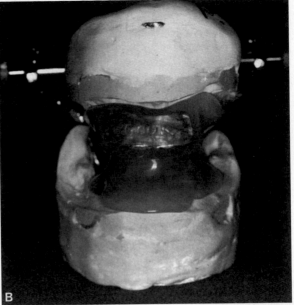

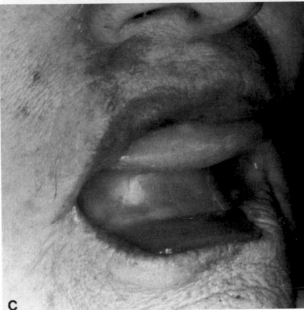

Figure 3.8 A 76-year-old woman presented with a lesion on the right side of the upper lip. On examination there was a slightly raised, erythematous lesion extending from the vermilion of the upper lip to the nasal ala, with upward retraction of the lip (**A**). The lesion was 2.2 cm in its largest dimension and involved almost the entire thickness of the lip. The inner mucosal lining was, however, intact. There were no palpable lymph nodes in the neck. A biopsy of this lesion showed basal cell carcinoma for which the patient received radiation therapy through an appositional 9-MeV electron field, which encompassed the tumor and a 1-cm margin of normal tissue. A lead cutout was used for skin collimation and a bolus of 1-cm thickness was placed over the skin to ensure an adequate dose at the surface of the tumor. Also, a bolus was placed in the right nostril to enhance the dose homogeneity. A dose of 50 Gy was given in 25 fractions, specified at the 90% isodose line, followed by an implant with radium needles. A stent was placed over the upper and lower alveolar processes to open the mouth and separate the lips, thereby excluding the lower lip from the radiation field (**B,C**). It also displaced the tongue posteriorly so that it was out of the range of the electron beam. To shield the gum, the part of the stent that was between the upper lip and the alveolar ridge was filled with cerrobend. Acrylic coating prevents overdosage to the mucosa of the upper lip by backscatter. At the completion of electron beam treatment, confluent mucositis occurred at the upper lip mucosa, whereas no appreciable reaction was observed on the mucosa of the gum. **A:** A woman with a slightly raised lesion extending from the vermilion of the upper lip to the nasal ala with upward retraction of the lip. **B:** The stent used mounted on an articulator. The upper part of the stent that separated the upper lip from the alveolar process contained cerrobend to shield the latter. **C:** The stent in treatment position. The lower flange held the lower lip away from the radiation field. (From Kaanders JH, Fleming TJ, Ang KK, et al. Devices valuable in head and neck radiotherapy. *Int J Radiat Oncol Bio Phys* 1992;23:639–645, with permission.)

the mask is put in position, or a geographic miss may result when the portals are planned. The final step is to choose the optimal site for isocenter and determine the portal size.

Determining Isocenter and Selecting Portal Size

The choice of the isocenter depends on the technique used for portal junction. For half-beam junction (or mono-isocentric) technique using asymmetric collimator jaw setting, the isocenter is placed on the desired junction location. For the conventional junction technique, which is used less frequently, the isocenter is placed near the center of the proposed field to reduce the size and weight of the customized blocks or to satisfy the need for setting the collimator jaw independently. Although the flexibility and automation available in modern equipment reduce these concerns, it

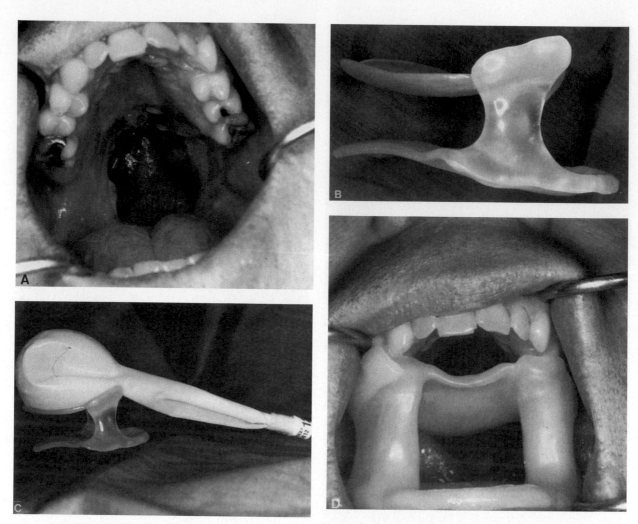

Figure 3.9   A 41-year-old man sought medical attention because of a 2-year history of a slowly enlarging soft palate mass. On physical examination he was found to have a 4-cm submucosal soft tissue mass involving the left side of the soft and hard palate, extending to the left maxillary tuberosity. The neck had no palpable nodes. The patient subsequently underwent a wide resection of the tumor with partial palatectomy and partial maxillectomy. Pathologic examination showed an adenoid cystic carcinoma measuring 3 cm in its largest diameter. The surgical margins were close and, therefore, he received postoperative radiotherapy. He was treated in the supine position with right and left lateral parallel–opposed 6-MV photon fields that encompassed the surgical bed and upper neck. A dose of 60 Gy, in 2-Gy fractions, was delivered to the isocenter. A field reduction was made after 44 Gy. A modification of the stent as described in Figure 3.7 was used. It served to open the mouth and depress most of the oral tongue out of the radiation field. The surgical procedure left a relatively large air cavity, which could compromise the dose homogeneity in the target volume (**A**). For this reason, a balloon filled with water (tissue equivalent for radiation absorption) was placed in the surgical defect. To support the balloon, a cradle was added on top of the tongue-depressing part (**B,C**). A space was provided between the upper incisors and the blade to insert the balloon (**D,E**). The position of the balloon can be verified by filling it with contrast material during simulation (**F**). **A:** Surgical defect after left partial palatectomy and partial maxillectomy in a patient with an adenoid cystic carcinoma. **B:** A balloon-supporting stent: The lower blade serves to depress the tongue and the cradle supports a water-filled balloon. **C:** Side view of the position of the balloon. **D:** Stent in position: A space was created to facilitate filling of balloon.

is still beneficial to get the setup right at the outset, because adjustments after simulation are a source of potential errors.

For parallel–opposed fields, the isocenter is generally placed at the midplane of the central axis. Appositional fields are generally treated using the source-to-surface distance technique. The isocenter for wedge pair or three-field technique is determined on the basis of the shape and size of the target volume.

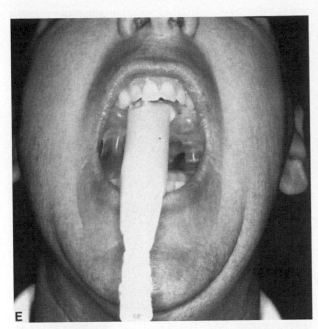
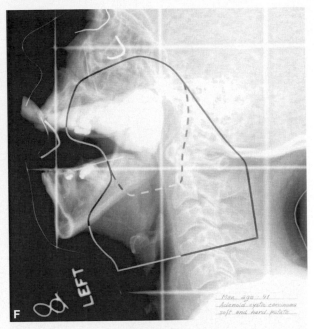

Figure 3.9 (*continued*) **E:** Stent and balloon in position. **F:** Simulation film—the tongue blade was marked by a radiopaque wire and the balloon was filled with contrast material to indicate the position of the device relative to the normal tissues; the lateral orbital canthi and oral commissures were also marked. The solid and dotted black lines represent the large and boost fields, respectively. (From Kaanders JH, Fleming TJ, Ang KK, et al. Devices valuable in head and neck radiotherapy. *Int J Radiat Oncol Bio Phys* 1992;23:639–645, with permission.)

Taking Simulation Film

To facilitate calculation of magnification factors (MF), the following conventions have been adopted for placement of simulation film cassettes:

- *For ^{60}Co irradiation:* source-to-axis distance (SAD) = 80 cm and skin–film distance (SFD) = 120 cm (MF: 1.5).
- *For 6- to 18-MV photon irradiation:* SAD = 100 cm and SFD = 140 cm (MF: 1.4).

Computed Tomography Simulation

CT scan simulation allows for defining the targets and digitally reconstructing the simulation films, and also offers the capability of virtual simulation. Following appropriate immobilization, the patient undergoes a planning CT scan on a CT scan simulator. At the time of the scan, either the true isocenter or the reference points are marked on the mask and/or patient. Following the scan, the target(s) and normal tissues are identified, and the field size, appropriate beam settings, and orientation are established. Blocks can be designed on the computer through virtual simulation or can be drawn on the digitally reconstructed radiographs.

TREATMENT PLANNING

There is increasing appeal to apply high-precision, conformal radiotherapy in the treatment of patients with head and neck cancer (see Fig. 3.10). Precision radiotherapy offers the possibility for reducing radiation exposure to normal tissues and thereby diminishing the morbidity of radiotherapy (e.g., xerostomia, fibrosis, and neuropathy). In advanced-stage cancer, the reduced toxicity in turn opens the opportunity to test whether therapy intensification—that is, escalation of the radiation dose or combination with chemotherapy—can improve local-regional tumor control without inducing more severe complications. However, expertise in the anatomy of the head and neck region and clinical examination, interpretation of diagnostic tumor imaging, and knowledge of pattern of tumor spread are crucial to minimize the likelihood of geographic miss, leading to marginal relapse.

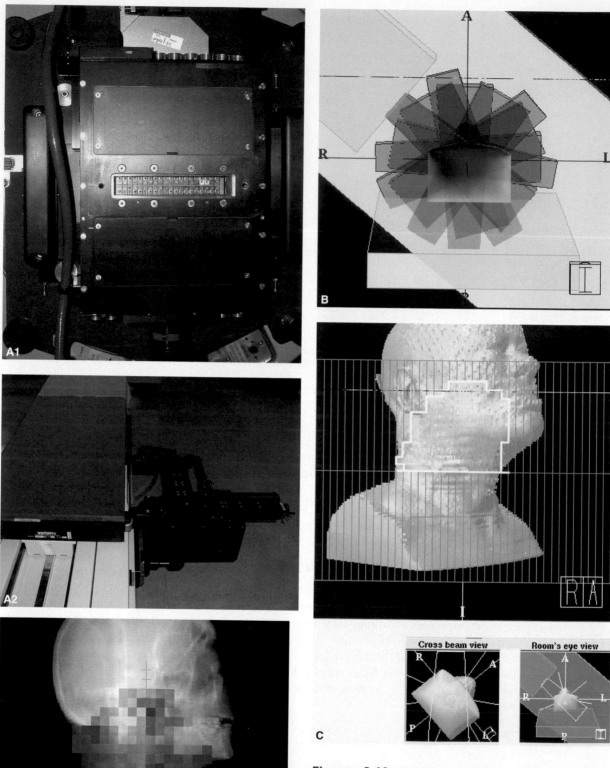

Figure 3.10 Intensity-modulated radiation therapy. **A:** Peacock multileaf intensity modulating collimator (*1*), MIMiC and crane (*2*) for couch indexing. **B:** Schematic of a nine-field beam orientation using DMLC-IMRT beams for the treatment of a patient with tonsillar carcinoma. **C:** Beam's-eye view of one of nine fields used to deliver DMLC-IMRT to the primary tumor and the upper neck nodes in a patient with tonsil carcinoma. The lower neck nodes receive radiation with an anterior portal through an isocentric match. **D:** The checkerboard-like pattern overlying the radiograph represent the fluence pattern of the field delivered with DMLC-IMRT as seen through a beam's-eye view.

Three-Dimensional Conformal Radiotherapy

Several conformal radiotherapy methods are presently available. The two main components of high-precision radiotherapy are the planning and the delivery systems. Generally, using a three-dimensional planning system, the target volumes and structures for avoidance are defined on thin-section CT scans. Two-dimensional beam's-eye views are used to visualize the targets and avoidance structures to select the optimal beam angles to best conform the radiation. In other words, the physician, physicist, and dosimetrist select what they believe are the ideal angles and number of beams, and then through an iterative process, select the appropriate weighting and wedging. This type of procedure is referred to as forward planning. Beam arrangements can be either coplanar or noncoplanar. To derive a plan that is highly conformal, it often necessitates the use of a large number of beams. When only custom-made cerrobend (Belmont Metal Inc, Brooklyn, NY) portal shaping is available, this can result in extremely long treatment sessions because therapists have to go in and out of the room to replace the blocks. The storage of these customized blocks inside a tight treatment vault can also be a problem.

The use of computer-driven multileaf collimation (MLC) facilitates treatment delivery by decreasing the time necessary for therapists to administer the multiple beams. Dynamic multileaf collimation (DMLC), which makes changing the beam shape while radiation is being delivered possible, provides the flexibility to design multiple portals to achieve the desired dose distribution. The newer model of an integrated MLC system can have a leaf resolution as small as 5 mm. Combining the wide travel range (up to 40 × 40 cm field size) and the ultra-high resolution and precision (usually less than 1 mm) in the leaf movement direction, the MLC can completely replace the cerrobend blocks. The ability to change the MLC-collimated field quickly adds further flexibility in designing treatment fields. For example, a field covering the target is designed. Within this field, a smaller field can be created to deliver additional dose to a portion of the target either to top-up the regions receiving lower than the desired dose or to achieve dose escalation. This manual beam patching technique is called the *field-in-field* technique, a forward planning and treatment technique used to achieve a more desirable dose distribution.

Intensity-Modulated Radiation Therapy

Although, technically, field-in-field technique can generate attractive dose distributions, for most people, conformal radiotherapy in the treatment planning is still a trial-and-error process. Most advanced conformal radiotherapy nowadays is planned using the *inverse* treatment planning systems. With these systems, treatment fields are automatically created using a complicated mathematical optimization process, using user-defined target dose prescription and normal tissue dose limits. This is also referred to as *intensity-modulated radiation therapy* (IMRT). Inverse planning actually requires that the treating physician explicitly define the desired doses to the target volumes and the acceptable doses to normal structures. Sometimes, the directions of the fields (beam angles) also require definition. Given these parameters, the computer optimizes the number of portals and the beam intensity pattern within each portal to generate the best dose distribution to fit the prescription. Because of the physics of radiation beams (e.g., the scatter and penumbra), sometimes these prescriptions cannot be fully satisfied. In such cases, prioritization of doses to tumor versus normal structures can be modified. For example, a lower tumor dose might be acceptable if the spinal cord dose could not otherwise be kept below the specification. Conversely, an ideal low dose to the parotid gland may not be acceptable if the desired dose cannot be delivered to an adjacent pathologic lymph node.

Once an IMRT plan is designed, several delivery methods are available. The most common method for IMRT treatment delivery is to use MLC at multiple (fixed) gantry positions. The treatment mode can either be static (i.e., step-and-shoot method) or dynamic (i.e., DMLC). In the step-and-shoot method, MLC leaves remain stationary during beam-on time and will move to the next set of leaf positions when the radiation beam is on hold. In the dynamic mode, MLC leaves can move during beam-on period, but the relation between leaf positions and the fractional dose delivered has to be maintained and synchronized. This will certainly call for a tighter specification on the MLC system.

The Peacock multileaf intensity modulating collimator (MIMiC) is the first dynamic IMRT system on the market. It is also referred to as *serial tomotherapy* because it uses continuous fan beams delivered through an arc treatment. The defined targets are treated slice by slice, in either 1- or 2-cm width. Each slice is delivered through the binary collimator composed of two rows of twenty 1×1 cm^2 (projection at isocenter) tungsten leaves. The leaves are pneumatically driven to open or close at each 5-degree of arc rotation. This allows each beam segment to have an intensity that can vary from 0% to 100% in 10% increments. Using an accurate couch indexing system, the couch is advanced to the next slice so that the next target position is treated. The newest form of this arc IMRT delivery system is the helical tomotherapy unit, which has recently been made available for clinical use. Tomotherapy is a highly integrated three-dimensional imaging and delivery system. The IMRT delivery system is similar to the Peacock MIMiC, except that the treatment couch advances continuously during the modulated arc beam delivery. In addition, there is a specially designed megavoltage CT scan imaging system, which can be used to perform a CT scan–guided treatment setup before tomotherapy treatment delivery.

PORTAL ARRANGEMENTS

Bilateral Irradiation

Opposed–lateral photon fields, with the patient immobilized in a supine position, are used for the treatment of most cancers of the oral cavity, larynx, and pharynx (see Figs. 3.11, 3.12). General principles for designing radiation portals follow.

The *superior border* is determined by the location of known disease and the likely spread pattern. Whenever possible, the optic pathways, part of the temporomandibular joints, temporal lobes, and auditory canals are excluded from the portals.

In the *anterior border,* a strip of anterior midline skin is shielded whenever possible to minimize lymph-drainage impairment after irradiation. This practice is not recommended when the primary tumor extends to the anterior subcutaneous tissues, large submandibular or jugular lymph nodes are present, the surgical scar (of neck dissection) approaches or crosses the midline, or histologic evidence of extracapsular nodal extension is present.

It is desirable to exclude the larynx proper from the lateral fields when this setup does not compromise the dose distribution to the primary tumor and/or involved neck nodes. Such a strategy is accomplished by placing the inferior border of the lateral fields just superior to the arytenoids.

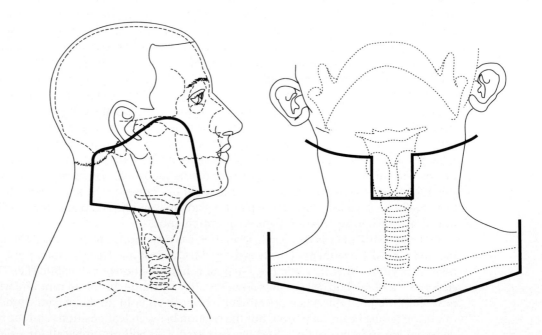

Figure 3.11   Schematic illustration of adjoining opposed–lateral fields and appositional anterior field above the arytenoids.

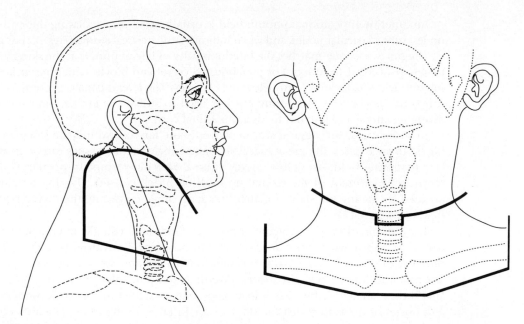

Figure 3.12   Schematic illustration of adjoining opposed–lateral fields and appositional anterior field below the larynx.

In patients who are able to hyperextend the head, an asymmetric jaw (half beam), isocentric-matching technique with the anterior lower-neck field can be achieved without collimator rotation. In patients who cannot hyperextend the head or when the primary tumor involves the vallecula, a slanted inferior border, at a maximal angle of 15 to 20 degrees (Fig. 3.11), can be used to avoid matching lateral portals and anterior lower-neck field at the sloping submental area. A preferred option now is to use isocentric matching with collimator rotation for lateral portals and to turn the couch 90 degrees and angle the gantry (superior tilt) to correspond to the angle of collimator rotation for the matching anterior field. When the larynx cannot be excluded, the inferior border is usually placed at the neck–shoulder junction (Fig. 3.12).

The location of the *posterior border* is dictated by the site of primary tumor and the extent of nodal disease.

- For N0 cases with low risk of subclinical spread to the posterior cervical nodes, the posterior border is placed just behind the insertion of the sternocleidomastoid muscle at the mastoid process.
- In N+ cases or primary tumors with substantial risk of subclinical spread to posterior cervical nodes (e.g., nasopharyngeal carcinoma), the posterior border is placed just behind the spinous processes, or even more posteriorly in the presence of large nodal masses. Once the prescribed spinal cord dose is reached, the posterior border is moved forward, usually to mid-vertebral body level. When the posterior pharyngeal wall or retropharyngeal nodes are part of the target volume, the border is placed closer to the posterior edge of the vertebral bodies. The posterior cervical strips that are no longer encompassed by the photon fields receive supplemental dose by lateral appositional electron fields. The electron beam energy is generally 9 MeV in the absence of palpable node, or higher (e.g., 12 MeV) in the presence of palpable nodes or in muscular patients. When electron energies of 12 MeV or greater are used to treat the posterior strips, CT scan dosimetry is crucial to compute the actual spinal cord dose.

After reaching the desired dose for the treatment of subclinical disease (most frequently 50 Gy/25 fractions), lateral fields are reduced to deliver the boost dose to the primary tumor and involved nodes. The field margins are determined by the extent of gross disease. Lateral or oblique photon fields, wedge-pair technique, or appositional electron fields can be used to deliver the boost dose, depending on the location and size of the primary lesion and nodes.

An anterior appositional photon field is usually used for irradiating the mid and lower neck nodes, supraclavicular nodes, and when indicated, the tracheal stoma (Figs. 3.11 and 3.12).

The *superior border* matches the inferior border of lateral portals at the skin by using asymmetric jaw (isocentric technique) or prefabricated cerrobend blocks with appropriate curvature. The *inferior border* is located 1 cm below the clavicles. The *lateral borders* encompass the medial two thirds of the clavicles. A midline block is used to shield the larynx and to prevent overlap of diverging lateral and anterior fields at the spinal cord.

In some cases, the surgical scar may overlie the larynx and may be shielded by the midline block. In such cases, the prelaryngeal skin and subcutaneous tissues can be treated with a separate matching field, using low-energy (6 to 8 MeV) electrons. In postlaryngectomy patients requiring treatment of the stoma, no midline block is used. Overlap on the spinal cord is avoided by having the slanted match line at an angle exceeding the divergence of the anterior field (see Fig. 3.13).

The combination of two lateral upper neck fields and a single anterior mid–lower neck field results in a somewhat lower dose to the mid-posterior cervical nodal region. Therefore, in the presence of posterior adenopathy it is necessary to use anterior and posterior portals to irradiate the mid and lower neck. The most convenient setup in such situations is the asymmetric jaw (half-beam) match. Otherwise, it may be prudent to adjust the superior border of both anterior and posterior fields to match the slope of the inferior border of the lateral fields by turning the treatment couch 90 degrees and angling the gantry accordingly.

Unilateral Irradiation

Well-lateralized tumors having a low risk of lymphatic spread to the contralateral neck nodes (e.g., retromolar trigone, buccal mucosa, salivary glands, and skin) receive treatment to the ipsilateral side only. In such cases, the patient is usually immobilized in the open neck position. General guidelines for designing radiation portals follow.

The primary tumor and upper neck are encompassed and irradiated through an appositional lateral field using electrons or a combination of electrons and photons. The depth of the primary tumor determines the energy of the electron beam. When high-energy electrons are needed, approximately 20% of the dose is given with megavoltage photons to reduce the skin dose, thereby avoiding occurrence of moist skin desquamation.

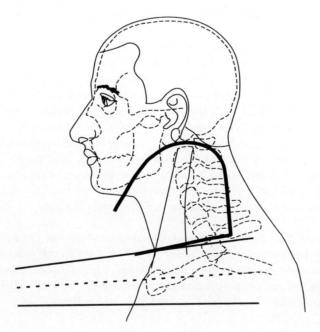

Figure 3.13   Schematic illustration of avoiding overlap on the spinal cord by choosing an appropriate angle of the match line.

The borders of the field are determined by the tumor location and extension (see Part II). The *inferior border* of the field is placed at or above the arytenoids whenever possible. The isodose constriction and greater dose perturbation by tissue inhomogeneity associated with electron beams must be taken into account in determining margins. Therefore, these cases require CT scan–based dosimetry with heterogeneity corrections.

The mid and lower neck nodes are irradiated with an adjoining appositional electron field when indicated. For a clinically negative neck, 9-MeV electrons are usually sufficient, except in patients with a large neck diameter. Palpable nodes may require higher energies, depending on their size and depth in the neck.

- *Superior border:* matches the inferior border of the primary field.
- *Anterior border:* is just short of fall-off.
- *Posterior border:* is at the edge of the trapezius muscle.
- *Inferior border:* is 1 cm below the clavicle.

PORTAL SHAPING

More than 90% of patients are treated with customized multileaf collimator or cerrobend blocks shaped to individual target volumes. Most modern linear accelerators come equipped with an MLC system for portal shaping through independent leaves driven by computer program (see Fig. 3.14). This system eliminates the need for custom-made cerrobend blocks. Within the primary rectangular shape field set by four collimator jaws, individual leaves can be adjusted to conform to the desired shape of the portal. Most current systems have leaves with a width of 0.5 to 1 cm (at isocenter), although equipment with 3-mm leaf widths is available.

In most situations, MLC should produce shaped portals equivalent to those achieved with customized blocks. MLC also is useful because it can easily produce smaller fields within a larger portal to compensate for underdosage to part of the target volumes because of differences in tissue thickness or heterogeneity. In rare occasions where millimeter precision is needed, the thickness of the leaves in most commercial systems may not be adequate.

Cerrobend blocks are manufactured using a standard commercial block-cutter system (Clark Research and Development Inc, Folsom, LA). The quality control program includes evaluation of the accuracy of Styrofoam, cut out with a verification light, and assessment of the size, shape, and precision of mounting on the tray by projecting the light field on the outline on the simulation film with a block verification unit (Med-Tech Inc, Tulsa, OK). Deviations of 2 mm or less are considered acceptable.

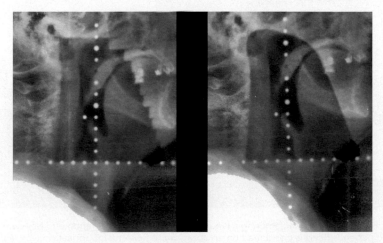

Figure 3.14 Comparison of multileaf-collimated **(left)** and cerrobend-blocked **(right)** portals. The patient received radiation treatment of T1 N3 squamous cell carcinoma of the glossopharyngeal sulcus. Off spinal cord fields are shown. Matching with the anterior lower–neck portal was by an isocentric (asymmetric jaw) technique. The isocenter is placed above the arytenoids so that the use of a 3-cm-wide block in the anterior portal can shield a large part of the larynx.

Shaping of electron field is done by secondary collimation. When necessary for treatment of tumors close to critical tissues, portal shaping can be accomplished by placing customized lead shield or mask directly on the patient's skin (skin collimation). The construction of appropriate lead mask takes several steps (see Fig. 3.15). First, the desired radiation field is drawn on the patient's skin. Then, an impression and mold are made (during this procedure, field borders are transferred automatically onto the impression). Subsequently, thin sheets of lead are cut, pounded into shape against the impression, and soldered together until the proper thickness is attained for the electron energy selected. The mask is then tried on the patient and final adjustments are made. When a shrinking-field technique is used, it is more practical to initiate treatment with the boost field because it is easier to enlarge the aperture of the mask by cutting out excess lead than to reduce its size.

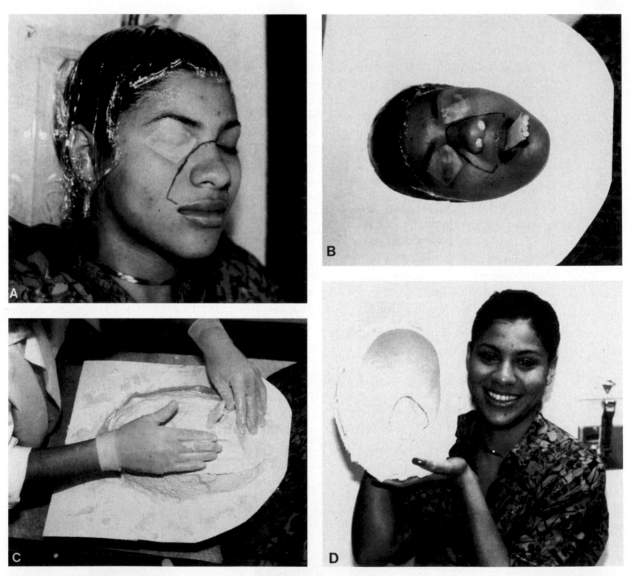

Figure 3.15   Procedure for manufacturing a lead mask for electron collimation and beeswax bolus. **A:** The field is outlined on the skin and the patient's head is positioned on an appropriate head rest. Lubrication jelly is put around the hairline, the hair is covered with plastic wrap, and the eyes are covered with gauze dressings (lubricate the edges for extra protection). **B:** A cardboard, with patient's face contour cut out, is placed at the desired position. The patient is informed that the impression mixture will be poured over the face. Therefore, it is necessary to fill the nostrils with lubricated cotton to keep out the impression mixture and to keep drinking straws in the mouth to allow breathing. **C:** The impression mixture is then poured over the area of interest, smoothed over, and allowed to set. Plaster strips are placed over the impression to hold it together (2 to 3 layers). **D:** After hardening (2 to 4 minutes), the impression is removed. The field outline that has transferred to the impression is touched up.

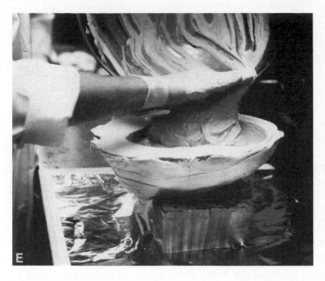

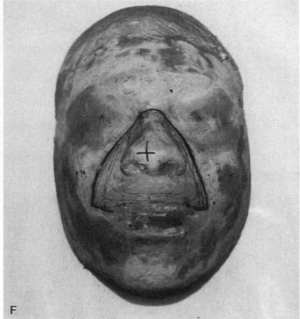

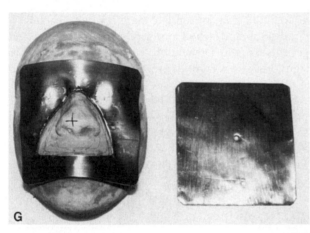

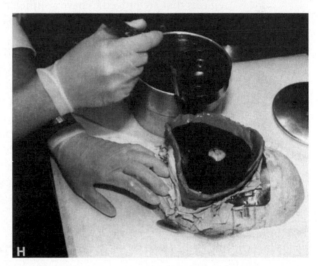

Figure 3.15 (*continued*) **E:** The impression is coated with lubricating jelly and dental stone (Labstone or Dentstone) is poured into it. The impression is vibrated for a few minutes to allow air bubbles to surface. **F:** The mold is removed the next day, and again the field outline is touched up. **G:** A thin sheet of lead is cut to the predetermined size. A hole is drilled through the center of the sheets. This is enlarged to approximate the radiation field. The sheets are then pounded onto the mold with a rubber hammer. The shape of the hole is then further trimmed to fit the field outline. This procedure is repeated until the required thickness is achieved. A thin foam is taped to the underside of the mask to improve wearer comfort. **H:** Customized beeswax bolus, when needed, is made directly on the mold. In this case, pottery clay is used to build a dam of the desired depth 1 cm beyond the field outline (to allow for wax shrinkage by drying and cooling). The stone mold is lubricated generously and a small amount of melted wax is poured into the dam and allowed to cool before another layer of wax is added. This step is repeated until the required thickness is achieved. A hot knife is then used to trim the bolus to the final dimension. (Courtesy Robert Gastorf and Michelle Rittichier, Department of Radiation Physics, M.D. Andersen Cancer Center. Described in detail by Gastorf et al. Quality assurance in the fabrication of radiation treatment aids. In: Starkschall G, Horton JL, eds. *Proceedings of an American College of Medical Physics Symposium.* Madison, WI: Medical Physics Publishing, 1991:239–245.)

DOSE SPECIFICATION

Photons

The radiation dose is prescribed at the isocenter when opposed–lateral portals are used. For three-field technique or wedge pair, the dose is prescribed to the isocenter or an appropriate isodose line encompassing the target volume, maintaining dose heterogeneity within the target volume to no more than $\pm 5\%$. The dose to the mid and lower neck given by an anterior appositional field is prescribed at D_{max} or 3-cm depth (D_{3cm}), depending on protocol specification.

Electrons

The dose for elective treatment of nodal areas is prescribed at D_{max}, and for therapeutic treatment of involved nodal areas is prescribed at 90% isodose line. The dose delivered through an appositional field for the treatment of cancer of the nasal vestibule or cavity, parotid gland, anterior faucial pillar, and retromolar trigone is prescribed at the desired isodose line (usually 90%). If medial coverage is inadequate, higher electron beam energy should be used, rather than specifying the dose to a lower isodose line. It is essential to obtain an isodose distribution with inhomogeneity corrections to ensure proper coverage of the target volume by the electron beam.

Intensity-Modulated Radiation Therapy

With IMRT, doses are prescribed to target volumes defined by clinicians. Both gross target volume (GTV) and clinical target volume (CTV) are delineated. The GTV encompasses all gross tumors detectable by physical and endoscopic examination and by CT scan and/or magnetic resonance imaging (MRI). The CTV comprises the GTV and the surrounding tissues judged to be at risk for microscopic contiguous and lymphatic disease spread. Typical margins around the GTV to encompass contiguous microscopic spread of primary tumor are 2 cm, although exceptions exist, such as a wider coverage for extensive perineural invasion.

GTV obviously does not exist after gross total tumor resection. The CTV in these cases include the operative bed and margins as judged individually. Additional CTVs are defined in undissected regions that are judged to have a sufficiently high probability of harboring microscopic disease to justify receiving elective irradiation. A patient may have several CTVs defined that differ in their assessment of risk and planned dose.

A planning target volume (PTV) is defined to provide an appropriate margin around each CTV, which accounts for variabilities in daily portal setup and, when applicable, organ motion and changes in anatomy due to tumor shrinkage. This margin is generally 5 mm, unless a center has studied and defined its own individual magnitude of uncertainty in portal setup or the tumor abuts a critical organ such as the spinal cord or the optic chiasma.

Currently, the Radiation Therapy Oncology Group (RTOG) is studying the feasibility of IMRT to provide adequate target coverage while sparing the contralateral parotid gland for patients with early stage oropharyngeal cancers. The dose prescription is specified to an isodose that encompasses at least 95% of the PTV. Other requirements are that no more than 20% of the PTV will receive greater than 110% of the prescribed dose, and no more than 1% of the PTV will receive less than 93% of the prescribed dose.

TECHNIQUES TO IMPROVE DOSE DISTRIBUTION

Compensating Filters

In situations where there is substantial variation in the tissue thickness within the treatment portals, photon beam dose homogeneity can be improved by the use of missing tissue compensating filters. Examples include treatment of the whole pharyngeal axis through opposed–lateral fields, especially in patients with thin necks, and irradiation of the neck and upper mediastinum through opposed AP to PA fields (see Fig. 3.16). The consequence of marked variation in tissue thickness reflects not only on an increase in total dose, but also in the dose per fraction ("double trouble") in the thinner region. However, because even small errors in mounting a compensating filter can produce an unsuspected hot or cold spot, *in vivo* dose verification with thermoluminescent dosimeters is essential whenever missing tissue compensators are used. Tissue compensators are best for patients in whom the change of tissue thickness is gradual. They are not well-suited for patients with sharp contour changes, such as a patient with significant tissue loss just inferior to the mandible.

The use of three-dimensional treatment planning enables the creation of CT scan–derived compensators to address missing external tissue and dose heterogeneity resulting, for example, from internal air cavity (e.g., in the pharynx, and paranasal sinuses).

As mentioned earlier, a more popular technique is to use multileaf collimator to improve dose distribution. With this technique, a large field is designed to encompass the target. Within this

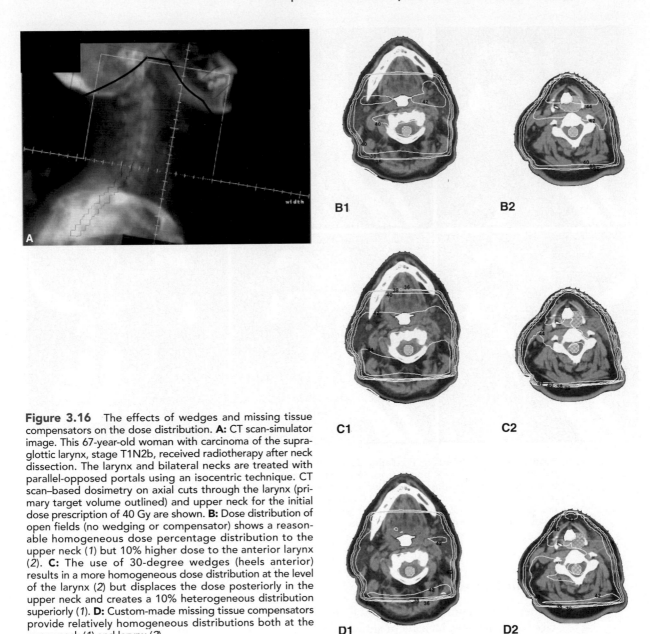

Figure 3.16 The effects of wedges and missing tissue compensators on the dose distribution. **A:** CT scan-simulator image. This 67-year-old woman with carcinoma of the supraglottic larynx, stage T1N2b, received radiotherapy after neck dissection. The larynx and bilateral necks are treated with parallel-opposed portals using an isocentric technique. CT scan–based dosimetry on axial cuts through the larynx (primary target volume outlined) and upper neck for the initial dose prescription of 40 Gy are shown. **B:** Dose distribution of open fields (no wedging or compensator) shows a reasonable homogeneous dose percentage distribution to the upper neck (*1*) but 10% higher dose to the anterior larynx (*2*). **C:** The use of 30-degree wedges (heels anterior) results in a more homogeneous dose distribution at the level of the larynx (*2*) but displaces the dose posteriorly in the upper neck and creates a 10% heterogeneous distribution superiorly (*1*). **D:** Custom-made missing tissue compensators provide relatively homogeneous distributions both at the upper neck (*1*) and larynx (*2*).

field, one or more smaller fields can be created to deliver additional doses to portions of the target receiving lower than the desired dose (see Fig. 3.17).

Electron Beam Bolus

Electron beam bolus may serve three functions. First, it can increase surface dose for low energy beams when skin sparing is not warranted. Second, it can attenuate the beam to protect underlying tissues in cases where a different depth of penetration is desired in different parts of the portal. Finally, it can be useful to "smooth" irregular surface contours, which perturbs electron beam dosimetry through uneven scatter.

For a simple skin dose buildup on a reasonably flat surface, a layer of superflab of appropriate thickness is sufficient. For surface contour modification, a custom-made beeswax bolus is preferred (Fig. 3.15). Care should be taken to ensure good contact between bolus material and the skin surface to minimize unintended perturbation of electron beam.

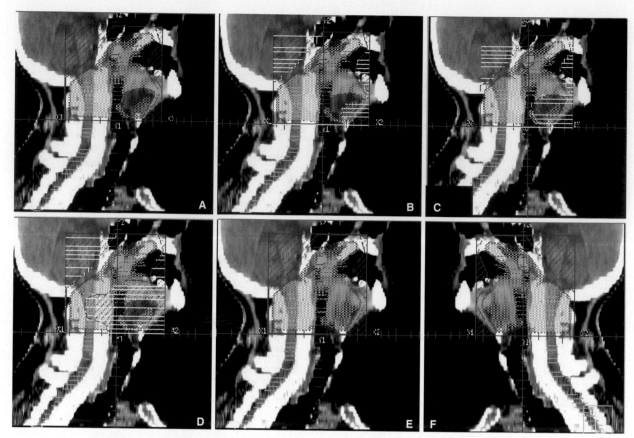

Figure 3.17 Distribution of radiation dose across the mid-sagittal plane, plotted in 5% gradients, of the initial large opposed–lateral portals encompassing the primary tumor and upper cervical nodal basins. Without beam modulation, the dose distribution varies from 95% (*blue color wash*) to 115% at the tongue base region (*dark sky-blue color wash*) **(A)**. Using MLC leaves (*white lines*) to shield the 115% isodose line from the right lateral field **(B)**, the 110% line from the left lateral field **(C)**, and finally the 105% line from the right portal **(D)** yields a dose distribution on the central plane to within 5% of the primary prescribed dose **(E, F)**.

Scatter Plates

Scatter plates mounted in the beam close to the skin surface can serve the same function as surface bolus, namely, increase of surface dose when required. They are preferred to surface bolus when the contour is curving, because they avoid the risk of excessive electron attenuation in the oblique trajectory through surface bolus (see Fig. 16.1).

The thickness of the scatter plate is adjusted according to the electron energy used and the desired surface dose. A one-quarter-inch-thick acrylic plate, for example, increases the surface dose of a 6-MeV electron beam from approximately 70% to approximately 95% and that of a 9-MeV beam from approximately 80% to approximately 90%.

Practical Aspects
of Brachytherapy

4

Traditionally, brachytherapy has played an important role in the radiotherapeutic management of cancers of the oral cavity. However, better reconstructive surgical techniques for filling defects that are left after tumor excision and for enhancing organ function have decreased the use of brachytherapy for these tumors. The availability of intensity-modulated radiation therapy (IMRT) may also reduce the application of brachytherapy.

Brachytherapy is used to boost residual infiltrative disease of the tongue base after external irradiation and to treat selected lesions involving the buccal mucosa, lip, oral commissure, nasal vestibule, and recurrent tumor of the nasopharynx. In addition, occasional patients with tumors of the oral tongue or floor of mouth who refuse surgery are treated primarily with brachytherapy.

TYPES OF BRACHYTHERAPY

Temporary Interstitial Brachytherapy

All temporary interstitial radiotherapy is given with iridium 192 (^{192}Ir) wires inserted into Teflon catheters or stainless steel needles, depending on the tumor site.

Permanent Interstitial Brachytherapy

Where a removable implant cannot be performed for technical or medical reasons, a permanent implant with gold 198 (^{198}Au) seeds can be done. It is not desirable to use iodine 125 (^{125}I) seeds for permanent implants for squamous cell carcinoma of the head and neck because the dose rate from such implants is too low in relation to the proliferative potential of tumor clonogens.

Endocavitary Brachytherapy

Either low dose rate (LDR) or high dose rate (HDR) brachytherapy can be used for the treatment of nasopharyngeal carcinoma. A Teflon ball with a high-intensity single cesium 137 (^{137}Cs) source is used for LDR brachytherapy. A high-activity ^{192}Ir stepping source is used for HDR. A remote-controlled HDR afterloader inserts the ^{192}Ir source into a flexible silicone applicator (e.g., the Rotterdam Nasopharyngeal Applicator).

Molds

A surface mold loaded with ^{192}Ir or ^{137}Cs is occasionally used, especially for lesions on the hard palate or the alveolar ridge.

DEFINITION OF THE IMPLANT TARGET VOLUME

The first step in preparation for brachytherapy is to determine the treatment volume so that the number, length, and intensity of radioactive sources can be appropriately planned in advance.

When patients are to receive brachytherapy after completion of external beam therapy, the patient is examined and the lesion is carefully documented before the tumor regresses or disappears.

PROTECTION OF NORMAL TISSUES

The most crucial aspect for reducing morbidity from brachytherapy is to provide separation between the radioactive sources and normal structures outside the target volume because distance is the primary means of protection with this mode of irradiation. In certain cases, special stents can be constructed to increase the distance. Occasionally, the stents may include shielding material (e.g., 2 mm of lead reduces the dose to shielded structures up to 50%). When stents cannot be made, gauze, dental roll, or other material may be used at the time of the procedure. Refinement of afterloading techniques and the availability of flexible radioactive wires improve the accuracy of implants, thereby reducing the volume of normal tissues exposed to high radiation doses.

Care should be taken to place radioactive sources at least 0.5 cm away from the mucoperiosteum of the mandible, whenever possible, to minimize the risk of radiation-induced bone exposure and osteoradionecrosis. In the absence of bone involvement, one source can be placed in the vicinity of the mandibular periosteum, when necessary, without excessive risk of inducing osteonecrosis.

OPERATING ROOM PROCEDURE FOR IMPLANTATION

The patient should be under general anesthesia and should be positioned appropriately for the implant. Care should be taken to minimize the trauma of needle placement to avoid massive edema. However, even if there appears to be little or no edema, patients receiving interstitial therapy to the tongue base may need a protective tracheotomy. Placement of needles or catheters is done primarily on the basis of disease extent rather than by attempting to follow prescribed geometric implant patterns. However, the basic concepts of source separation and active length must be kept in mind. In general, the higher the dose to be delivered with brachytherapy, the more closely the implantation rules need to be followed to prevent unwanted "hot" or "cold" spots.

Proper radiation protection measures should be applied in the operating room. Most temporary implants can be afterloaded, thereby obviating radiation exposure to operating room personnel. When active sources are being implanted, the best protection for the operator and operating room personnel is to minimize the time of exposure. Everything should be kept in readiness before the implant is begun, and delays should be avoided. Personnel not actively involved in the implant should stand away from the sources.

DOSIMETRY

For afterloading techniques, catheters are loaded with dummy wires for obtaining orthogonal x-rays. The computer-generated dose distribution is then obtained on the basis of specific activity of available interstitial sources, and a plan for afterloading is developed. Because of the decay of iridium sources, it is desirable to keep wires with varying linear intensities. Sources are chosen that will deliver dose rates of 30 to 50 cGy per hour at the periphery of the implant. As a general rule, for single plane implants, the required activity is 0.5 to 0.7 mCi per cm radium equivalent for 1 cm spaced sources. In choosing an isodose contour that will cover the tumor volume, care is taken to ensure that the "hot spots" around the sources are not too large.

Dosimetry for patients receiving permanent [198]Au seed implants is purely for the purpose of documentation, because no adjustment is possible.

MANAGEMENT OF PATIENT DURING IMPLANT

Most patients with head and neck implants in place require nasogastric or gastric tube feeding for the duration of the implant. Adequate analgesia is also provided, although pain is usually not a problem after the first day. The patients must be nursed in shielded rooms with restricted access.

REMOVING INTERSTITIAL IMPLANTS

Most implants can be removed without general anesthesia, except for tumor of the posterior oral tongue and base of the tongue. Adequate provision is made for the possibility of hemorrhage when an interstitial implant is removed, especially from the tongue or pharynx. Upon removal of an implant, all sources must be accounted for and a radiation survey of the room performed after the sources are returned to the safe.

Practical Aspects of Endocavitary Beam Therapy

Endocavitary beam therapy is a valuable method of delivering boost doses to well-circumscribed lesions in the oral cavity and anterior oropharynx as an alternative to brachytherapy or higher doses of external beam therapy. We use an orthovoltage x-ray beam of 125 to 250 kVp for this mode of therapy.

PATIENT SELECTION

Ideal candidates for endocavitary beam therapy are those with a well-circumscribed lesion that is visible and accessible by cone through the mouth and does not involve the mucoperiosteum of the mandible (e.g., cancer of the soft palate or anterior faucial pillar). Patients with an exaggerated gag reflex are not suitable for this type of treatment.

PROCEDURE

A patient selected for endocavitary beam (intraoral cone) therapy generally receives this treatment component before external beam therapy for better tumor localization. Patient tolerance to intraoral cone therapy is also better before manifestation of mucositis induced by external beam irradiation. Once a cone of appropriate size is selected, it is sometimes possible to manufacture a stent for automatic cone positioning (Fig. 9.1). Intraoral cone therapy is delivered under direct supervision of radiation oncologists. After placing the cone in the desired treatment position, the x-ray unit is docked to the cone. A periscope is then used to verify tumor location within the cone aperture.

In lateral lesions, the cone is angled to avoid irradiation of the spinal cord during the endocavitary beam therapy. This is not possible, however, when the tumor arises from the midline. In this case, the dose contribution to the spinal cord should be calculated and taken into account in planning the external beam therapy component.

Patient Care Before and During Radiotherapy

DENTAL CARE

Evaluation, treatment, and prevention of any pre-existing oral or dental pathology are an integral part of management of patients with head and neck cancer because complications vary with dental status, the type of malignancy, and the therapeutic approach. Underlying pre-existing silent pathology can become prominent in a patient receiving radiation, and particularly so in combined therapy. Mild problems of the oral cavity can develop into severe complications that can either compromise cancer therapy or cause considerable morbidity. Oral complications can be minimized, and in some cases eliminated, if identified and addressed early by a dental team. It is, therefore, important to assess the patients' access to dental care and their commitment to daily oral hygiene procedures.

A comprehensive head and neck evaluation includes an oral and dental clinical examination supplemented by intraoral radiologic evaluation. Selected dental radiographs are essential in evaluating potential areas of infection that are not obvious on clinical examination (e.g., periodontal–periapical tooth pathology, residual cysts, and impacted or partially erupted exfoliating teeth). From this information, the dentist can plan oral treatment to bring the dental problem under control, thereby meeting immediate needs before radiation therapy. Oral treatment plans should be designed to correct restoration overhangs, rough or sharp edges in teeth, and any other defects likely to cause soft tissue irritation. Patients should be instructed to avoid abrasive food that could traumatize soft tissues. Ill-fitting intraoral prostheses should not be worn during radiation therapy. Dental implants should be carefully assessed, and their removal should be considered if maintenance of peri-implant health cannot be reasonably anticipated or if integration is poor. Any potential source of oral infection should be identified and eliminated.

In general, patients with good dental status, including those who need routine restoration of a few cavities, are instructed to maintain oral hygiene and undergo brush training. They also receive custom-made carriers for fluoride prophylaxis, to prevent caries and hypersensitivity of teeth; and mouth guards, made of flexible plastic material, to prevent biting irradiated tissues that may become edematous. Edentulous patients are instructed to maintain oral hygiene and to avoid trauma and premature use of prosthesis. In patients undergoing surgical therapy, the oral cavity should also be prepared for appropriate prosthetic rehabilitation to correct surgical deficits.

When there are findings of periapical pathosis, questionable periodontal status, unrestorable teeth with advanced caries, supererupted teeth, and, possibly, unopposed dentition, the teeth involved should be considered for extraction. Endodontic therapy is a viable alternative for pulpal necrosis, provided that the treatment can be expeditiously performed before the initiation of cancer therapy. To ensure bone coverage and adequate wound healing, extractions should be performed 2 to 3 weeks before initiation of cancer therapy. Extractions and associated alveoloplasty should be performed with minimal trauma and should include smoothing of sharp surrounding hard tissue, appropriate irrigation, and primary closure in order to promote rapid healing. In general, periodontal surgical procedures should be avoided because prolonged healing and meticulous oral hygiene are needed to achieve the desired results.

The decrease in saliva production that often results from radiation to the head and neck region reduces the natural lavage of food and microbial debris from the oral cavity, which can lead to the development of dental caries. The change in the composition of saliva and reduced pH and buffering capacity also create a cariogenic oral environment, particularly in patients ingesting a diet high in carbohydrates or sucrose. Increased gingival recession may occur without signs or symptoms of periodontal inflammation. Therefore, special oral care is needed to prevent complications.

Good oral hygiene during and after therapy is essential for improving oral comfort and for reducing the risk of oral pathology. Bacterial and fungal superinfection can occur but are less likely to induce septicemia in patients undergoing radiotherapy alone than in those receiving chemotherapy or concurrent radiation and chemotherapy. Oral rinsing with a solution of 1 tablespoon of sodium bicarbonate dissolved in 12 oz of water many times each day reduces oral microorganisms and aids in maintaining mucosal hydration. This measure, along with the elimination of secondary sources of irritation, such as alcohol, smoking, coarse or hot foods, alcohol- or phenol-containing mouth rinses, and sodium products, can help in minimizing mucositis.

The daily use of a fluoride gel can help minimize dental decay. The common formulations used are either 1.0% sodium fluoride gel or 0.4% stannous fluoride gel. Compared with sodium fluoride, stannous fluoride is slightly more acidic, but its uptake into the enamel matrices is four times greater. In adults with xerostomia, fluoride is released from the enamel within 24 hours; therefore, the fluoride regimen must be performed daily for optimal protection. The most efficient method of fluoride application is to use a custom-made polypropylene fluoride carrier that completely covers and extends slightly beyond the tooth surface. Patients fill the carriers with fluoride gel and place them onto the dentition daily for 10 minutes. Patients who receive low doses of radiation and are expected to have a slight degree of xerostomia can use a toothbrush to apply the fluoride gel. Sensitivity and pain are common side effects of fluoride and may necessitate a change in the fluoride concentration or the method of application. A daily fluoride program can decrease hypersensitivity, help mineralize cavitated enamel matrices, and, more important, inhibit caries-forming organisms.

Conventional oral physiotherapy is recommended during and after radiation, especially if the pterygoid muscles are within the radiation portals. Fibrosis of this musculature leads to trismus, which may be irreversible. Therefore, patients should be encouraged to perform mouth-stretching exercises before, during, and after radiation therapy. When needed, sophisticated means of oral opening exercises with opening devices may be recommended.

Radiation diminishes cellular elements of bone, thereby reducing its ability to heal after infection, trauma, or surgical procedure (e.g., dental extraction, alveoloplasty), which may result in osteoradionecrosis (ORN). Therefore, periodontal surgical intervention should be planned carefully and the use of parenteral antibiotics and hyperbaric oxygen should be considered.

NUTRITIONAL SUPPORT

Assessment and Guidance

Nutritional care is crucial in the radiation treatment of most patients with head and neck cancer. Patients receive dietary advice to help maintain their weight and nitrogen balance during the course of radiotherapy and the ensuing recovery period. Good nutritional support minimizes the need for therapy modifications (interruptions or dose reduction due to worsening of general condition and/or excessive reactions) that would compromise tumor cure probability.

It is essential that the dietitian establishes a good rapport with the patient and provides basic instructions during the first week of treatment before the onset of acute reactions. It is prudent to counsel the patient's family members because the patient, who is under stress after learning the diagnosis and experiencing discomfort and pain, may not fully comprehend the instructions. Follow-up meetings are scheduled once a week, or more often when interim problems occur, and data of weekly interviews are recorded along with the patient's initial and follow-up body weight.

The attending physician and nutritionist should review the chart and recommend dietary adjustments when necessary.

Patients receiving radiation treatment of cancers of the oral cavity, oropharynx, nasopharynx, and hypopharynx are particularly prone to develop difficulties with food intake because of irradiation of a large area of mucous membranes and salivary glands. Therefore, they are encouraged to take supplemental calories at the beginning of treatment before the onset of reactions. The first problem encountered by this group of patients relates to alteration in salivary function, resulting in mucoid thick saliva. Moistened foods and increased fluid intake frequently facilitate mastication and deglutition during the first week.

Taste distortion (metallic flavor), loss of appetite, and burning sensation in the throat when swallowing citrus juices and acidic or spicy food become prominent during the second and third weeks. Helpful measures include the use of bland fruit nectars or fruit-flavored drinks fortified with vitamin C, elimination of highly seasoned foods, addition of food aroma, and serving meals at room temperature.

Mucosal edema and denudation, resulting in dysphagia and pain, dominate the latter part of the treatment. At this time, the patient and family need constant support from the medical team. During this period, the diet should contain sufficient calories and supplementary protein to promote normal tissue regeneration. It is important to adjust the diet individually in terms of texture, consistency, and portion size. In general, soft diet (blended meat and vegetable) and frequent intake of small meals are recommended. Analgesics taken before meals can ease the pain.

Tube Feeding

If weight reduction exceeds 5%, feeding through a gastrostomy tube, inserted by percutaneous fluoroscopic or endoscopic procedure, is usually recommended. Occasionally, a Dobhoff nasogastric feeding tube is used. Several commercially prepared canned products are available for tube feeding. These formulas have a known nutritional composition and are convenient to use and store. Lactose-free and low osmolarity products are also available to minimize diarrhea.

Examples of commonly used formulas include Isocal HN (1 cal per mL or 250 cal per can) and Protain XL (contains fiber and 237 cal per can). Isosource (contains fiber and 1.5 cal per mL or 375 cal per can) is more suitable for heavy patients. Tube feeding by gravity drip method begins with a half can on the day of gastric tube placement and increases gradually to six to eight cans per day, or more for heavier patients, generally divided into four or more sessions, depending on the estimated caloric requirement. Feedings are generally given over 1 hour for each session with a gravity drip and a bag. It is important to flush the gastric tube with 120 mL of water after feeding to prevent clogging. Depending on the fluid balance, supplemental water intake may be advised.

In case patients or their family members wish to prepare the tube feeding formula at home, guidelines for adding minerals and vitamins are provided because these elements may be destroyed by food processing and by repeated heating. Patients receiving concurrent radiation and chemotherapy may need hospital admission for rehydration and feeding.

Diet after Completion of Radiotherapy

Instructions for future meal plans are provided at discharge. Generally, nutritional problems continue for 2 to 3 weeks after completion of radiotherapy. The recovery period can be longer after altered fractionation or combination of radiation and chemotherapy. Subsequently, the patient can progress gradually to a normal diet except for the adaptation required to circumvent dryness of the mouth. It is advantageous for patients to visit the dieticians again during follow-up visits to reassess their nutritional status.

Swallowing Assessment and Rehabilitation

Both acute and late effects of radiation can disrupt a patient's ability to swallow. Early assessment by speech pathologists with expertise in swallowing rehabilitation is desirable, preferably before initiation of radiation, for planning strategies for the prevention of chronic dependence on feeding tubes or swallowing dysfunction that can lead to aspiration. Specific swallowing exercises designed to potentially prevent the debilitating effects of post-radiation fibrosis, when recommended, need to be implemented as early as possible.

Patients with postirradiation swallowing difficulties are also referred to speech pathologists for rehabilitative purposes. A modified barium swallow, a study designed to examine the oropharyngeal movement while swallowing various food consistencies, provides information on bolus movement patterns, motility problems, and the cause of aspiration. A specific rehabilitation program can be implemented based on the findings.

SYMPTOMATIC MANAGEMENT OF REACTIONS

Careful management of acute reactions manifesting during treatment is important for decreasing discomfort and for avoiding interruption of radiotherapy, which is shown to compromise local–regional control of head and neck carcinoma.

Acute Mucositis

Treatment of acute mucositis is mainly symptomatic. In addition to pain management (see following text), patients receive instruction and encouragement to maintain good oral hygiene and to rinse and gargle with baking soda solution (1 teaspoon dissolved in 1 quart of water) after and between meals, at least five to six times a day, to minimize secondary infection. When oral candidiasis occurs, it is treated with nystatin suspension (100,000 U per mL, 4 to 6 mL, swish and swallow, four times per day) or clotrimazole (Mycelex) troche (one troche orally, five times per day).

It has been suggested that mucositis is in part mediated by endotoxins mainly produced by gram-negative oral bacteria that are able to penetrate the radiation-injured mucous membrane. Therefore, prevention of superinfection by gram-negative bacteria and candida is thought to be effective in reducing the acute reactions. Data on the efficacy of oral rinses or troches with a combination of polymyxin B, tobramycin, and clotrimazole or amphotericin in decreasing the severity of radiation-induced mucositis are rather conflicting. A recently completed randomized study testing the efficacy of IB-367 (iseganan), a broad spectrum, topical antimicrobial peptide, did not show beneficial effects.

The role of amifostine or WR-2721 (Ethyol), a radioprotector, in reducing the incidence of mucositis is not yet clearly defined. The data of a small French trial using a highly accelerated radiation fractionation schedule that resulted in an extremely high rate of confluent mucositis suggested an amelioration of the intense mucosal reactions with the administration of amifostine. These conflicting results may be due to the requirement of higher amifostine doses to protect mucosa than to protect salivary glands.

The role of systemic or topical administration of growth factors or prostaglandins for the prevention of mucositis remains investigational. Antiulcer medications such as sucralfate (Carafate) rinse have been used, but numerous randomized trials have not shown its benefit in reducing the incidence of mucositis or in diminishing the duration of mucositis.

Analgesics

Almost all patients receiving head and neck radiotherapy need pain management to get through a period of acute radiation reactions. Various combinations of acetaminophen with hydrocodone, codeine, or oxycodone can be used. For easing mild-to-moderate pain starting to manifest 10 to 14 days into a course of radiotherapy, a frequently prescribed analgesic is acetaminophen 500 mg and hydrocodone bitartrate 7.5 mg tablets (Lortab 7.5/500) or elixir (15 mL contains about the same dose as one 500/7.5 tablet). The usual dosing is one to two tablets or 15 to 30 mL elixir every 4 to 6 hours. Other frequently used analgesics include acetaminophen 300 mg and codeine phosphate 30 mg (Tylenol with codeine No. 3), one to two tablets every 4 to 6 hours; acetaminophen 325 mg and oxycodone hydrochloride 5 mg (Percocet); and acetaminophen 325 mg and propoxyphene napsylate 50 mg (Darvocet-N 50), one to two tablets orally every 4 to 6 hours.

Severe and refractory pain, which can occur during the second half of the radiotherapy regimen, may necessitate therapy with stronger opioids. Examples include morphine sulphate (10 or 20 mg per 5 mL elixir, 10 to 30 mg orally every 4 to 6 hours); hydromorphone tablets (Dilaudid; 2 to 4 mg every 4 to 6 hours) or oral liquid (5 mg per 5 mL every 4 to 6 hours); or suppositories (3 mg every 4 to 6 hours).

Sustained-release opioids may help in maintenance therapy for severe pain. Examples include morphine sulfate tablets (MSContin; 30 mg, 60 mg, or higher dose, every 12 hours) and fentanyl transdermal patch (Duragesic; 25, 50, 75, 100 μg per hour, every 3 days).

In general, topical anesthetics should be used sparingly because of their tendency to induce hypersensitivity reactions. When indicated, lidocaine gel 2% can be prescribed for topical application or swish-and-swallow/spit, up to four times a day. Frequently, minor oral or pharyngeal pain can be ameliorated with a solution of viscous lidocaine, diphenhydramine hydrochloride (Benadryl), and aluminum hydroxide/magnesium hydroxide (Maalox) (Xyloxylin; Magic Mouthwash).

Prevention and Treatment of Constipation

It is prudent to inform patients that analgesics tend to cause constipation and to prescribe sennoside tablets (Senokot; two tablets, up to four times a day) or docusate sodium capsules (Colace; 100 mg, one to two capsules every day) to prevent this side effect. Patients receiving tube feeding can take docusate sodium syrup (15 mL, 20 mg per 5 mL) plus sennoside syrup (Senokot; 5 mL, 8.8 mg per 5 mL) two to three times per day via the gastric tube.

Antiemetics

Depending on the site and size of radiation portals, a variable proportion of patients experiences nausea and occasional vomiting. Useful medications include prochlorperazine maleate (Compazine; 5 or 10 mg tablets every 6 to 8 hours, 5 mg per 5 mL syrup 1 to 2 teaspoons every 6 to 8 hours, or 25 mg suppositories twice daily) and metoclopramide hydrochloride (Reglan; 10 mg tablet or 1 to 2 teaspoons syrup, 5 mg per 5 mL, before meals and at bedtime). Capsules containing 0.34 mg lorazepam, 25 mg diphenhydramine, and 2 mg haloperidol (ABH capsules) or suppositories (containing 1 mg lorazepam, 12.5 mg diphenhydramine, and 2 mg haloperidol) are effective when given every 4 to 6 hours.

Serotonin 5-HT3 receptor antagonists such as ondansetron hydrochloride (Zofran; 8 mg tablets or sublingual preparation every 8 to 12 hours) are also effective, especially for patients receiving concurrent chemotherapy. However, nausea and vomiting are often secondary to poor oral fluid intake, resulting in dehydration and, therefore, intravenous fluids rather than antiemetics are required to correct the problem.

Skin Reactions

With megavoltage radiotherapy, skin care generally consists of prevention of local irritation by encouraging the use of soft clothing and avoiding sunlight exposure. Small areas of moist skin desquamation that occur occasionally require cleaning with a diluted 1% hydrogen peroxide solution to prevent secondary infection. Larger areas of moist skin desquamation can be managed with hydrogel sheet (e.g., CoolMagic) wound dressing.

Aquaphor ointment is routinely prescribed for topical application after completion of radiotherapy. Patients are also instructed to use sunblock over the irradiated skin surface.

Prevention and Management of Xerostomia

The salivary glands are relatively radiosensitive. The dose of radiation causing irreversible damage to the salivary glands was thought to be approximately 35 Gy, although the volume of gland irradiated and the variation of the baseline individual flow affect the severity of radiation-induced xerostomia. Xerostomia compromises quality of life because it necessitates a change in lifestyle and eating habits, which can be devastating to some patients. Efforts to alleviate this problem involve both prevention and symptom management.

Prevention of xerostomia has taken two directions: Reducing radiation dose to the salivary glands and using chemical protectors. Advances in intensity-modulated radiation therapy technology enable sparing of the salivary gland even in patients not suitable for receiving unilateral irradiation. This approach has been studied in a number of centers and by the Radiation Therapy Oncology Group and is being implemented in many centers. Data obtained so far suggest that maintaining a mean dose of less than 25 to 26 Gy to one parotid gland can prevent complete xerostomia.

Amifostine has been studied extensively for prevention of various radiation side effects, particularly xerostomia. A randomized trial comparing intravenous amifostine, 200 mg per m^2 daily before each radiation fraction, to no treatment demonstrated a reduction of the incidence of grade 2 xerostomia from approximately 50% to 30%. The study demonstrated no obvious "tumor protection" because the disease-free and overall survival rates were no different between the two treatment arms. There was a significant increase in the incidence of nausea in patients receiving the drug along with a low incidence of amifostine-induced hypotension. Based on the results of this trial, the US Food and Drug Administration approved the use of amifostine for prevention of xerostomia in patients receiving postoperative radiotherapy.

Intravenous administration before daily fractionated radiation is cumbersome for patients and the radiation support personnel. Therefore, studies have been undertaken to investigate the efficacy of subcutaneous administration, with the expectation that this route of delivery is logistically easier and has a lower toxicity profile.

The role of pilocarpine (Salagen), a cholinergic agonist, in the treatment of xerostomia has been studied extensively. A large randomized trial compared 5 to 10 mg of pilocarpine, given three times a day, against placebo in patients with documented radiation-induced xerostomia. Both objective and subjective test endpoints demonstrated a benefit of the drug. A recently completed randomized trial of the Radiation Therapy Oncology Group revealed that pilocarpine administered during the course of radiotherapy increased the salivary flow at 3 months after treatment, but without detectable improvement in quality of life end points.

Sialogogues and saliva substitutes are available and may benefit occasional patients. Caution is recommended regarding some sialogogues, particularly candies, because the limited subjective benefit can be countered by rapid dental decay.

Other Supportive Care

Moisturizing nasal spray (e.g., Ocean Spray, Nose Better) is recommended during the period of confluent mucositis occurring in the nasal cavity to prevent crusting and bleeding. Topical antibiotic (Neosporin ointment) is prescribed when infection develops.

Antitussive expectorant without suppressant (e.g., guaifenesin 600 mg, one to two tablets twice daily [Humibid-LA]) or with suppressant (e.g., guaifenesin and dextromethorphan, 600/30, one to two tablets twice daily [Humibid-DM]) can relieve symptoms in a number of patients. Other options in lieu of hydrocodone bitartrate and aspirin include 5 mL syrup containing 10 mg hydrocodone bitartrate and 8 mg chlorpheniramine maleate (Tussionex), which can be a good cough suppressant for nighttime relief.

SUGGESTED READINGS

Brizel DM, Wasserman TH, Henke M, et al. Phase III randomized trial of amifostine as a radioprotector in head and neck cancer. *J Clin Oncol* 2000;18:3339.

Trotti A, Garden A, Warde P, et al. A multinational, randomized phase III trial of iseganan HCl oral solution for reducing the severity of oral mucositis in patients receiving radiotherapy for head-and-neck malignancy. *Int J Radiat Oncol Biol Phys* 2004;58:674.

PART

Site-Specific Indications and Techniques

The second part of this manual systematically presents the treatment approach and technique of radiotherapy applied in each disease site. A uniform presentation format is followed to facilitate review. First, the treatment strategies for various tumor stages are summarized. A large number of clinical studies, including most of those cited in the previous edition, have been completed in the interim stage and some have yielded data that change our standard of care. Therefore, the treatment strategy and recommendations for a number of cancers have been updated. The staging system used for treatment recommendations for individual sites is based on the 6th edition manual of the American Joint Committee on Cancer, published in 2002, unless otherwise specified.

Subsequently, the technical details of radiation treatment (target volumes, field setup and arrangements, and dose prescription and fractionation) are described. Case illustrations (i.e., history, simulation film with portal design, target volumes, and other relevant materials) are provided for common disease varieties. This is intended to allow readers to follow each step of treatment planning and delivery in day-to-day practice. With the impressive progress in computer technology, there have been substantial technologic advances in dosimetric planning and treatment delivery since the publication of the second edition. High-precision radiotherapy has become an appealing and practical technique ready for clinical testing. There is increasing interest in applying conformal radiotherapy in the treatment of patients with head and neck cancers in attempts to reduce troublesome complications (e.g., xerostomia and fibrosis), to increase tumor control by improving target volume coverage, or both. Since intensity-modulated radiation therapy (IMRT) is relatively new, we have added many illustrative examples.

Finally, background clinical data are referenced. It is not the intention to provide a comprehensive review of the literature but rather to present data that have contributed to the development of our institutional standard and the results that have been obtained by applying such strategies. The stages presented in the clinical background data sections are obviously according to the staging system used by the authors during the respective study periods. Therefore, it is not prudent to make a direct comparison between data of different series because the characteristics of the study populations are not equivalent among most series.

Site-Specific Indications and Techniques

Oral Cavity

7

LIP

Treatment Strategy

Surgery is generally preferred in medically operable patients in the following situations:

- T1 lesions (up to 2 cm in diameter) that do not involve the oral commissure. Excision of such lesions is simple (V or W excision with primary closure or flap reconstruction), and the functional and cosmetic outcome is satisfactory.
- Younger patients who will have prolonged sunlight exposure (e.g., those engaged in outdoor work).
- Diffuse, superficial lesion of the vermilion or the presence of severe actinic keratosis adjacent to the carcinoma. A lip shave with oral mucosa advancement closure generally yields a good control rate with satisfactory cosmetic outcome.

Radiation is a good option for lesions larger than 2 cm or those involving the commissure, in which surgical resection results in microstomia or oral incontinence. Radiotherapy can be delivered by external beam irradiation, brachytherapy, or a combination of both, depending on the location and size of the lesion.

A combination of surgery and radiotherapy is frequently required for advanced destructive lesions, that is those invading the bone or nerve, or with nodal involvement.

Primary Radiotherapy

Target Volume
Initial Target Volume
- *T2 N0:* primary tumor with 2-cm margins. Elective neck irradiation is not given routinely for well-differentiated carcinomas.
- *T3 N0:* primary tumor with 2-cm margins and submental, submandibular, and subdigastric nodes.
- *T2, T3, N+:* primary tumor with 2-cm margins and submental, submandibular, subdigastric, mid- and low jugular nodes.

A boost volume encompasses the primary lesion with 1-cm margins and, when present, involved nodes.

Setup and Field Arrangement for External Beam Irradiation
An intraoral stent containing cerrobend is used to displace the tongue posteriorly and, if feasible, shield the alveolar ridge. The patient is immobilized in a supine position. An appositional field is used to treat the primary tumor. Field borders are determined clinically by bimanual palpation. Treatment can be given with orthovoltage x-rays or electrons. Electron energy is chosen on the basis of thickness of the lesion. The upper neck nodes are treated with lateral parallel–opposed photon fields:

- *Anterior border:* 1 cm in front of the mandibular arch.
- *Superior border:* splitting the horizontal ramus of the mandible.
- *Posterior border:* midvertebral body.
- *Inferior border:* just above the arytenoids.

Moustache field for upper lip lesion: appositional electron fields (usually approximately 15-degree gantry angle) are used to treat the facial lymphatics.

- *Medial border:* matches the lateral border of the anterior field (primary tumor).
- *Anterior border:* extends down from oral commissure to midmandible.
- *Posterior border:* from the upper edge of the anterior field to just above the angle of the mandible.
- *Inferior border:* splitting the horizontal ramus of the mandible and adjoining the upper neck field.
- This field is set up clinically after designing the primary tumor and upper neck portals.

Patients with palpable node(s) receive irradiation to mid- and lower neck nodes through an anterior portal. The primary lesion receives boost dose through an appositional field with orthovoltage x-rays or electrons. Nodal metastases receive boost dose with appositional electrons or glancing photon fields.

Brachytherapy

Brachytherapy is usually accomplished by afterloading iridium 192 (^{192}Ir)-wire implants. Whenever possible, a custom-made plastic device is placed between the lip and gum to increase the distance between the radioactive sources and alveolar structures to decrease radiation exposure to normal tissues. Occasionally, cerrobend can be incorporated in the device to provide additional protection.

Dosage

- *Small lesions (less than 1.5 cm):* 50 Gy in 25 fractions, in addition to 6 to 10 Gy in three to five fractions boost by external irradiation or 60 to 65 Gy over 5 to 7 days by implants.
- *Larger lesions:* 50 Gy in 25 fractions, in addition to 10 to 16 Gy in five to eight fractions boost by external beam or 20- to 25-Gy boost by implants.
- *Elective treatment of facial (moustache area) and upper neck nodes:* 50 Gy in 25 fractions.
- Palpable nodes receive boost dose to a total dose of 66 to 70 Gy depending on the size.

Dose Specification

In external beam irradiation, the dose to the primary lesion is administered at D_{max} for orthovoltage x-rays and at 90% for electrons. This accounts for the difference in relative biologic effectiveness between the two beam modalities.

For brachytherapy, the dose is administered at the isodose line encompassing the lesion.

Moustache fields are irradiated with 6-MeV electrons and the dose is prescribed at D_{max}.

Postoperative Radiotherapy

Indications for postoperative irradiation are advanced lesions (bone involvement, extensive perineural invasion), positive margins, and multiple nodes or extracapsular extension (ECE).

In general, the radiation setup is the same as that for primary radiotherapy, but should be tailored individually depending on the location of the primary lesion (upper vs. lower lip) and on the extent of nerve and lymphatic coverage.

The dose prescription is 60 Gy in 30 fractions to areas with high-risk features, 56 Gy per 28 fractions to the surgical bed, and 50 Gy in 25 fractions to electively irradiated regions.

Background Data

TABLE 7.1

CONTROL OF PRIMARY LIP LESION BY TREATMENT METHOD

Initial Treatment to Primary Lesion	Nodal Involvement on Admission	No. of Cases	Percentage of Patients with Primary Controlled by	
			Initial Treatment	Later Treatment
Radiotherapy alone	Absent	2,415	85.3	8.3
	Present	243	68.7	7.4
Radiotherapy + surgery	Absent	158	88.0	5.7
	Present	7	57.1	14.3
Surgery alone	Absent	21	71.4	14.3
	Present	5	60.0	—
All methods	Absent	2,598	85.2	8.2
	Present	256	68.0	7.4

Data from the Ontario Cancer Treatment and Research Foundation.
From MacKay EN, Sellers AH. A statistical review of carcinoma of the lip. *Can Med Assoc J* 1964;90:670–672, with permission.

TABLE 7.2

CANCER OF THE LIP IN PREVIOUSLY UNTREATED PATIENTS

Size of Lesion (cm)	Treatment	No. of Patients	No. Controlled	No. Salvaged	Total No. Controlled
0–1	Radiotherapy	30	30	—	30
	Surgery	239	233	6	239
1–2	Radiotherapy	36	34	1	35
	Surgery	116	113	1	114
>2	Radiotherapy	7	7	—	7
	Surgery	7	4	0	4
Massive	Radiotherapy	1	1	—	1
	Surgery	8	7	0	7

Data from M.D. Anderson Cancer Center.
Modified from MacComb WS et al. Intra-oral cavity. In: MacComb WS, Fletcher GH, eds. *Cancer of the head and neck.* Baltimore: Williams & Wilkins, 1967.

FLOOR OF MOUTH AND ORAL TONGUE

Treatment Strategy

Surgical resection is generally preferred in medically operable patients. Depending on the size, depth of invasion, and grade of differentiation of the primary tumor and nodal status, surgery may include a modified neck dissection.

Postoperative radiotherapy is recommended in the following situations (see Figs. 7.1 to 7.3): large primary tumor (e.g., T3 or T4); close or positive surgical margins; presence of perineural spread,

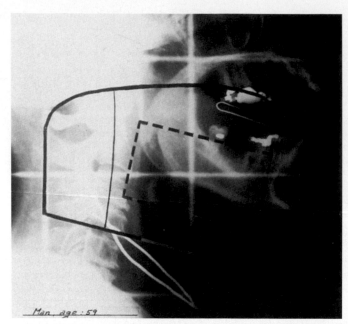

Figure 7.1   A 59-year-old man presented with a 1-month history of sore mouth. On physical examination, a 2.5-cm ulcerative, mobile lesion was noted in the right anterior part of the floor of mouth. The tumor involved the frenulum of the tongue, but did not cross the midline. The mobility of the tongue was normal. A 1.5-cm mobile lymph node was palpated at the right submandibular area. Biopsy of the primary tumor showed moderately differentiated squamous cell carcinoma. Stage: T2 N1 M0. This patient underwent a wide local excision of the primary tumor and bilateral supraomohyoid neck dissections. The defect in the floor of mouth was repaired with a split-thickness skin graft. At the time of surgery, the tumor was found to involve the sublingual gland and the deep musculature. The initial deep margin was positive, but was converted to negative by further excision of the muscle. Of the five nodes recovered from the right neck specimen, one submandibular node measuring 2 cm was involved with carcinoma with evidence of extracapsular extension (ECE). Seven lymph nodes recovered from the left side were all free of tumor. Pathologic stage: p T4 N1. The patient was placed on the postoperative radiotherapy protocol. The primary site and upper neck were treated with parallel opposed–lateral photon fields. By using a tongue depressor, the hard palate and part of the soft palate and upper gums could be excluded from the radiation field. The mid- and lower neck nodes were treated with an anterior appositional photon field with a midline block to shield the larynx. This block was placed just above the surgical scar in the neck, which is marked with a wire. The primary tumor bed and uninvolved nodal areas received 57.6 Gy in 32 fractions. Because of the presence of ECE, the involved nodal area was boosted to 63 Gy in 35 fractions. The boost dose to the right upper neck was delivered with an appositional electron field. He had no evidence of disease and was free of complications 2 years after treatment.

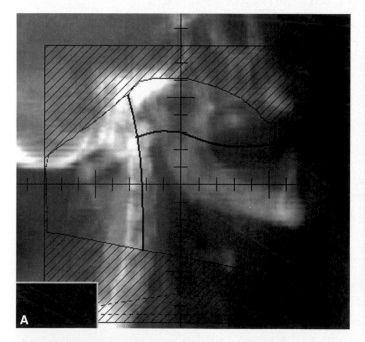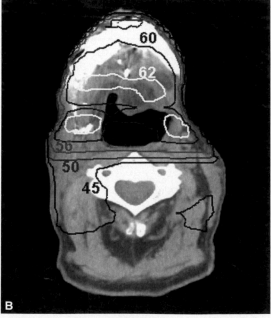

Figure 7.2   A 54-year-old man underwent a partial glossectomy for a small oral tongue carcinoma. The surgical margins were negative and there were no adverse features for recommending adjuvant radiation. He re-presented 2 years later with a large recurrent tumor (biopsy positive for squamous cell carcinoma) with extension into the anterior floor of mouth and base of tongue as well as to the lateral pharyngeal wall. He underwent a composite resection and neck dissection. Final section margins were negative, and two lymph nodes contained metastatic squamous cell carcinoma. Stage: recurrent. He received adjunctive postoperative radiotherapy given in 2 Gy per day. An off–spinal cord reduction was made at 42 Gy and the boost cone-down at 56 Gy to bring the total dose to 60 Gy. He was treated with a mouth-opening stent depressing the remaining oral tongue and floor of mouth tissues. A digitally reconstructed radiograph with the primary, off–spinal cord, and boost portals is shown (**A**) along with the isodose distribution through an axial cut in the oral cavity (**B**). Following the off–spinal cord reduction, the posterior cervical strips were supplemented with electrons (not shown). Large-field irradiations were delivered with cobalt-60 beam, whereas the off–spinal cord and boost fields were irradiated with 6 MV photons. The low neck is treated with a matching supraclavicular field.

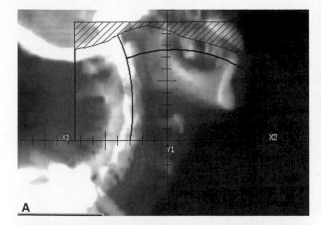

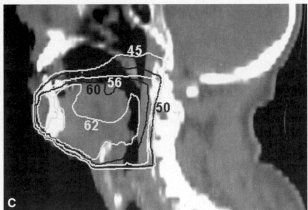

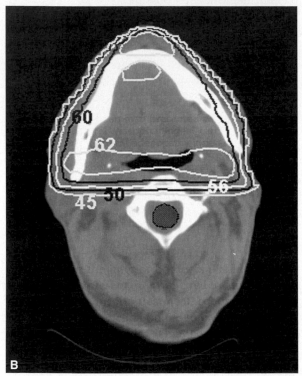

Figure 7.3 A 65-year-old man presented with ill-fitting dentures and oral pain. Physical examination revealed a 4-cm tumor on the right lateral tongue, an enlarged submandibular gland, and a 3-cm right upper jugular node. Stage T2 N2b M0. He underwent a partial glossectomy and selective right neck dissection. Pathologic examination showed a squamous cell carcinoma of the tongue with negative section margins but presence of perineural invasion. Five of 40 dissected nodes were positive and there was extracapsular extension. He received adjunctive postoperative radiotherapy delivered with 6 MV photons for the entire treatment using an isocentric technique. A 3-mm tissue-equivalent bolus was placed over the scar. A digitally reconstructed radiograph with the fields is shown **(A)**. An off–spinal cord reduction was made at 42 Gy and a boost cone-down at 56 Gy. The posterior cervical strips were supplemented with 9 MeV electrons, 18 Gy to the right strip and 8 Gy to the left strip. Axial **(B)** and sagittal **(C)** isodoses through the tongue are shown. The supraclavicular field had a larynx (and spinal cord safety) block. Both sides of the lower neck received 50 Gy. The right mid- and lower neck received 6 Gy boost dose. These fields were further reduced off the inferior border to take the right neck at risk to 60 Gy.

vascular invasion, or both; or presence of multiple positive nodes or ECE. Patients considered at high risk, such as those having positive section, margins or ECE, are now recommended to receive concurrent radiation with cisplatin when there is no medical contraindication.

Primary radiotherapy is generally reserved for patients who refuse surgery or those who are borderline operable.

Postoperative Radiotherapy

Target Volume

Initial Target Volume

The entire surgical bed—site of the primary tumor, dissected neck (in most cases, neck dissection is part of the surgical treatment), and dissected draining lymphatics. Elective nodal irradiation is given in conjunction with postoperative radiotherapy to the primary tumor bed in N0 patients who are not undergoing nodal dissection.

Boost Volume

In areas of original tumor and involved nodes, a second cone-down may be made to deliver additional boost dose to the region carrying the highest risk of recurrence (e.g., sites of extracapsular nodal disease or positive margins).

Setup and Field Arrangement

The patient is immobilized in a supine position with a thermoplastic mask. For tumors of the oral tongue or floor of mouth that extend close to or into the tongue, an intraoral stent is used to open the mouth, depress the tongue, and protrude the lower lip. This device allows exclusion of a large area of the buccal mucosa, lower lip, and oral commissure from the radiation portals. For tumors of the floor of mouth not extending into the oral tongue, a stent that opens the mouth and elevates the tip of the tongue beyond the field is used to exclude as much of the tongue (tip, dorsum) from the radiation portal as possible. Marking of surgical scar and oral commissures before obtaining a simulation film may facilitate portal design.

Parallel opposed–lateral photon fields are used to treat the primary tumor bed and upper neck nodes.

- *Anterior border:* just in front of the mandible for anterior tumors or 2 cm in front of the scar for posterior oral cavity lesions. The lower lip is shielded whenever possible.
- *Superior border:* 1 to 1.5 cm superior to the dorsum of the tongue or the scar if part of the oral tongue can be spared. In the event of positive nodes, this border should encompass the high jugular nodes to the jugular fossa.
- *Posterior border:* usually is dictated by the surgical scar. The level II nodes are systematically irradiated. Therefore, the posterior border is placed behind the spinous processes or farther back to cover an extended scar.
- *Inferior border:* just superior to the arytenoids.

An anterior appositional field is used to treat the mid- and lower neck nodes. Field borders are indicated in the section "General Principles."

To deliver the boost dose to the primary tumor and upper neck nodes, the size of lateral fields is reduced to encompass the known disease locations. To boost the upper neck without the primary site, a lateral appositional electron field is used. To deliver the boost to the mid- or lower neck, a lateral appositional electron field or glancing photon fields are used.

Dose

- A dose of 60 Gy in 30 fractions is administered to areas with high-risk features, that is close or microscopically positive margins, perineural extension, vascular invasion, positive nodes, or extranodal extension. An additional boost dose of 6 Gy in three fractions may be given when indicated, such as when multiple adverse features are present or when the interval between surgery and radiation is much longer than 6 weeks.
- A dose of 56 Gy in 28 fractions to the surgical bed.
- A dose of 50 Gy of elective irradiation in 25 fractions to undissected regions.

Intensity-Modulated Radiation Therapy Planning

Conformal radiotherapy can eliminate sequential portal cone-down because the difference in dose prescription to the tumor bed and to regions at risk for harboring microscopic disease is achieved by varying the fraction size. When using intensity-modulated radiation therapy (IMRT) in the postoperative setting, treatment is given in 30 fractions. The target volumes to receive various levels of doses are delineated and dosimetric plans are generated by the iterative process. Generally, the tumor bed target volume receives 60 Gy, the operative bed receives 57 Gy, and undissected regions receive 54 Gy. Various situations where IMRT are used are given in Figures 7.4–7.6.

Smaller target volumes considered to be at extra-high risk, often determined in collaboration with the surgeon and based on pathologic findings, receive 64 to 66 Gy (Fig. 7.6).

The patient is immobilized in a supine position, with an extended thermoplastic mask covering head and shoulder. Thin-cut computed tomography (CT) images are obtained in treatment position and target volumes are outlined for dosimetric planning.

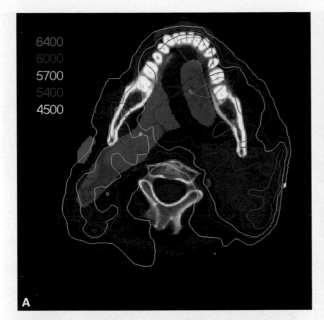

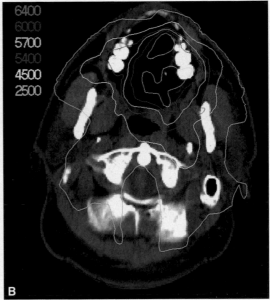

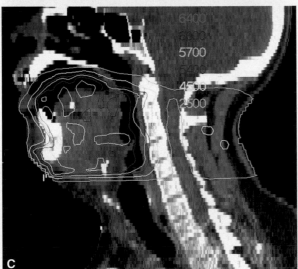

Figure 7.4   A 38-year-old man treated with a limited resection of an oral tongue squamous cell carcinoma presented 2 years following surgery with a recurrence. He underwent a left partial glossectomy with a radial forearm graft reconstruction and left neck dissection. The tumor had 1.3-cm depth of invasion, section margins were negative (deep margin 0.6 cm) and nodes were not involved. Due to the recurrent nature and depth of invasion, he was treated with postoperative radiation using intensity-modulated radiation therapy. **A:** Axial view with contours. The green volume represents the preoperative disease and blue volume the clinical target volume to receive 60 Gy. The purple volume represents the remaining operative bed (including a wired scar), planned to 57 Gy, while the yellow contour represents the remaining tongue and contralateral neck nodes planned to 54 Gy. **B:** Superior axial cut. **C:** Sagittal view of isodose distribution through midplane. The patient remains well 2 years from all therapy with good speech and oral comfort.

Timing of Postoperative Radiotherapy

It is desirable to commence postoperative radiotherapy as soon as possible after healing of surgical wounds. With good communication between surgical, radiation, and dental oncologists, simulation can usually take place 3 to 4 weeks after surgery, and radiotherapy can start a few days later in most patients. When delayed wound healing postpones commencement of postoperative radiation to beyond 5 to 6 weeks, we administer accelerated fractionation, such as concomitant boost, by delivering twice-a-day irradiations for 1 week, usually at the end of the radiation course, to reduce the potential hazard of prolonged cumulative treatment time.

Dose Specification: See "General Principles"

Primary Radiotherapy

Target Volume
Initial Target Volume
- *A well-differentiated, superficial lesion of 1 cm or less with no palpable lymphadenopathy (T1 N0):* primary tumor with 2-cm margins.

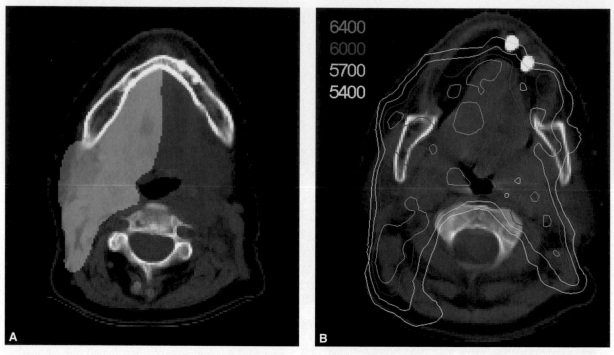

Figure 7.5   A 62-year-old woman presented with 2 months of oral pain was found to have a biopsy-proven squamous cell carcinoma of the right lateral oral tongue, clinically staged T1 N0. She underwent a right partial glossectomy and right neck dissection. Histologic examination revealed a 2.5-cm tumor with negative section margins but perineural invasion, and two positive level II nodes. She was treated with postoperative intensity-modulated radiation therapy. **A:** The right tongue and neck were identified as clinical target volume 60 (*green*), whereas the univolved contralateral tongue and neck were CTV 54 (*blue*). **B:** Axial isodose distribution. She remains without disease 30 months post-treatment.

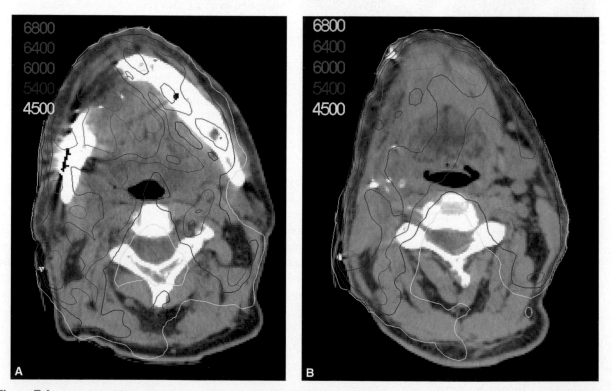

Figure 7.6   A 61-year-old man presented with a mass on his right alveolar ridge, biopsy of which revealed squamous cell carcinoma. There was no clinical lymphadenopathy but there was bone invasion—stage T4 N0. He underwent a gingival resection with marginal mandibulectomy and right neck dissection. Pathology revealed a positive final margin and, despite clinically N0 status, six positive nodes with extracapsular spread. He was treated postoperatively with concurrent chemotherapy and intensity-modulated radiation therapy. Axial isodose distributions through the mandible **(A)** and the floor of mouth **(B)** are shown. A high-risk target volume, the area of positive margin (reviewed with the surgeon), received 65 Gy while the remaining operative bed received 60 Gy. The patient is 18 months out from treatment, without local recurrence, but had developed pulmonary metastases 1 year after his radiation.

- *Floor of mouth (mostly anterior) lesion of 1- to 4-cm maximal diameter without palpable lymphadenopathy (T1-2 N0):* primary tumor with at least 2-cm margins and level I (submental and submandibular) and Level II (subdigastric only) nodes.
- *Oral tongue tumor greater than 1 cm thick with no palpable lymphadenopathy:* primary tumor with at least 2-cm margins and level I–IV (submental–submandibular, subdigastric, and mid- and lower jugular) nodes.
- Presence of lymphadenopathy (N+) at diagnosis calls for irradiation of the entire cervical nodal basins.

A boost volume encompasses the primary tumor (1- to 2-cm margins) and involves lymph nodes.

Setup and Field Arrangement

For small T1 N0 lesions, the entire treatment is given with an intraoral cone or by implant (if the risk for anesthesia is low).

For all other stages, the patient is immobilized in a supine position with a thermoplastic mask. Use of stent is as in postoperative cases. Inserting a seed at the anterior border of the tumor and marking the oral commissures before obtaining simulation film facilitates shaping of the radiation portal. Parallel–opposed lateral photon fields are used to treat the primary tumor and upper neck nodes. Field borders are, in general, similar to postoperative irradiation. The *anterior border* should be at least 2 cm in front of the tumor depending on the growth pattern. The *posterior border* depends on the nodal status (see "General Principles"). An anterior appositional photon field is used to treat the mid- and lower neck and supraclavicular nodes when indicated.

The boost dose to the primary tumor is preferably delivered by interstitial implant. If the patient cannot undergo anesthesia, boost dose is given with orthovoltage x-rays through an intraoral cone when accessible; in this case, the boost is delivered before the start of the external beam therapy while the tumor is clearly visible and palpable. In rare cases when neither implant nor intraoral cone is feasible, the boost is delivered using an external beam encompassing the tumor with 1- to 2-cm margins.

The technique for delivering the boost dose to palpable nodes depends on the strategy selected for the treatment of the primary lesion. It could be an interstitial implant, electron beams, or photons (included in the primary boost field or with separate fields, depending on the location).

Dose

Initial Target Volume

This volume receives 40 Gy in 20 fractions if this is followed by an interstitial implant, or 50 Gy in 25 fractions if the boost is delivered by intraoral cone or external beam.

Boost

The boost dose to the primary lesion delivered by an interstitial implant is 40 Gy, specified at an isodose line approximately 0.5 cm from the tumor margin; the boost dose by intraoral cone is 15 Gy in 3-Gy fractions or 20 to 25 Gy in 2.5-Gy fractions, and by external beam is 20 Gy in 10-Gy fractions for T1 lesions or 22 to 24 Gy in 2-Gy fractions for T2 to T3 lesions.

The dose to involved lymph nodes is in general 66 to 70 Gy for less than 3-cm nodes, or even higher for larger nodes if neck dissection is not contemplated because of anesthesia risk.

Small (less than 1 cm), superficial lesions may be treated with the intraoral cone (40 Gy in 10 fractions) or by an implant only (60 Gy in approximately 6 days).

Dose Specification: See "General Principles"

Background Data

TABLE 7.3

FLOOR OF MOUTH CANCER: FAILURE TO CONTROL THE PRIMARY LESION BY MODALITIES OF IRRADIATION—JANUARY 1948 THROUGH DECEMBER 1968

Stage	Failure Rate	External Irradiation	Interstitial Irradiation Only	External + Interstitial Irradiation Only
T1	2.0% (1/49)	0/10	1/31 (3%)	0/8
T2	11.5% (9/77)	5/23 (22%)	3/34 (9%)	1/20 (5%)
T3	23.0% (14/60)	9/25 (36%)	3/17 (18%)	2/18 (11%)
T4	79.0% (19/24)	13/16 (81%)	2/4	4/4

Data from M.D. Anderson Cancer Center.
Modified from Chu A, Fletcher GH. Incidence and causes of failures to control by irradiation the primary lesions in squamous cell carcinomas of the anterior two-thirds of the tongue and floor of mouth. *AJR Am J Roentgenol* 1973;117:502, with permission.

TABLE 7.4

CAUSES OF DEATH IN 116 PATIENTS WITH T1 (46 PATIENTS) OR T2 (70 PATIENTS) EPIDERMOID CARCINOMAS OF THE FLOOR OF THE MOUTH TREATED BY INTERSTITIAL RADIOTHERAPY

Stage	Disease-Related			Others			
	Tumor Failure	Neck Failure	Metastases	2nd Treatment	Cancer	Intercurrent	Unknown
T1 N0	1	2	—	—	10	7	6
T2 N0	10	2	1	2	12	2	5
T2 N1-3	7	5	2[a]	1	4	1	1

Cause of death is assigned in an orderly Tumor Neck Metastases fashion when more than one site of failure was present.
[a]Patients not treated to the neck because of rapid onset of metastatic disease after curietherapy.
Modified from Mazeron JJ, Grimard I, Raynal M, et al. Comparison of curietherapy versus external irradiation combined with curietherapy in stage II squamous cell carcinomas of the mobile tongue. *Int J Radiat Oncol Biol Phys* 1990;18:1299, with permission.

TABLE 7.5

ORAL CAVITY CANCERS TREATED WITH SURGERY AND POSTOPERATIVE IRRADIATION: INFLUENCE OF MARGIN STATUS ON LOCAL CONTROL (LITERATURE REVIEW)

Margin Status	Oral Tongue		Floor of Mouth	
	No. Controlled/Total (%)		No. Controlled/Total (%)	
	MSKCC	U of FL[a]	MSKCC	U of FL[a]
Negative	7/9 (78%)	9/12 (75%)	9/9 (100%)	10/13 (77%)
Close	10/16 (62%)	7/11 (64%)[b]	6/8 (75%)	8/9 (89%)[b]
Positive	2/4 (50%)	1/4 (25%)	4/5 (80%)	8/13 (62%)
Total	19/29 (66%)	17/27 (63%)	19/22 (86%)	26/35 (74%)

MSKCC, Memorial Sloan Kettering Cancer Center (Zelefsky MJ, Harrison LB, Fass DE, et al. 1993); University of Florida (Parsons JT, Mendenhall WM, Springer Sp, et al, 1997).
[a]Local–regional control.
[b]Includes close and initially positive.

TABLE 7.6

ORAL CAVITY CANCERS TREATED WITH SURGERY AND POSTOPERATIVE RADIATION: DISEASE CONTROL BY SITE, MARGIN STATUS, AND NODAL EXTENT

	No. of Patients	Local Control	Nodal Control	Control Above Clavicles	Distant Metastases
Oral tongue	137	78%	74%	65%	23%
Floor of mouth	107	70%	82%	60%	27%
Mandibular gingiva	28	81%	77%	63%	21%
Positive margin	32	73%	80%	58%	38%
Nodal ECE	110	72%	62%	48%	35%
Multiple nodes	158	67%	69%	51%	35%
Overall results	272	75%	77%	63%	27%

Unpublished data from M.D. Anderson Cancer Center, 1970–1995.
ECE, extracapsular extension.
All rates are 5-year actuarial.

TABLE 7.7

SITES AND FREQUENCY OF NODAL INVOLVEMENT[a] AT PRESENTATION IN 602 PATIENTS WITH CANCER OF THE MOBILE TONGUE

Site[b]	Ipsilateral	Contralateral
Submaxillary and submental	60 (10%)	13 (2%)
Subdigastric: upper jugular	130 (22%)	7 (1%)
Midjugular	110 (18%)	5 (1%)
Lower jugular: supraclavicular	34 (5%)	1 (.1%)

[a]Node either positive on aspiration cytology or on histologic examination or the node is 3 cm or more in dimension.
[b]Patients may have more than one site involved.
Modified from Decroix Y, Ghossein NA. Experience of the Curie Institute in treatment of cancer of the mobile tongue, I. Treatment policies and results. *Cancer* 1981;47:503.

TABLE 7.8

SQUAMOUS CELL CARCINOMAS OF THE ORAL TONGUE, TREATMENT WITH INTERSTITIAL IRRADIATION ALONE: INCIDENCE OF CLINICAL APPEARANCE OF NECK NODES BY STAGE AND TOPOGRAPHICAL LOCATION, JANUARY 1954–DECEMBER 1978 (ANALYSIS MARCH 1981)

Stage	No. of Patients	Neck Node Location				Incidence of Failure
		SM	UJ	MJ	LJ	
T1	44	2	9	3	—	32% (14/44)
T2	28	—	11	1	—	43% (12/28)
T3	4	—	—	1	—	25% (1/4)

SM, submandibular; UJ, upper jugular; MJ, midjugular; LJ, lower jugular.
Data from the M.D. Anderson Cancer Center.
From Meoz RT, Fletcher GH, Lindberg RD. Anatomic coverage in elective irradiation of the neck for squamous cell carcinoma of the oral tongue. *Int J Radiat Oncol Biol Phys* 1982;8:1881, with permission.

TABLE 7.9

PRIMARY CONTROL OF ORAL TONGUE CARCINOMA BY T-STAGE AND MODE OF RADIOTHERAPY

Method of Treatment	T1	T2	Total
Interstitial only	7/8 (88%)	4/9 (44%)	11/17 (65%)
Interstitial + external <40 Gy	2/2 (100%)	21/23 (92%)	23/25 (92%)
Interstitial + external = 40 Gy	4/6 (66%)	25/39 (64%)	29/45 (64%)
External only	—	2/7 (29%)	2/7 (29%)
Total	13/16 (81%)	52/78 (67%)	65/94 (69%)

Data from M.D. Anderson Cancer Center.
Modified from Wendt CD, Peters LJ, Delclos L, et al. Primary radiotherapy in the treatment of stage I and II oral tongue cancers: importance of the proportion of therapy delivered with interstitial therapy. *Int J Radiat Oncol Biol Phys* 1990;18:1287–1292, with permission.

TABLE 7.10

PRIMARY FAILURE RATE BY TREATMENT METHOD: STAGE T1 N0 AND T2 N0 SQUAMOUS CELL CARCINOMAS OF THE ORAL TONGUE

Method of Treatment	Number	At Risk <24 mo	Primary Failure	Primary Salvage (Salv/attempted)	Ultimate Primary Control
Interstitial only	18	1	6	5/6	16/17 (94%)
Interstitial + external <40 Gy	31	6	2	0/2	23/25 (92%)
Interstitial + external = 40 Gy	46	1	16	9/16	38/45 (84%)
External only	8	1	5	2/4	4/7 (57%)

Data from M.D. Anderson Cancer Center.
Modified from Wendt CD, Peters LJ, Delclos L, et al. Primary radiotherapy in the treatment of stage I and II oral tongue cancers: importance of the proportion of therapy delivered with interstitial therapy. *Int J Radiat Oncol Biol Phys* 1990;18:1287–1292, with permission.

TABLE 7.11

CONTROL OF SUBCLINICAL NECK DISEASE IN PATIENTS WITH PRIMARY CONTROL: STAGE I AND II ORAL TONGUE CANCERS

Method of Treatment	In-Field Failure	Out-Field Failure	% 2-yr Control with Initial Treatment[a]	No. Salvaged	Ultimate 2-yr Control[a] No. (%)
None (n = 16)	0	7	56	6	15/16 (94%)
<40 Gy to upper neck (n = 22)	6	2	63	6	20/22 (91%)
>40 Gy to upper neck (n = 15)	2	2	73	0	11/15 (73%)
>40 Gy to whole neck (n = 13)	1	0	93	1	13/13 (100%)

Data from M.D. Anderson Cancer Center.
[a]Excludes patients who died NED less than 2 years and those who had primary failure before or with neck failure.
Modified from Wendt CD, Peters LJ, Delclos L, et al. Primary radiotherapy in the treatment of stage I and II oral tongue cancers: importance of the proportion of therapy delivered with interstitial therapy. *Int J Radiat Oncol Biol Phys* 1990;18:1287–1292, with permission.

RETROMOLAR TRIGONE AND ANTERIOR FAUCIAL PILLAR

Treatment Strategy

Primary radiotherapy is indicated for relatively early tumors (T1–T2 and selected cases of T3 without deep ulceration or bone exposure) (see Fig 7.7). Larger tumors are treated with either combination of radiation and chemotherapy or surgery and postoperative radiotherapy.

Primary Radiotherapy

Target Volume
Initial Target Volume
- A *well-lateralized tumor without lymphadenopathy:* primary lesion (at least 2-cm margins) and ipsilateral level IB (submandibular) and level II (subdigastric) nodes.
- A *well-lateralized tumor with a single small ipsilateral node (N1):* primary lesion and the entire ipsilateral neck (including supraclavicular nodes).
- *Other cases (larger tumors and/or more advanced N-stage):* primary lesion and bilateral neck.

Boost Volume
The coned-down boost volume encompasses the primary tumor (1- to 2-cm margins) and, when present, the involved node. A limited planned neck dissection is carried out in rare occasions where a residual neck mass is present 6 weeks after completion of radiotherapy.

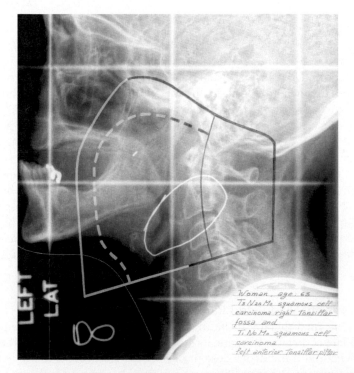

Figure 7.7 A 69-year-old man sought medical attention because of soreness in the left tonsillar area. An ulcerative tumor was observed on the left anterior tonsillar pillar extending to the edge of the retromolar trigone. The largest diameter of the tumor was 2.5 cm. There were no palpable neck nodes. A biopsy showed squamous cell carcinoma. Stage: T2 N0 M0. The patient was treated with an ipsilateral field encompassing the primary tumor and upper neck nodes. Metal seeds were inserted to indicate the medial and posterior borders of the tumor. A combination of 20 MeV electrons and 6 MV photons, in 4:1 proportion, was used. A dose of 50 Gy was delivered to the 90% isodose line and an off-cord reduction was made after 44 Gy. Subsequently, a field reduction was made to deliver a total dose of 66 Gy to the primary tumor.

Setup and Field Arrangement

For unilateral treatment only, generally a combination of electrons and photons, in a ratio of 4:1, is used. Insertion of metal seed(s) at tumor border(s), when feasible, and marking of ipsilateral oral commissure may facilitate portal design. An intraoral stent is used to shield the tongue and to displace it to the contralateral side (see Fig. 3.4). The patient is immobilized in an open-neck position. An appositional lateral field encompasses the primary tumor and upper neck nodes:

- *Anterior border:* at least 2 cm anterior to the tumor.
- *Superior border:* includes the pterygoid plates when the tonsillar fossa is involved (this border is at least 1 to 1.5 cm rostral to the hard palate).
- *Posterior border:* just behind the mastoid process (N0) or behind the spinous processes (N+).
- *Inferior border:* just above the arytenoids.

When indicated, an adjoining appositional electron field is added to irradiate the mid- and lower neck (see "General Principles"). To deliver the boost dose to the primary tumor and, if necessary, upper neck, the field size is reduced to encompass the known disease locations with 1- to 2-cm margins.

For bilateral treatment, metal seeds are inserted, when feasible, to help delineate the primary lesion, and oral commissures are wired to aid in shaping the portal. The patient is immobilized in a supine position. Parallel–opposed lateral photon fields are used to treat the primary tumor and upper neck. Field borders are similar to that of ipsilateral treatment. An anterior appositional photon field is used to treat the mid- and lower neck borders (see "General Principles"). The lateral portals are reduced to deliver the boost dose to the primary tumor and the upper neck node(s). The boost dose to the involved mid- or lower neck nodes can be given through an appositional electron field or anterior photon portal.

Dose

The initial target volume receives 50 Gy in 25 fractions or 54 Gy in 30 fractions when a concomitant boost regimen is prescribed. Delivering the boost with intraoral cone is preferred when feasible for relatively small, superficial, and accessible lesions to reduce morbidity by limiting the dose to the mandible and salivary glands. In such situations, a boost dose of 15 Gy is delivered in five to six fractions before the external beam irradiation (see Fig. 9.1).

The external beam boost is 16 Gy in eight fractions for T1 and small, superficial T2 lesions; 18 Gy in 12 fractions (given as second daily fractions according to concomitant boost regimen) for large T2 and T3 tumors.

Conformal radiotherapy eliminates sequential portal cone-down because the difference in dose prescription to the gross tumor and regions at risk for harboring microscopic disease is achieved by varying the fraction size. In other words, the gross target volume (GTV) receives a larger fraction size than does the clinical target volume (CTV) (e.g., 2.2 Gy vs. 1.8 Gy). Currently recommended doses range from 66 Gy to 70.4 Gy to the primary tumor and involved node(s), depending on the tumor size, and 54 to 57.6 Gy to the subclinical disease PTV administered in 30 to 32 fractions over 6 to 6.5 weeks.

Intensity-Modulated Radiation Therapy Planning

Conformal therapy including IMRT is an alternative for patients requiring either unilateral or bilateral therapy. For patients in whom unilateral therapy is sufficient, conformal therapy may be beneficial if the depth dose profiles of the electron beam are insufficient for tumor coverage or hotspots on the mandible can be avoided because osteoradionecrosis is a risk for these patients. In those patients requiring bilateral treatment, conformal therapy can exclude a large portion of the contralateral parotid gland from the high-dose volume without compromising the coverage of the primary tumor and draining lymphatics.

The patient is immobilized in a supine position with an extended thermoplastic mask covering head and shoulder. Thin-cut CT images are obtained in treatment position. The GTV, CTV, and PTV are outlined for dosimetric planning. We generally prescribe a dose of 66 Gy in 30 fractions for T1-T2 tumors or N1 node. A dose 70 Gy in 32 to 33 fractions is prescribed for larger lesions or N2-N3 nodes. The uninvolved nodal regions receive 54 Gy in 30 fractions or approximately 56 Gy in 32 to 33 fractions.

Dose Specification: See "General Principles"

Postoperative Radiotherapy

Target Volume
Initial target volume is the entire surgical bed (see Fig 7.8). Guidelines for ipsilateral versus bilateral treatment and for treatment of nodal areas are the same as those for primary radiotherapy. Extension of the surgical scar well over the midline is another indication for bilateral irradiation.

For the boost volume, the same principle applies as for postoperative radiotherapy for the oral tongue and floor of the mouth.

Setup and Field Arrangement: See "Primary Radiotherapy"
Marking the external surgical scar may facilitate portal design. The *anterior* and *superior field borders* are determined by the local spread of the primary tumor as well as by the extent of surgery (guided by the scar).

Dose
- A dose of 60 Gy in 30 fractions to areas with high-risk features: close or microscopically positive margins, perineural extension, vascular invasion, positive nodes, or extranodal extension.

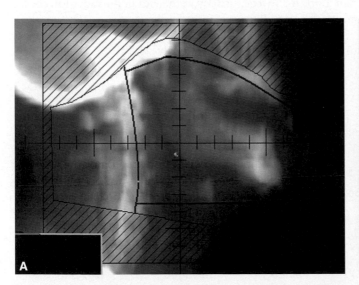
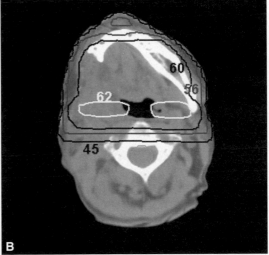

Figure 7.8 A-59-year-old man presented with toothache, dysphagia, 30-pound weight loss, and right otalgia. A tumor in the right retromolar trigone region was found, and a biopsy showed squamous cell carcinoma. Computed tomography scan revealed the lesion with invasion of the mandible as well as upper jugular adenopathy. He underwent resection of the tumor, including partial glossectomy, pharyngectomy, palatectomy, and hemimandibulectomy. Section margins were negative, and the surgical pathology otherwise confirmed the clinical findings. The defect was repaired with a pectoralis major rotational flap. A right modified radical neck dissection revealed six of 26 nodes positive with extracapsular extension. Stage: p T4 N2b. He had a Zubrod performance status 2. His nutritional support was through a percutaneous gastrostomy tube. Adjunctive postoperative radiotherapy was delivered to a dose of 60 Gy in 30 fractions. Digitally reconstructed radiograph with portal design **(A)** and an axial isodose distribution **(B)** of the photon beams are shown (note the missing portion of the mandible secondary to the surgery). The patient began his therapy with cobalt-60 beam to 42 Gy. The off–spinal cord and boost fields (16 Gy and 4 Gy, respectively) were delivered with 6 MV photons. The posterior cervical strips were treated with 9 MeV electrons, 18 Gy to the right side and 8 Gy to the clinically uninvolved left side. A matching anterior supraclavicular field with larynx block was treated to 50 Gy. Because the neck dissection scar was in close proximity to the larynx block, the skin over the larynx was treated with 6 MeV electrons to a dose of 42 Gy in 14 fractions. The right neck received additional irradiation with cone-down portal with an appositional 9-MeV electron beam to a total of 60 Gy.

An additional boost dose of 6 Gy in three fractions may be given when indicated, such as when multiple adverse features are present or when the interval between surgery and radiation is much longer than 6 weeks.

- A dose of 56 Gy in 28 fractions is given to the surgical bed.
- A dose of 50 Gy of elective irradiation in 25 fractions is given to undissected regions.

Intensity-Modulated Radiation Therapy Planning

When using IMRT in the postoperative setting, treatment is given in 30 fractions. The target volumes to receive various levels of doses are delineated and dosimetric plans are generated by iterative process. Generally, the tumor bed target volume receives 60 Gy, the operative bed 57 Gy, and undissected regions 54 Gy. Smaller volumes considered to be at extra-high risk, often determined in collaboration with the surgeon and based on pathologic findings, are to receive 64 to 66 Gy.

The patient is immobilized in a supine position with an extended thermoplastic mask covering head and shoulder. Thin-cut CT images are obtained in treatment position and target volumes are outlined for dosimetric planning.

Timing of Postoperative Radiotherapy

It is desirable to commence postoperative radiotherapy as soon as possible after healing of surgical wounds. With good communication between surgical, radiation, and dental oncologists, generally simulation can take place 3 to 4 weeks after surgery and radiotherapy can start a few days later in most patients. When delayed wound healing postpones commencement of postoperative radiation to beyond 5 to 6 weeks, we prescribe accelerated fractionation, such as concomitant boost, by delivering twice-a-day irradiations for 1 week, usually at the end of the radiation course, to reduce the potential hazard of prolonged cumulative treatment time.

Dose Specification: See "General Principles"

Background Data

TABLE 7.12

LOCAL CONTROL RATES IN EVALUABLE PATIENTS (ANTERIOR FAUCIAL PILLAR–RETROMOLAR TRIGONE): JANUARY 1966–AUGUST 1981 (ANALYSIS JANUARY 1986)

			Evaluable Patients[a]		
Stage	All Patients Under Local Control	Local Control (%)	Treatment of Primary Failure	No. of Patients Salvaged	Ultimate Control Rate No. (%)
T1	15/20 (75%)	12/17 (71%)	Surgery (5)[b]	5/5	17/17 (100%)
T2	69/93 (74%)	57/81 (70%)	No treatment (2) Surgery (21) Surgery + XRT (1)	19/24[c]	76/81 (94%)
T3	30/36 (83%)	19/25 (76%)	Surgery (5) Surgery + Chemo (1)	4/6[c]	23/25 (92%)
T4	8/10 (80%)	3/5	Surgery (1) Chemo (1)	1/2[c]	4/5 (80%)

Data from M.D. Anderson Cancer Center.
XRT, radiotherapy; Chemo, chemotherapy.
[a]31 patients who died in less than 2 years with no evidence of local disease are not evaluable.
[b]Numbers in parentheses indicate number of patients.
[c]Five T2, one T3, and one T4 patients died in less than 2 years with no evidence of local disease.
Modified from Lo K, Fletcher GH, Byers RM, et al. Results of irradiation in the squamous cell carcinomas of the anterior faucial pillar—retromolar trigone. *Int J Radiat Oncol Biol Phys* 1987;13:969–974, with permission.

TABLE 7.13

INCIDENCE OF NECK FAILURES BY N STAGE AND AREAS OF THE NECK IRRADIATED (AFP-RMT): JANUARY 1966–AUGUST 1981 (ANALYSIS JANUARY 1986)

Area of Neck Irradiated	NX	N0	N1	N2A	N2B	N3B	Total
Ipsilateral upper	—	10/87 (4)	0/6	—	—	—	10/93 (4)
Ipsilateral upper and lower	—	2/11 (1)	1/8	—	—	—	3/19 (1)
Ipsilateral upper + contralateral upper	—	0/3	0/2	0/1	—	0/1	0/7
Ipsilateral upper and lower + contralateral upper	—	0/1	—	—	—	—	0/1
All areas	0/1	1/14 (1)	1/9 (1)	0/6	0/6	1/3 (1)	3/39 (3)
Total	0/1	13/116 (6)	2/25 (1)	0/7	0/6	1/4 (1)	16/159 (8)

Data from M.D. Anderson Cancer Center.
Number in parentheses indicate number of ultimate failures after salvage treatment.
From Lo K, Fletcher GH, Byers RM, et al. Results of irradiation in the squamous cell carcinomas of the anterior faucial pillar—retromolar trigone. *Int J Radiat Oncol Biol Phys* 1987;13:969–974, with permission.

BUCCAL MUCOSA

Treatment Strategy

For T1 to T2 lesions, surgery or primary radiotherapy is selected, depending on the thickness and location of the lesion, anticipated functional/cosmetic outcome, and patient preference (see Fig. 7.9).

For T3 to T4 lesions, surgery followed by postoperative radiotherapy is generally recommended.

Primary Radiotherapy

Target Volume
Initial Target Volume
- *T1 to T2 N0:* primary tumor and ipsilateral level IB (submandibular) and level II (subdigastric) nodes.
- *T1 to T2 N1:* primary tumor and entire ipsilateral neck.
- *N2 to N3:* bilateral irradiation.

Boost volume encompasses the primary tumor and, when present, involves lymph nodes.

Setup and Field Arrangement
Tumor borders are marked by seeds or wires, whenever possible, along with the ipsilateral oral commissure to help shape the field. An intraoral stent is used to displace the tongue toward the contralateral side and to shield it (Figs. 3.4, 3.5, and 3.6). The patient is generally placed in an open-neck position for ipsilateral irradiation with combination of electrons and photons (usually in a ratio of 4:1).

- An appositional field is used to irradiate the primary lesion and upper neck nodes.
- *Anterior and superior borders*: at least 2-cm margins from the visible–palpable tumor borders.
- *Posterior and inferior borders*: same as for those for retromolar trigone primary.

The commissure and lips are shielded whenever possible to reduce morbidity. Care should be taken to exclude the eyes from the radiation field.

An appositional electron field is used (see "General Principles") to irradiate mid- and lower neck when indicated. For delivering the boost dose with external beam, the field is reduced to encompass the tumor with at least 1-cm margins and, when present, involved upper neck nodes.

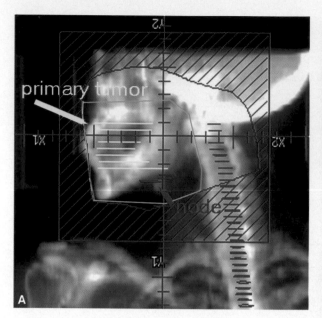

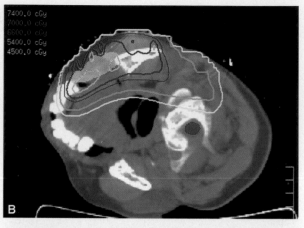

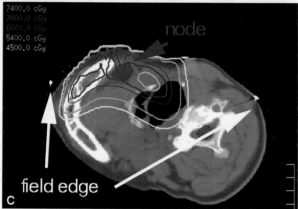

Figure 7.9   A 50-year-old woman presented with a tumor of the left buccal mucosa since 1 year. She had no associated symptoms. A biopsy was positive for moderately differentiated squamous cell carcinoma. Examination revealed a 2.5-cm, superficial tumor in the left buccal mucosa, with extension posteriorly toward the mucosa overlying the ascending ramus of the mandible. There was a 2-cm level 1 lymph node palpable. Stage T2 N1 M0. It was elected to treat her with chemoradiation consisting of conventional fractionation with cisplatin (100 mg per m^2 i.v. on days 1, 22 and 43). An appositional field was used with the patient in an open-neck position to deliver a dose of 50 Gy specified to the 90% isodose line using a combination of 16 MeV electrons and 6 MV photons, loaded 4:1. A boost was delivered to both the primary tumor and gross nodal disease with 12 MeV electrons to an additional 18 Gy also specified at the 90% line. A digitally reconstructed radiograph of the initial field covering the primary tumor and upper neck is shown **(A)** along with the axial isodoses through the primary tumor **(B)** and neck node **(C)**. The low neck was treated to 50 Gy, at D_{max}, with a matching appositional 9-MeV electron portal.

Superficial, circumscribed lesions receive boost dose with brachytherapy. Field borders for bilateral treatment are the same as those for unilateral irradiation; however, the patient is immobilized in a supine position.

Dose

The initial target volume receives 50 Gy in 25 fractions. The boost dose depends on the size of the primary tumor and on the technique used. For external beam technique, 16 Gy in eight fractions for T1 and 20 Gy in ten fractions for T2 lesions are administered. For brachytherapy, 25 to 30 Gy is administered.

Dose Specification: See "General Principles"

Postoperative Radiotherapy

Target Volume

The initial target volume is the entire surgical bed, including primary site and ipsilateral submandibular and subdigastric nodes, and the ipsilateral mid- and lower neck (see Fig. 7.10). The boost volume encompasses areas of known disease locations. Occasionally, IMRT may be preferable.

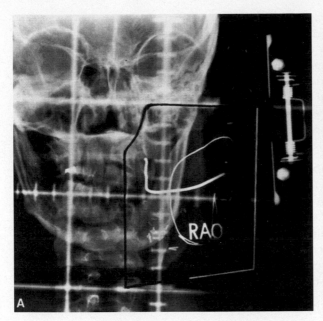 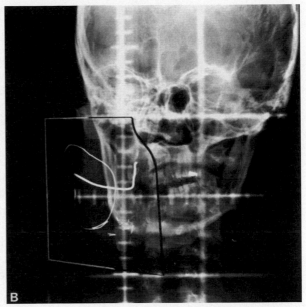

Figure 7.10   A 33-year-old man, who had a long history of chewing tobacco and betel nuts, sought medical attention because of a persistent ulcer in the left buccal mucosa. Biopsy of this lesion showed an infiltrating, poorly differentiated carcinoma. Physical examination revealed a 5 × 3-cm ulcerative lesion extending from the left oral commissure back and downward to the gingivobuccal sulcus. The lesion infiltrated the subcutaneous tissues of the cheek but there was no palpable lymphadenopathy. Further head and neck exam was unremarkable (Stage: T3 N0 M0). He underwent a wide excision of the primary lesion that involved a through-and-through removal of a large part of the left cheek and a small part of the upper and lower lips, a left supraomohyoid neck dissection, and reconstruction of the cheek with a free myocutaneous flap. Pathologic examination showed good section margins, except the inferior border, which was only 2 mm, and involvement of one of seven submental–submandibular lymph nodes with extracapsular extension (Stage p T3 N1 M0). Postoperative radiotherapy was recommended because of these findings. It was initially planned to treat the primary tumor bed and ipsilateral neck nodes. However, physical examination after surgery showed that the graft was 4 to 5 cm thick. Irradiating the primary tumor bed with electrons would have required the use of the 20-MeV beam. This would have resulted in delivering high doses to the lips and part of the oral and nasal cavities. Therefore, it was decided to treat the patient with photons. Parallel–opposed oblique fields were used to irradiate the primary tumor bed and ipsilateral upper neck nodes. Figure 7.6 outlines the right anterior oblique **(A)** and left posterior oblique **(B)** radiation fields relative to the facial structures. The thin wire taped on the cheek indicated the size of the graft. One end of the thick wire was inserted in the oral cavity and brought in contact with the surface of the reconstructed mucosa and the other end was twisted at the commissure and taped on the skin to define the thickness of the graft and to facilitate portal design. This setup prevented irradiation of most of the lips and oral and nasal cavities. A total dose of 60 Gy was given in 30 fractions through the oblique fields. The ipsilateral lower neck received 50 Gy in 25 fractions through an abutting anterior appositional field.

The most common scenario is in patients with T4 disease who require large surgical reconstructions, and the flap thickness precludes efficient use of electron beams.

Setup and Field Arrangement
This is similar to that of primary radiotherapy. Marking the external surgical scar facilitates portal design. The anterior and superior field borders are determined by the contiguous spread pattern of the primary tumor and by the extent of surgery (scar, flap).

Dose
- A dose of 60 Gy in 30 fractions is given to areas with high-risk features, i.e., close or microscopically positive margins, perineural extension, vascular invasion, positive nodes, or extranodal extension. An additional boost dose of 6 Gy in three fractions may be given when indicated, such as when multiple adverse features are present or when the interval between surgery and radiation is much longer than 6 weeks.
- A dose of 56 Gy in 28 fractions is given to the surgical bed.
- A dose of 50 Gy of elective irradiation in 25 fractions is given to undissected regions.

Intensity-Modulated Radiation Therapy Planning

When using IMRT in the postoperative setting, treatment is given in 30 fractions. The target volumes to receive various levels of doses are delineated and dosimetric plans are generated by iterative process. Generally, the tumor bed target volume receives 60 Gy, the operative bed 57 Gy, and undissected regions 54 Gy. Smaller volumes considered at extra-high risk, often determined in collaboration with the surgeon and based on pathologic findings, are to receive 64 to 66 Gy.

The patient is immobilized in a supine position with an extended thermoplastic mask covering head and shoulder. Thin-cut CT images are obtained in treatment position and target volumes are outlined for dosimetric planning.

Timing of Postoperative Radiotherapy

It is desirable to commence postoperative radiotherapy as soon as possible after healing of surgical wounds. With good communication between surgical, radiation, and dental oncologists, generally simulation can take place 3 to 4 weeks after surgery and radiotherapy can start a few days later in most patients. When delayed wound healing postpones commencement of postoperative radiation to beyond 5 to 6 weeks, we prescribe accelerated fractionation, such as concomitant boost, by delivering twice-a-day irradiations for 1 week, usually at the end of the radiation course, to reduce the potential hazard of prolonged cumulative treatment time.

Dose Specification: See "General Principles"

Background Data

TABLE 7.14

RESULTS OF RADIOTHERAPY IN CANCER OF THE BUCCAL MUCOSA: SITE OF FAILURE BY UICC, T AND N STAGES

Stage	Primary Failure No. (%)	Nodal Failure No. (%)	Total Failure No. (%)
T1 N0	0/13 (0%)	0/13 (0%)	0/13 (0%)
T2 N0	13/49 (27%)	7/49 (14%)	18/49 (37%)
T3 N0	15/49 (31%)	1/49 (2%)	15/49 (31%)
T4 N0	6/12 (50%)	1/12 (8%)	7/12 (58%)
Any T & N1	51/94 (54%)	48/94 (51%)	55/94 (59%)
Any T & N3	12/17 (71%)	15/17 (88%)	14/17 (82%)

Modified from Nair MK, Sankaranarayanan R, Padmanabhan TK. Evaluation of the role of radiotherapy in the management of carcinoma of the buccal mucosa. *Cancer* 1988;61:1326 with permission.

TABLE 7.15

FIVE-YEAR SURVIVAL RATES IN 119 PATIENTS WITH SQUAMOUS CELL CARCINOMA OF THE BUCCAL MUCOSA

Variable	5 yr Survival Rate (%)
AJCC Stage I	78
AJCC Stage II	66
AJCC Stage III	62
AJCC Stage IV	50
Node negative	70
Node positive	49
No extracapsular spread	69
Extracapsular spread	24

Data from M.D. Anderson Cancer Center
AJCC, American Joint Committee on Cancer.
Modified from Diaz EM Jr, Holsinger FC, Zuniga ER, et al. Squamous cell carcinoma of the buccal mucosa: one institution's experience with 119 previously untreated patients. *Head Neck* 2003;25: 267–273, with permission.

HARD PALATE AND UPPER ALVEOLAR RIDGE

This section deals with true hard palate and alveolar ridge cancers. Most hard palate and alveolar ridge tumors are manifestations of maxillary sinus cancers.

Treatment Strategy

Surgery is the treatment of choice in most cases. Postoperative radiotherapy is delivered when indicated (see "Floor of Mouth and Oral Tongue") (see Fig. 7.11).

Primary radiotherapy is indicated for small, superficial squamous cell carcinomas (SCC).

Postoperative Radiotherapy

Target Volume

Initial Target Volume

The entire surgical bed is encompassed. In most cases, the location of the primary lesion, the extent of surgery, or both, necessitates treatment with opposed–lateral fields. Ipsilateral irradiation (wedge pair) may suffice in well-lateralized lesions of the alveolar ridge.

Elective irradiation of upper neck nodes is given to patients with SCC. All cervical nodal areas are irradiated in N+ patients regardless of histologic type. Boost volume encompasses areas of known disease.

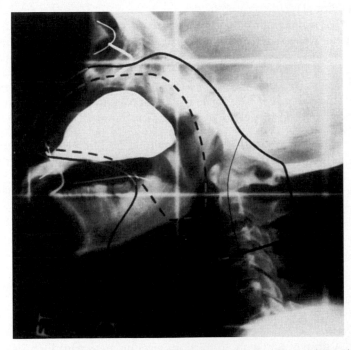

Figure 7.11   A 42-year-old woman noticed a tumor on the left side of her palate. Physical examination revealed a 4 × 3-cm exophytic tumor on the left side of the hard palate. The lesion extended posteriorly to involve the anterior part of the soft palate, laterally onto the left upper alveolar ridge, medially approaching the midline, and anteriorly to the level of the first premolar. There was no palpable adenopathy in the neck. A computed tomography scan confirmed the physical findings and also showed involvement of the floor of the maxillary sinus with bone destruction. A biopsy showed moderately differentiated squamous cell carcinoma. Stage: T4 N0 M0. This patient underwent a left intraoral palatectomy and maxillectomy. Pathologic examination showed involvement of bone and extension to the mucosa of the floor of the maxillary sinus and floor of the left nasal cavity. There was perineural spread along the greater palatine nerve. All margins of resection were negative. She received postoperative radiotherapy with lateral parallel–opposed photon fields encompassing the surgical bed and the course of the palatine and maxillary nerves to the gasserian ganglion, to a dose of 54 Gy in 30 fractions. The tumor bed was then boosted to a total dose of 63 Gy. Ten months after completion of radiotherapy, she started to experience left-sided back pain. Physical examination showed no evidence of local–regional disease. However, chest x-rays revealed a paravertebral mass at the level of the third intercostal space. A fluoroscopic-guided fine needle aspiration showed squamous cell carcinoma consistent with metastatic deposit from the palate lesion. Palliative radiotherapy was given, which diminished the back pain. She expired a month later.

Setup and Field Arrangement

For bilateral irradiation, an intraoral stent is used to open the mouth and, for an anterior lesion, to protrude the upper lip. If the surgical defect is large enough, a water-containing balloon is used to fill the surgical defect (see Fig. 3.9). Otherwise the mouth-opening stent is fabricated with the palatal prosthesis in place. Marking the external surgical scar, oral commissures, and lateral canthi may facilitate portal design. The patient is immobilized in a supine position.

The initial target volume encompasses parallel–opposed fields to treat the primary tumor bed and, when indicated, the upper neck nodes.

- *Anterior and superior borders:* at least 2 cm beyond the surgical bed. If disease extended into the maxillary sinus, the entire sinus is included up to the floor of the orbit.
- *Posterior border:* at midvertebral bodies for non-SCC and N0; behind the mastoid process for SCC and N0; behind the spinous processes for N+ (or more posteriorly to cover large surgical bed).
- *Inferior border:* just above the arytenoids for squamous cell carcinoma with no nodal involvement, or 2 cm below the surgical margin for low-grade minor salivary gland tumors.

In the presence of positive nodes, an anterior photon field is used for irradiation of the mid- and low cervical nodes.

For boost volume, the fields are reduced to encompass the tumor volume with at least 1-cm margins; involved upper neck nodes are included in the lateral fields or in a separate appositional electron field; involved mid- and lower neck nodes are irradiated with an appositional electron field or glancing photon fields.

For ipsilateral irradiation, the patient is immobilized in a supine position. Anterior and ipsilateral wedge-pair photon fields are used to treat the primary tumor bed (usually with 45-degree wedges).

- *Lateral field: borders* are the same as those for bilateral treatment.
- *Anterior field: medial border* is 2 cm beyond the surgical margin; *lateral border* is short of falling-off; and *superior* and *inferior borders* correspond to those of the lateral field.

A lateral appositional electron field is used for elective treatment of the submandibular and subdigastric nodes when ipsilateral treatment is adopted for SCCs.

- *Superior border:* matches the inferior border of the photon fields (a small triangle over the cheek may be spared).
- *Anterior border:* just short of fall-off.
- *Posterior border:* behind the mastoid process.
- *Inferior border:* at the thyroid notch.

For boost irradiation, photon fields are reduced to encompass the tumor volume with at least a 1-cm margin.

Dose

- A dose of 60 Gy in 30 fractions given to areas with high-risk features, that is, close or microscopically positive margins, perineural extension, vascular invasion, positive nodes, or extranodal extension. An additional boost dose of 6 Gy in three fractions may be given when indicated, such as when multiple adverse features are present or when the interval between surgery and radiation is much longer than 6 weeks.
- A dose of 56 Gy in 28 fractions given to the surgical bed.
- 50 Gy of elective irradiation in 25 fractions given to undissected regions.

Intensity-Modulated Radiation Therapy Planning

IMRT may be used in lieu of a wedge-pair technique. In the postoperative setting, treatment is given in 30 fractions. Generally, the tumor bed target volume receives 60 Gy, the operative bed 57 Gy, and undissected regions 54 Gy (see Fig. 7.12). In patients with no clinical evidence of involved nodes, elective irradiation is limited to level II and level I (for anterior nodes).

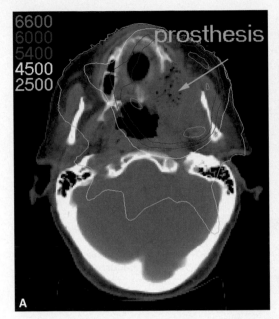 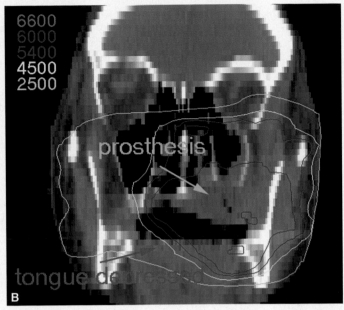

Figure 7.12 A 59-year-old woman presented with a 3-year history of an ill-fitting maxillary denture. When she finally sought medical attention, a mass in the left lateral hard palate was noted and biopsy revealed polymorphous low-grade adenocarcinoma with perineural invasion. She underwent palatectomy, infrastructure maxillectomy, and alloderm reconstruction. This was followed by postoperative intensity-modulated radiation therapy. The defect was not large enough to support a balloon, so a mouth-opening stent was used with the palatal prosthesis. The clinical target volume planned for 60 Gy was delineated based on the clinical and operative findings of the tumor extent, broadly encompassing the palatal defect with margin, the inferior maxillary sinus, the pterygoids, and buccal space. An additional 1-cm margin and the entire left maxilla were included in the 54 Gy CTV. Because the tumor was low grade, the neck nodes did not receive elective irradiation. Axial **(A)** and coronal **(B)** isodose distributions are shown. She remains well more than 3 years from completion of therapy.

Smaller volumes considered to be at extra-high risk, often determined in collaboration with the surgeon and on the basis of pathologic findings, are to receive 64 to 66 Gy.

Timing of Postoperative Radiotherapy

It is desirable to commence postoperative radiotherapy as soon as possible after healing of surgical wounds. With good communication between surgical, radiation, and dental oncologists, generally simulation can take place 3 to 4 weeks after surgery and radiotherapy can start a few days later in most patients. When delayed wound healing postpones commencement of postoperative radiation to beyond 5 to 6 weeks, accelerated fractionation, such as concomitant boost, by delivering twice-a-day irradiations for 1 week, is prescribed, usually at the end of the radiation course, to reduce the potential hazard of prolonged cumulative treatment time.

Dose Specification: See "General Principles"

The dose delivered by anterior and lateral wedge-pair photon fields is specified at the appropriate isodose line encompassing the target volume.

Primary Radiotherapy

Target Volume

- *Initial target volume:* primary tumor with 2-cm margins (no elective neck irradiation for small, superficial lesions).
- *Boost volume:* primary tumor with 1-cm margins.

Setup and Field Arrangement

This is similar to that of postoperative radiotherapy. The boost dose is preferably delivered with a surface mold.

Dose

The initial target volume receives 50 Gy in 25 fractions.

The boost dose is 15 to 20 Gy at 0.5-cm depth when delivered by surface mold and 16 Gy in eight fractions (T1) or 20 Gy in ten fractions (T2) when delivered by external beam.

Dose Specification: See "General Principles"

The dose delivered by intraoral cone is specified at D_{max}.

Background Data

TABLE 7.16

HARD PALATE CARCINOMA TREATED WITH RADIOTHERAPY

	Number of Patients	5 yr Actuarial Survival Rate (%)	Crude Local Recurrence Rate (%)
T1 and T2	17	54	18
T3 and T4	14	55	57
Node negative	24	65	37
Node positive	7	19	29
Squamous cell carcinoma	19	48	32
Salivary gland carcinoma	12	63	42

Data from Christie Hospital, Manchester UK
Modified from Yorozu A, Sykes AJ, Slevin NJ. Carcinoma of the hard palate treated with radiotherapy: a retrospective review of 31 cases. *Oral Oncol* 2001;37:493–497, with permission.

SUGGESTED READINGS

Akine Y, Tokita N, Ogino T, et al. Stage I-II carcinoma of the anterior two-thirds of the tongue treated with different modalities: a retrospective analysis of 244 patients. *Radiother Oncol* 1991;21:24.

Barker JL, Fletcher GH. Time dose and tumor relationships in megavoltage irradiation of squamous cell carcinomas of the retromolar trigone and anterior tonsillar pillar. *Int J Radiat Oncol Biol Phys* 1977;2:407.

Beauvois S, Hoffstetter S, Peiffert D, et al. Brachytherapy for lower lip epidermoid cancer: tumoral and treatment factors influencing recurrences and complications. *Radiother Oncol* 1994;33:195.

Benk V, Mazeron JJ, Grimard L, et al. Comparison of curietherapy versus external irradiation combined with curietherapy in stage II squamous cell carcinomas of the mobile tongue. *Radiother Oncol* 1990;18:339.

Byers RM, Anderson B, Schwarz EA, et al. Treatment of squamous carcinoma of the retromolar trigone. *Am J Clin Oncol* 1984;7:647.

Chaudhary AJ, Pande SC, Sharma V, et al. Radiotherapy of carcinoma of the buccal mucosa. *Semin Surg Oncol* 1989;5:322.

Chu A, Fletcher GH. Incidence and causes of failures to control by irradiation the primary lesions in squamous cell carcinomas of the anterior two thirds of the tongue and floor of mouth. *AJR Am J Roentgenol* 1973;117:502.

Chung CK, Johns ME, Cantrell RW, et al. Radiotherapy in the management of primary malignancies of the hard palate. *Laryngoscope* 1980;90:576.

Dearnaly DP, Dardoufas C, A'Hearn RP, et al. Interstitial irradiation for carcinoma of the tongue and floor of mouth: Royal Marsden Hospital experience. *Radiother Oncol* 1991;21:183.

Decroix Y, Ghossein NA. Experience of the Curie Institute in treatment of cancer of the mobile tongue, I. Treatment policies and results. *Cancer* 1981;47:496.

Delclos L. Afterloading interstitial irradiation techniques. In: Levitt SH, Khan FM, Potish RA, eds. *Technological basis of radiation therapy*, 2nd ed. Philadelphia, PA: Lea & Febiger, 1992.

Delclos L, Lindberg RD, Fletcher GH. Squamous cell carcinoma of the oral tongue and floor of mouth. Evaluation of interstitial radium therapy. *AJR Am J Roentgenol* 1976;126:223.

Diaz EM Jr, Holsinger FC, Zuniga ER, et al. Squamous cell carcinoma of the buccal mucosa: one institution's experience with 119 previously untreated patients. *Head Neck* 2003;25:267.

Dixit S, Vyas RK, Toparani RB, et al. Surgery versus surgery and postoperative radiotherapy in squamous cell carcinoma of the buccal mucosa: a comparative study. *Ann Surg Oncol* 1998;5:502–510.

Eicher SA, Overholt SM, el-Naggar AK, et al. Lower gingival carcinoma. Clinical and pathologic determinants of regional metastases. *Arch Otolaryngol Head Neck Surg* 1996;122:634.

Fletcher GH. Oral cavity and oropharynx. In: Fletcher GH, ed. *Textbook of radiotherapy*, 3rd ed. Philadelphia, PA: Lea & Febiger, 1980.

Fu KK, Lichter A, Galante M. Carcinoma of the floor of the mouth: an analysis of treatment results and the sites and causes of failures. *Int J Radiat Oncol Biol Phys* 1976;1:829.

Genden EM, Ferlito A, Shaha AR, et al. Management of cancer of the retromolar trigone. *Oral Oncol* 2003;39:633.

Gerbaulet A, Pernot M. Squamous cell carcinoma of the internal surface of cheek: a report of 248 cases. *J Eur Radiother* 1985;6:1.

Greenberg JS, El Naggar AK, Mo V, et al. Disparity in pathologic and clinical lymph node staging in oral tongue carcinoma. Implication for therapeutic decision making. *Cancer* 2003;98:508.

Guillamondegui O, Oliver B, Hayden R. Cancer of the anterior floor of mouth. Selective choice of treatment and analysis of failures. *Am J Surg* 1970;120:505.

Hicks WL Jr, Loree TR, Garcia RI, et al. Squamous cell carcinoma of the floor of mouth: a 20-year review. *Head Neck* 1997;19:400.

Hinerman RW, Mendenhall WM, Morris CG, et al. Postoperative irradiation for squamous cell carcinoma of the oral cavity: 35-year experience. *Head Neck* 2004;26:984.

Ildstad ST, Bigelow ME, Remensnyder JP. Intra-oral cancer at the Massachusetts General Hospital: squamous cell carcinoma of the floor of the mouth. *Ann Surg* 1983;197:34.

Kligerman J, Lima RA, Soares JR, et al. Supraomohyoid neck dissection in the treatment of T1/T2 squamous cell carcinoma of oral cavity. *Am J Surg* 1994;168:391.

Lefebvre JL, Coche-Dequeant B, Castelain B, et al. Interstitial brachytherapy and early tongue squamous cell carcinoma management. *Head Neck* 1990;12:232.

Lo K, Fletcher GH, Byers RM, et al. Results of irradiation in the squamous cell carcinomas of the anterior faucial pillar—retromolar trigone. *Int J Radiat Oncol Biol Phys* 1987;13:969.

Lydiatt DD, Robbins KT, Byers RM, et al. Treatment of stage I and II oral tongue cancer. *Head Neck* 1993;15:308.

Maciejewsky B, Withers HR, Taylor JM, et al. Dose fractionation and regeneration in radiotherapy for cancer of the oral cavity and oropharynx. Part 2. Normal tissue tolerance and late effects. *Int J Radiat Oncol Biol Phys* 1990;18:101.

Maciejewsky B, Withers HR, Taylor JM, et al. Dose fractionation and regeneration in radiotherapy for cancer of the oral cavity and oropharynx. Part 1. Tumor dose-response and repopulation. *Int J Radiat Oncol Biol Phys* 1989;16:831.

Marks JE, Lee F, Smith PG, et al. Floor of mouth cancer: patient selection and treatment results. *Laryngoscope* 1983;93:475.

Mazeron JJ, Grimard L, Raynal M, et al. Iridium-192 curietherapy for T1 and T2 epidermoid carcinomas of the floor of the mouth. *Int J Radiat Oncol Biol Phys* 1990;18:1299.

Mazeron JJ, Simon JM, Le Pechoux C, et al. Effect of dose rate on local control and complications in definitive irradiation of T1-2 squamous cell carcinomas of mobile tongue and floor of mouth with interstitial iridium-192. *Radiother Oncol* 1991;21:39.

Meoz RT, Fletcher GH, Lindberg RD. Anatomic coverage in elective irradiation of the neck for squamous cell carcinoma of the oral tongue. *Int J Radiat Oncol Biol Phys* 1982;8:1881.

Million RR, Cassisi NJ. Oral cavity. In: Million RR, Cassisi NJ, eds. *Management of head and neck cancer: a multidisciplinary approach.* Philadelphia, PA: JB Lippincott Co, 1985.

Nair MK, Sankaranarayanan R, Padmanabhan TK. Evaluation of the role of radiotherapy in the management of carcinoma of the buccal mucosa. *Cancer* 1988;61:1326.

Northrop M, Fletcher GH, Jesse RH, et al. Evaluation of neck disease in patients with primary squamous cell carcinoma of the oral tongue, floor of mouth, and palatine arch, and clinically positive neck nodes neither fixed nor bilateral. *Cancer* 1972;29:23.

Pernot M, Hoffstetter S, Peiffert D, et al. Epidermoid carcinomas of the floor of mouth treated by exclusive irradiation: statistical study of a series of 207 cases. *Radiother Oncol* 1995;35:177.

Pernot M, Malissard L, Aletti P, et al. Iridium-192 in the management of 147 T2N0 oral tongue carcinomas treated with irradiation alone: comparison of two treatment techniques. *Radiother Oncol* 1992;23:223.

Pierquin B, Wilson JF, Chassagne D, eds. *Modern brachytherapy.* New York: Masson Publishing, 1987.

Pop L, Eijkenboom WM, de Boer MF, et al. Evaluation of treatment results of squamous cell carcinoma of the buccal mucosa. *Int J Radiat Oncol Biol Phys* 1989;16:483.

Rodgers LW Jr, Stringer SP, Mendenhall WM, et al. Management of squamous cell carcinoma of the floor of mouth. *Head Neck* 1993;15:16.

Richaud P, Tapley N. Lateralized lesions of the oral cavity and oropharynx treated in part with the electron beam. *Int J Radiat Oncol Biol Phys* 1979;5:461.

Shah JP, Candela FC, Poddar AK. The patterns of cervical lymph node metastases from squamous cell carcinoma of the oral cavity. *Cancer* 990;66:109.

Shaha AR, Spiro RH, Shah JP, et al. Squamous carcinoma of the floor of the mouth. *Am J Surg* 1984;148:455.

Smith GI, O'Brien CJ, Clark J, et al. Management of the neck in patients with T1 and T2 cancer in the mouth. *Br J Oral Maxillofac Surg* 2004;42:494.

Vegers JW, Snow GB, van der Waal I. Squamous cell carcinoma of the buccal mucosa. A review of 85 cases. *Arch Otolaryngol* 1979;105:192.

Wang CC, Kelly J, August M, et al. Early carcinoma of the oral cavity: a conservative approach with radiation therapy. *J Oral Maxillofac Surg* 1995;53:687.

Wendt CD, Peters LJ, Delclos L, et al. Primary radiotherapy in the treatment of stage I and II oral tongue cancers: importance of the proportion of therapy delivered with interstitial therapy. *Int J Radiat Oncol Biol Phys* 1990;18:1287.

White D, Byers RM. What is the preferred initial method of treatment for squamous carcinoma of the tongue? *Am J Surg* 1980;140:553.

Yorozu A, Sykes AJ, Slevin NJ. Carcinoma of the hard palate treated with radiotherapy: a retrospective review of 31 cases. *Oral Oncol* 2001;37:493.

Zelefsky MJ, Harrison LB, Fass DE, et al. Postoperative radiation therapy for squamous cell carcinomas of the oral cavity and oropharynx: impact of therapy on patients with positive surgical margins. *Int J Radiat Oncol Biol Phys* 1993;25:17.

Nasopharynx

8

TREATMENT STRATEGY

The Phase III intergroup trial on nasopharyngeal carcinoma (NPC), in demonstrating the benefit of the combination of radiation with concurrent cisplatin plus adjuvant cisplatin-fluorouracil chemotherapy over radiation alone on overall survival and local-regional control, used
the staging criteria of the fourth edition of American Joint Committee on Cancer (AJCC) Cancer Staging Manual, published in 1992. The fifth edition of AJCC Cancer Staging Manual, published in 1998, introduced a substantial change in the staging classification for NPC. By the criteria of the fifth and sixth editions, tumors involving more than one nasopharyngeal wall but not extending beyond the nasopharynx, formerly considered T2, were reclassified as T1. Therefore, the current stage I group includes former stage I and stage II groups. Correspondingly, tumors that were classified T3 (which represented a subset of stage III group) were downgraded to T2 (stage II group).

Accounting for the changes in the staging system, the current standard treatment for stage I NPC is radiotherapy. The standard treatment for stage II to IV NPC is combination of radiation and chemotherapy. Outside protocol study setting, the recommended chemotherapeutic regimen in the United States was established through an intergroup Phase III trial. This regimen consists of 100 mg per m^2 of cisplatin given during weeks 1, 4, and 7 of radiation, followed 3 to 4 weeks later by three courses of adjuvant therapy comprising 80 mg per m^2 of cisplatin given on day 1 and 1,000 mg/m^2/day of fluorouracil on days 1 to 4, repeated every 4 weeks.

Neck dissection is indicated in a very small number of patients who have a residual neck mass 6 to 10 weeks after completion of radiotherapy.

DETAILS OF RADIOTHERAPY

Target Volume

Initial Target Volume
The initial portals encompass the primary tumor and contiguous routes of spread, and the retropharyngeal and cervical nodes. For T1 lesions, the following structures are to be treated (see Figs. 8.1 and 8.2): nasopharynx, floor of sphenoid sinus, clivus, pterygoid fossa, parapharyngeal space, retropharyngeal nodes, and bilateral cervical nodes, including level V (spinal accessory and supraclavicular) nodes. The extent of nasal cavity and/or oropharynx coverage depends on the contiguous spread of the primary tumor.

For T2 lesions, adjust the target volume to encompass the disease extension to the nasal cavity and/or oropharynx. For T3 to T4 tumors, adjust the target volume to encompass the disease extension to the clivus, cranial fossa, infratemporal fossa, or hypopharynx. It is important to have a generous coverage of the base of skull and known intracranial extension up to the tolerance

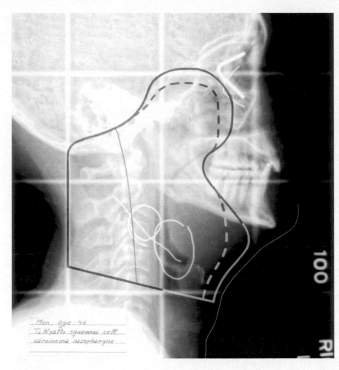

Figure 8.1 A 46-year-old man presented with a 3-week history of sinusitis, nasal congestion, and a left neck mass. An excisional biopsy of this neck mass showed squamous cell carcinoma. He was referred to our institution for workup and treatment. Physical examination revealed an erythematous mass in the nasopharynx centered on the right posterolateral wall and extending across the midline. The left posterior oropharyngeal wall was swollen consistent with enlarged retropharyngeal nodes. The nasal cavities were unremarkable. Neck examination showed a well-healed scar in the left subdigastric region with underlying residual adenopathy. A 3.5 × 2.5 cm node and a 2-cm node were palpated in the right subdigastric area. A computed tomography (CT) scan confirmed the physical findings and showed that the base of skull was uninvolved. A biopsy from the nasopharyngeal lesion showed poorly differentiated squamous cell carcinoma. Stage: T1 N2 M0. This patient received primary radiotherapy according to the concomitant boost schedule. The primary tumor and upper neck nodes were treated with lateral-opposed photon fields. The lateral orbital canthi and external auditory canals were marked along with the upper neck scar and palpable neck nodes. The mid and lower neck nodes were treated through an anterior appositional photon field with a midline block to shield the larynx and spinal cord. The dose to the primary tumor and involved neck nodes was taken to 72 Gy in 42 fractions over 6 weeks. Areas of subclinical disease received 54 Gy in 30 fractions over 6 weeks. Because the nodal biopsy site on the palpable left and the nodes on the right side were partly in the electron fields supplementing the posterior cervical areas, these fields were also taken to a total dose of 72 Gy. To deliver an adequate dose to the involved nodal areas, 12 MeV electrons were used and the dose was specified at the 90% isodose line.

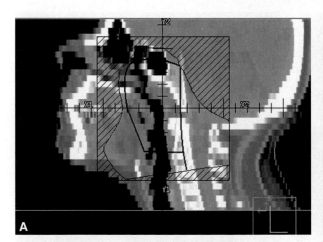

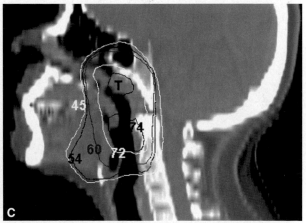

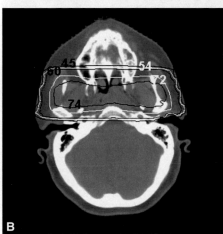

Figure 8.2 A 52-year-old woman presented with pressurelike sensation in her left ear. Further workup revealed a polypoid mass centered and confined to the roof of the nasopharynx. A biopsy was positive for World Health Organization (WHO) type-3 nasopharyngeal carcinoma. There was no adenopathy. Staging workup included magnetic resonance imaging (MRI), which confirmed the lesion was confined to the nasopharynx. Stage: T1 N0 M0. This patient received primary radiotherapy according to the concomitant boost schedule. The primary tumor and upper neck nodes were treated with lateral–opposed photon fields using 6 MV photons. A digitally reconstructed sagittal view through the nasopharyngeal mass is shown (**A**) overlaid by a representation of the lateral primary, off–spinal cord, and boost portals. The initial fields were reduced off the spinal cord at 41.4 Gy. The off–spinal cord fields continued to 54 Gy. The posterior cervical strips were treated with 9 MeV electrons to 54 Gy. The boost was delivered as second daily fractions with 18 MV photons to 18 Gy in 12 fractions, bringing the total dose to the tumor to 72 Gy. Isodose distributions of the lateral photon fields through the nasopharynx are shown in both axial (**B**) and sagittal (**C**) views. The mid and lower neck nodes were treated through an anterior appositional photon field with a midline block to shield the larynx and spinal cord. Areas of subclinical disease received 54 Gy in 30 fractions over 6 weeks.

dose of normal tissues. Intensity-modulated radiation therapy (IMRT) may allow better coverage of the primary tumor or retropharyngeal nodes while maintaining normal tissues below unacceptable dose levels (see Figs. 8.3 and 8.4).

Boost Volume

The boost portals cover gross disease sites with 0.5- to 1-cm margins, depending on the type of adjacent normal tissues. In case of tumor extension through the clivus, the margin on the brain stem can be only a few millimeters to avoid delivery of greater than 60 Gy to this critical structure.

Setup and Field Arrangement

The patient is immobilized in a supine position. Marking of lateral canthi, external auditory canals, and palpable nodes may facilitate portal design. With conventional technique, the primary tumor and upper neck nodes are irradiated with lateral–opposed photon fields.

- *Anterior border:* posterior one third to one half of the nasal cavities, depending on the size of the lesion (or 2 cm beyond tumor extension). Usually, most of the oral cavity can be shielded by shaping the field with a notch below the soft palate.
- *Superior border:* at the floor of the pituitary fossa and just above the clivus for T1 to T2 lesions. An initial margin of 2 cm is taken beyond tumor extension into the clivus or intracranially for T3 to T4 disease.
- *Posterior border:* just behind the spinous processes, or more posteriorly when large spinal accessory nodes are present.

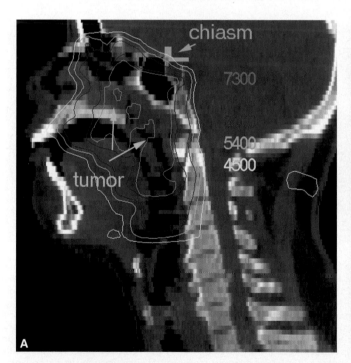
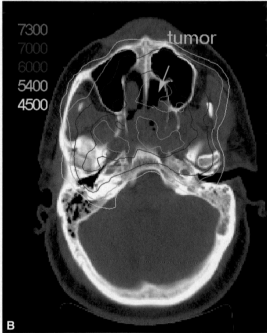

Figure 8.3 A 44-year-old man presented with nasal obstruction. He was found to have a rather bulky nasopharyngeal tumor extending into and obstructing the nasal cavity without clinical lymphadenopathy (Stage T2 N0). A biopsy revealed nasopharyngeal carcinoma, World Health Organization (WHO) type-2. He received concurrent intensity-modulated radiation therapy (IMRT) and cisplatin followed by adjuvant chemotherapy. Isodose distributions on a sagittal **(A)** and axial **(B)** image are shown. The primary tumor with margin received 70 Gy, whereas a wider margin including the clivus and neck nodes received 60 Gy all given in 33 fractions. The lower neck was treated with a matching anterior portal to 50 Gy in 25 fractions. At the completion of his external beam therapy, he had questionable residual disease. Therefore, 2 high dose rate brachytherapy applications, each delivering 5 Gy, were delivered. He remains without evidence of disease more than 2 years after completion of therapy.

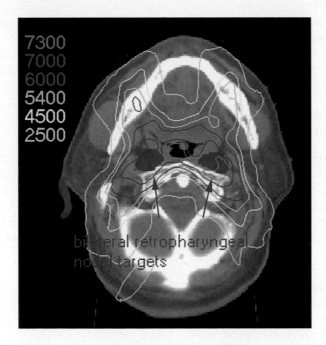

Figure 8.4 A 53-year-old Asian man presented with otitis media, which was secondary to a left-sided, biopsy-proven, undifferentiated nasopharyngeal carcinoma. Magnetic resonance imaging (MRI) staging revealed clival invasion and bilateral adenopathy including bilateral retropharyngeal nodes. He was treated with taxane-based chemotherapy followed by concurrent intensity-modulated radiation therapy (IMRT) and cisplatin. An axial slice with isodose curves is shown at the level of C1 highlighting the retropharyngeal region. He is alive without evidence of disease 3 years later.

■ *Inferior border:* the inferior border is placed just above the arytenoids. When more advanced neck disease is present, it is preferred to junction therapy through the nodes above the larynx.

■ After off-cord reduction treatment, continue with the *posterior border* placed over the posterior one third of the vertebral bodies to ensure adequate coverage of the posterior pharyngeal wall and retropharyngeal nodes. It may be necessary to use oblique lateral fields in the presence of retrostyloid parapharyngeal extension of primary disease or large retropharyngeal node(s). Patients with bilateral retrostyloid parapharyngeal extension present a particularly difficult technical problem in covering the extent of the disease without overdosing the medulla and upper cervical spinal cord without the use of conformal techniques.

An anterior appositional portal is used for the mid neck and lower neck. If there is nodal disease in the posterior midcervical chain, a posterior field is added to supplement the dose to this area (see "General Principles").

For the boost volume, lateral fields are reduced to include the primary tumor and involved upper neck nodes.

■ *Superior border:* adjusted to exclude the optic nerves, chiasm, and tracts after a dose of 54 Gy.

■ *Anterior border:* 1 to 1.5 cm beyond gross disease.

■ *Posterior border:* over the posterior one third of the vertebral bodies. Proper margins for the boost volumes are taken to encompass all clinically or radiologically apparent disease extension. These margins may be extremely tight posteriorly for tumors invading through the skull base or brain to avoid brain stem injury.

■ *Inferior border:* depends on the nodal status. If N0, the inferior border is at the level of the mid-tonsillar fossa (more inferior if the oropharynx is involved). If upper neck nodes are involved, the border is above the arytenoids.

- As with the initial off-cord reduction, it may be necessary to use oblique lateral fields to cover retropharyngeal or parapharyngeal disease.
- Electron fields or glancing photon fields are used to boost the nodes in the mid and lower neck. In case where both the posterior strip and the mid neck need to be boosted, a single L-shape electron field is typically used.

Intensity-Modulated Radiation Therapy

IMRT is gaining popularity for the treatment of NPC. With this technique, thin-cut planning computed tomography (CT) scans are obtained for outlining the gross target volume (GTV), clinical target volume (CTV), and planning target volume (PTV), which are necessary for dosimetric planning (see Figs. 8.3 to 8.7). Most planning systems are CT based, but it is crucial to incorporate diagnostic MRI images into the planning process, preferably by fusion, because MRI generally is preferred for displaying the disease extent, particularly at the skull base region. Careful target volume delineation is crucial for IMRT.

Gross Target Volume

GTV represents all areas determined from clinical examination and imaging studies to contain gross disease. Any cervical lymph node greater than 1 cm or retropharyngeal lymph node greater than 0.5 cm is considered to contain a tumor.

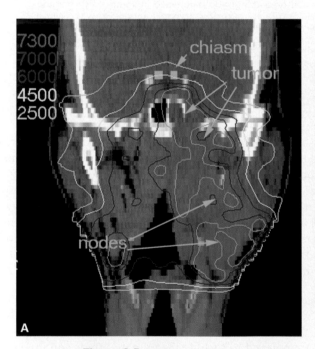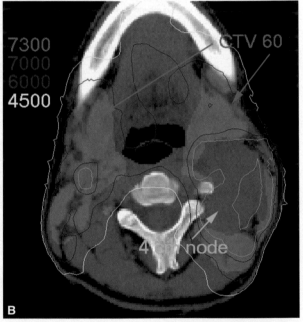

Figure 8.5 A 30-year-old Asian man presented with a left neck mass and headaches. Examination revealed a 4-cm left neck node and a nasopharyngeal mass that involved the left torus tubarius, fossa of Rosenmüller, posterior wall, and roof. A biopsy was positive for undifferentiated nasopharyngeal carcinoma, World Health Organization (WHO) type-3. Magnetic resonance imaging revealed a large, left-sided nasopharyngeal tumor with destruction of the ipsilateral clivus, floor of the sella, and floor of the medial portion of middle fossa, with tumor extending into the adjacent sphenoid sinus. There was minimal asymmetrical plaquelike thickening along the left parasellar dura suggesting intracranial tumor invasion. The left petrous apex was irregularly eroded. The tumor infiltrated the left prevertebral muscle and was associated with large left lateral retropharyngeal lymphadenopathy. The clinically apparent 4-cm lymph node in the upper jugular region was seen along with multiple additional nodes suspicious for metastatic lymphadenopathy. Stage: T4 N1 M0. The treatment consisted of a combination of concurrent cisplatin and radiation. Intensity-modulated radiation therapy (IMRT) with nine separate beam angles was delivered with "step and shoot" collimation. A separate isocentrically matched anterior field treated the low neck and supraclavicular fossa to 50 Gy. Isodoses on a coronal **(A)** and axial **(B)** image through the primary tumor and neck are shown. The primary nasopharynx tumor and gross neck disease received 70 Gy, and subclinical disease in the contralateral neck received 57 Gy. The brain stem and optic chiasm doses were limited to 54 Gy and the spinal cord to 45 Gy. He is without disease 42 months out from treatment with grade-1 xerostomia.

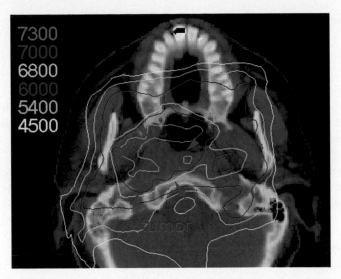

Figure 8.6   A 52-year-old woman presented with right adenopathy. Before finding the primary tumor, she underwent a right modified neck dissection, which revealed squamous cell carcinoma poorly differentiated in 10 lymph nodes. Subsequent workup revealed a nasopharynx tumor extending posteriorly and superiorly to involve the clivus and abut the right carotid vessel and prevertebral space. She was treated with intensity-modulated radiation therapy (IMRT) and concurrent cisplatin. The clinical target volume 1 (CTV1) received 70 Gy in 33 fractions. An axial isodose distribution at the level of the jugular fossa is shown. To respect the brainstem/spinal cord, the posterior margin was rather tight. Thus, the isodose demonstrates the 70 Gy line breaks up, but the 68 Gy line encompasses the tumor. The right neck received 63 Gy within the intensity-modulated radiation therapy volume. The mid and low neck were treated with an anterior portal, with a posterior beam on the right mid neck to supplement dose posteriorly to tissues considered at risk. The right mid neck received 60 Gy in 30 fractions. Following completion of her IMRT, there was suspicion of residual disease at the nasopharynx. She was treated with stereotactic radiation boost, 10 Gy in three fractions. She was without disease at follow-up 2 years later.

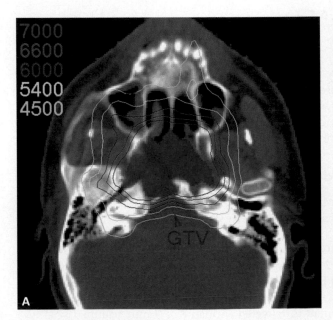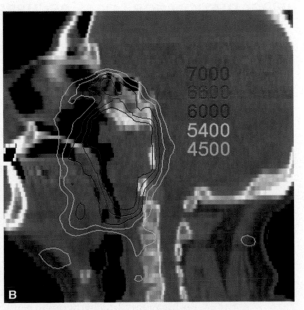

Figure 8.7   A 40-year-old man diagnosed with poorly differentiated squamous carcinoma of the nasopharynx, stage T3 N2 M0. He received concurrent radiation and chemotherapy. The sagittal and axial images demonstrate the full thickness destruction of the clivus (note the absence of bone). The tumor extent necessitated taking the edge of the brainstem to 60 Gy. The isodose distribution demonstrates the ability of intensity-modulated radiation therapy (IMRT) to provide conformal coverage in this difficult case. The patient was without disease at the follow-up visit 3 years out from therapy.

Clinical Target Volume

Two clinical target volumes (CTVs) are generally delineated.

- CTV1 delineates volumes to receive the highest dose, usually 70 Gy (therefore also referred to as CTV_{70}). This includes the primary and nodal GTVs with 5 to 10 mm margins. The entire nasopharynx is encompassed unless the tumor is well lateralized.
- CTV2 delineates volumes to receive an intermediate dose, usually 60 Gy (therefore also referred to as CTV_{60}). The general guidelines for delineating CTV2 are as follows:
    - *Anterior:* posterior third of the nasal cavity and maxillary sinuses.
    - *Posterior:* retropharyngeal regions and clivus.
    - *Lateral:* parapharyngeal regions extending to the middle of the pterygoid muscles.
    - *Superior:* inferior third of the sphenoid sinus, and adjacent skull base.
    - *Inferior:* 1 cm margin beyond the nasopharynx or inferior to CTV1.

Elective Nodal Irradiation

In the absence of clinical nodal involvement, levels II to V receive elective irradiation. In the presence of involved nodes, level IB of the involved side also receives elective dose.

Dose

With the conventional technique, 50 Gy is given in 25 fractions to regions at risk for harboring subclinical disease, followed by a boost dose of 16 to 20 Gy in eight to ten fractions to the primary tumor and involved node(s), depending on the size.

With IMRT, 66 to 70 Gy is given to the primary tumor and involved node(s), and 54 to 57.6 Gy is given to regions at risk for harboring subclinical disease in 30 to 33 fractions. The fraction size varies from 1.8 Gy to the subclinical region to 2.2 Gy to the gross disease. The preferred fractionation for patients receiving concurrent chemo-radiation is 70 Gy in 33 fractions (2.12 Gy per fraction) to gross disease and margin. Subclinical sites receive 60 Gy.

Dose Specification: See "General Principles"

REIRRADIATION FOR LOCAL RECURRENCE

Eligibility

In our center, retreatment with curative intent after previous high dose irradiation is restricted to patients with locally recurrent disease that is confined to the nasopharynx or with a limited extension to the adjacent parapharyngeal space, base of skull, or both (see Fig. 8.8). Conformal radiotherapy is now used to maximize the tolerance to reirradiation by limiting the volume of normal tissues exposed to the second course of radiotherapy (see Fig. 8.9).

Target Volume, Setup, and Field Arrangement

Superficial thin, recurrent tumors are treated with combinations of conformal external beam irradiation and brachytherapy, whereas thicker lesions receive conformal external beam irradiation alone.

External beam component: The GTV encompasses the clinically and radiologically detectable recurrent disease with 1- to 2-cm margins. When combined with brachytherapy, the external beam component is delivered first with the aim of flattening the lesion to allow better placement of the intracavitary source and to improve brachytherapy dose distribution.

Endocavitary brachytherapy component is delivered with an 8×3 mm cesium 137 (^{137}Cs) source afterloaded in a Teflon ball placed into the nasopharynx under general anesthesia. Four sizes of Teflon balls (diameters: 1.5, 2.0, 2.5, and 3.0 cm) are available. The largest Teflon ball that can be inserted snugly is chosen to improve the depth dose distribution.

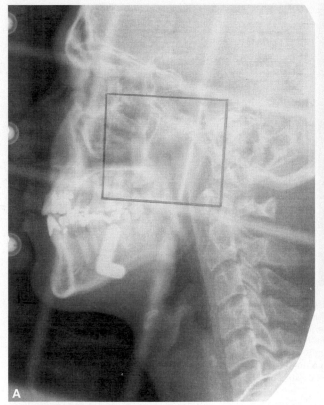

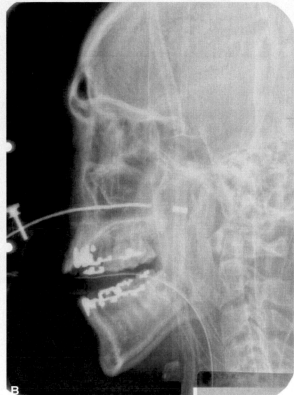

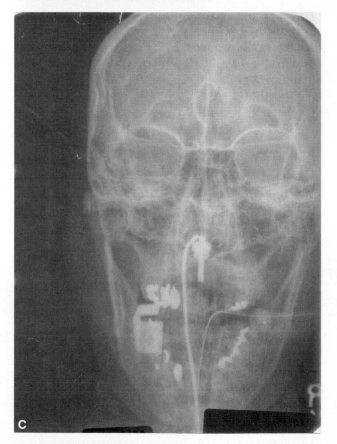

Figure 8.8 A 34-year-old man underwent radiation treatment for a T1 N0 M0 lymphoepithelioma of the nasopharynx. He received 64.8 Gy in 36 fractions to the primary tumor and 45 Gy in 25 fractions to the cervical nodes. He did well until a year later when he presented with epistaxis. Physical examination showed a small lesion in the left lateral wall, biopsy of which revealed a lymphoepithelioma. He was referred to our center for workup and treatment. Examination at this time revealed a superficial lesion confined to the left lateral wall. There was no palpable lymphadenopathy. Workup for metastatic disease was negative. He received external beam irradiation with 25 MV x-rays through lateral–opposed portals **(A)** to a dose of 25 Gy in 12 fractions. This was followed by an intracavitary insertion of ^{137}Cs source (18.75 mg radium equivalent) into a Teflon ball **(B, C)** for 35.6 hours to deliver a dose of 50 Gy to the mucosal surface (23 Gy at 0.5 cm depth). This patient was alive without evidence of disease and without late complications from this treatment 10 years later.

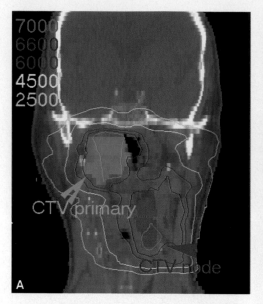
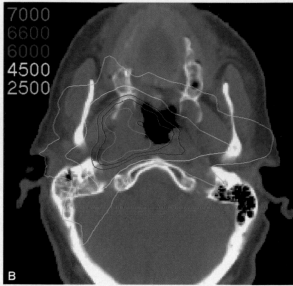

Figure 8.9   A 67-year-old man was diagnosed with nasopharynx carcinoma, World Health Organization type-3. He received a combination of radiation and chemotherapy, but discontinued therapy at 50 Gy due to toxicity. He developed a recurrence in the right nasopharynx and left neck. He received reirradiation with intensity-modulated radiation therapy (IMRT) and concurrent cisplatin. The clinical target volume 1 (CTV1) received 66 Gy in 33 fractions. Isodose distributions are shown on a coronal **(A)** and axial **(B)** image. The spinal cord was kept to a maximal dose of 20 Gy in 33 fractions. He had no evidence of disease at last follow-up 2 years after retreatment.

Dose

For external beam irradiation, prescribed dose is 20 to 30 Gy in ten to 15 fractions, depending on the thickness of the recurrent lesion and the previous radiation dose. In general, the cumulative external beam dose is kept to 100 Gy or less and, particularly, the cumulative dose to the temporal lobes is kept below 105 Gy to minimize the risk of brain necrosis.

For endocavitary brachytherapy, prescribed dose is 40 to 50 Gy surface dose delivered at a dose rate of 0.4 to 0.6 Gy per hour.

Background Data

TABLE 8.1
FAILURES AT THE PRIMARY SITE IN TUMORS OF THE NASOPHARYNX

Stage (1992 AJCC System)	No. of Patients	10-yr Actuarial Local Control (%)
T1	55	87
T2	138	75
T3	67	63
T4	118	45
Total	378	66

AJCC, American Joint Committee on Cancer.
Data from M.D. Anderson Cancer Center.
Adapted from Sanguineti G, Geara FB, Garden AS, et al. Carcinoma of the nasopharynx treated by radiotherapy alone: determinants of local and regional control. *Int J Radiat Oncol Biol Phys* 1997;37:985–996, with permission.

TABLE 8.2
FAILURES AT THE PRIMARY SITE IN TUMORS OF THE NASOPHARYNX

Histologic Findings	No. of Patients	10-yr Actuarial Local Control (%)
Squamous cell carcinoma	193	54
Lymphoepithelioma	154	71
Undifferentiated carcinoma	31	79

Data from M.D. Anderson Cancer Center.
Adapted from Sanguineti G, Geara FB, Garden AS, et al. Carcinoma of the nasopharynx treated by radiotherapy alone: determinants of local and regional control. *Int J Radiat Oncol Biol Phys* 1997;37:985–996, with permission.

TABLE 8.3
NODAL RECURRENCE BY LYMPH NODE STAGE AND HISTOLOGY

Stage (1992 AJCC System)	No. of Patients	10-yr Actuarial Regional Control (%)
N0	80	95
N1	32	94
N2a	38	91
N2b	50	80
N2c	80	77
N3	70	71

AJCC, American Joint Committee on Cancer.
Data from M.D. Anderson Cancer Center.
Adapted from Sanguineti G, Geara FB, Garden AS, et al. Carcinoma of the nasopharynx treated by radiotherapy alone: determinants of local and regional control. *Int J Radiat Oncol Biol Phys* 1997;37:985–996, with permission.

TABLE 8.4
REVIEW ON SQUAMOUS CELL CARCINOMA OF THE NASOPHARYNX: SURVIVAL AND CUMULATIVE INCIDENCE (%) OF PERSISTENCE AND RELAPSE

Author	No. of Cases	Persistence			Relapse			Survival	
		L	R	M	L	R	M	5 yr	10 yr
Baker	99	—	—	—	32	34	38	24	—
Cellai et al.	138	20	18	—	17	12	18	40	—
Hagbhin et al.	79	—	—	—	25	4	24	33	19
Hoppe et al.	82	—	—	—	21	9	18	62	55
Mesic et al.	251	—	—	—	20	13	29	52	—
Moench and Phillips	146	—	—	—	38	14	22	38	—
Rahima et al.	91	—	—	—	35	30	35	62	42
Sham and Choy	759	—	—	—	18	21	24	—	—
Stein et al.	49	—	—	—	22	8	14	42	—
Vikram et al.	107	—	—	—	31	4	17	56	—
Yamashita et al.	77	—	—	—	58	39	16	25	—
Lee et al.	5,037	13	13	6	18	17	30	52	42

L, local; R, regional; M, distant metastases.
From Lee AWM, Poon YF, Foo W, et al. Retrospective analysis of 5037 patients with nasopharyngeal carcinoma treated during 1976–1985. Overall survival and patterns of failure. *Int J Radiat Oncol Biol Phys* 1992;23:261, with permission.

TABLE 8.5

RESULTS OF COMBINED CHEMOTHERAPY AND RADIATION: RANDOMIZED TRIALS[a] (LITERATURE REVIEW)

First Author	Chemotherapy: No. of Cycles	Radiation (Gy)	No. of Patients Randomized	Survival
Rossi	VCA:×6 after RT	60–70	229	RT: 67% RTC: 59% (4Y-A)
Chan	CF:×2 before, ×4 after RT	66	82	RT: 81% RTC: 80% (2Y-A)
Chua	CE:×2–3 before RT	66–74	334	RT: 71% RTC: 78% (3Y-A)
INCSG	BEC:×3 before RT	65–70	339	RT: 45% RTC: 67% (Crude-DFS)
Ma	CBF:×2–3 before RT	68–72	456	RT: 56% RTC: 63% (5Y-A)
Al-Sarraf	C:×3 during RT CF:×3 after RT	70	193	RT: 47% RTC: 78% (3Y-A)

INCSG, International Nasopharynx Cancer Study Group; VCA, vincristine, cyclophosphamide, adriamycin; CF, cisplatin, 5-FU; CE, cisplatin, epirubicin; BEC, bleomycin, epirubicin, cisplatin; CBF, cisplatin, bleomycin, 5-FU; C, cisplatin; RT, radiation alone; RTC, radiation and chemotherapy; Y-A, year actuarial; DFS, disease-free survival.
[a]All trials randomized patients to radiation alone or radiation and chemotherapy.
Adapted from Rossi A, Molinari R, Boracchi P, et al. Adjuvant chemotherapy with vincristine, cyclophosphamide, and doxorubicin after radiotherapy in local-regional nasopharyngeal cancer: results of a 4-year multicenter randomized study. *J Clin Oncol* 1988;6:1401–1410; Chan AT, Teo PM, Leung TW, et al. A prospective randomized study of chemotherapy adjunctive to definitive radiotherapy in advanced nasopharyngeal carcinoma. *Int J Radiat Oncol Biol Phys* 1995;33:569–577; Chua DT, Sham JS, Choy D, et al. Preliminary report of the Asian-Oceanian Clinical Oncology Association randomized trial comparing cisplatin and epirubicin followed by radiotherapy versus radiotherapy alone in the treatment of patients with locoregionally advanced nasopharyngeal carcinoma: Asian-Oceanian Clinical Oncology Association Nasopharynx Cancer Study Group. *Cancer* 1998;83:2270–2283; *INCSG*. Preliminary results of a randomized trial comparing neoadjuvant chemotherapy (cisplatin, epirubicin, bleomycin) plus radiotherapy vs radiotherapy alone in stage IV (N2, M0) undifferentiated nasopharyngeal carcinoma: a positive effect on progression-free survival. *Int J Radiat Oncol Biol Phys* 1996;35:463–469; Ma J, Mai HQ, Hong MH, et al. Results of a prospective randomized trial comparing neoadjuvant chemotherapy plus radiotherapy with radiotherapy alone in patients with locoregionally advanced nasopharyngeal carcinoma. *J Clin Oncol* 2000;19:1350–1357; and Al-Sarraf M, LeBlanc M, Giri PG, et al. Chemoradiotherapy versus radiotherapy in patients with advanced nasopharyngeal cancer: Phase III randomized intergroup study 0099. *J Clin Oncol* 1998;16:1310–1317, with permission.

TABLE 8.6

RESULTS OF IMRT IN THE TREATMENT OF NASOPHARYNGEAL CARCINOMA (LITERATURE REVIEW)

Authors	Patient No.	Median Follow-up	% Local Control	% Nodal Control
Lee et al.	67	31 mo	97% (4-yr)	98%
Kam et al.	63	29 mo	92% (3-yr)	98%
Kwong et al.	33	24 mo	100% (3-yr)	100%

IMRT, Intensity-modulated radiation therapy.
Adapted from Lee N, Xia P, Quivey JM, et al. Intensity-modulated radiation therapy in the treatment of nasopharyngeal carcinoma: an update of the UCSF experience. *Int J Radiat Oncol Biol Phys* 2002;53:12–22; Kam MK, Teo PM, Chau RM, et al. Treatment of nasopharyngeal carcinoma with intensity-modulated radiation therapy: the Hong Kong experience. *Int J Radiat Oncol Biol Phys* 2004;60:1440–1450; and Kwong DL , Pow EH , Sham JS , et al. Intensity-modulated radiation therapy for early-stage nasopharyngeal carcinoma: a prospective study on disease control and preservation of salivary function. *Cancer* 2004;101:1584–1593, with permission.

TABLE 8.7

RESULTS OF REIRRADIATION OF RECURRENT NASOPHARYNGEAL CARCINOMA (LITERATURE REVIEW)

Institutions	No. of Patients	Survival (5 yr)	% With Severe Complications
Stanford (Hoppe et al.)	13	Median: 13 mo.	Not stated
UCSF (Fu et al.)	42	Overall: 41%	9
Beijing (Yan et al.)	219	Overall: 18%	29
MGH (Wang et al.)	51	T1, T2: 38%; T3, T4: 15%	2
MDACC (Pryzant et al.)	53	Confined to nasopharynx: 32%; larger: 9%	8

From Pryzant RM, Wendt CD , Delclos L , et al. Re-treatment of nasopharyngeal carcinoma in 53 patients. *Int J Radiat Oncol Biol Phys* 1992;22:941, with permission.

SUGGESTED READINGS

Al-Sarraf M, LeBlanc M, Giri PG, et al. Chemoradiotherapy versus radiotherapy in patients with advanced nasopharyngeal cancer: phase III randomized intergroup study 0099. *J Clin Oncol* 1998;16:1310.

Chan AT, Teo P, Huang DP. Pathogenesis and treatment of nasopharyngeal carcinoma. *Semin Oncol* 2004;31:794.

Chan ATC, Teo PM, Leung TW, et al. A prospective randomized study of chemotherapy adjunctive to definitive radiotherapy in advanced nasopharyngeal carcinoma. *Int J Radiat Oncol Biol Phys* 1995;33:569.

Chen KY, Fletcher GH. Malignant tumors of the nasopharynx. *Radiology* 1971;99:165.

Chen WZ, Zhou DL, Luo KS. Long-term observation after radiotherapy for nasopharyngeal carcinoma (NPC). *Int J Radiat Oncol Biol Phys* 1989;16:311.

Chua DT, Ma J, Sham JS, et al. Long-term survival after cisplatin-based induction chemotherapy and radiotherapy for nasopharyngeal carcinoma: a pooled data analysis of two phase III trials. *J Clin Oncol* 2005;23:1118.

Delclos L, Moore BE, Sampiere VA. A disposable "afterloadable" nasopharyngeal applicator for radioactive point sources. *Endocur Hypertherm Oncol* 1994;10:43.

Fletcher GH, Million RR. Nasopharynx. In: Fletcher GH, ed. *Textbook of radiotherapy*, 3rd ed. Philadelphia: Lea & Febiger, 1980.

Geara FB, Sanguineti G, Tucker SL, et al. Carcinoma of the nasopharynx treated by radiotherapy alone: determinants of distant metastasis and survival. *Radiother Oncol* 1997;43:53.

Hunt MA, et al. Treatment planning and delivery of intensity-modulated radation therapy for primary nasopharynx cancer. *Int J Radiat Oncol Biol Phys* 2001;49:623.

International Nasopharynx Cancer Study Group. Preliminary results of a randomized trial comparing neoadjuvant chemotherapy (cisplatin, epirubicin, bleomycin) plus radiotherapy vs. radiotherapy alone in stage IV (≥N2, M0) undifferentiated nasopharyngeal carcinoma: a positive effect on progression-free survival. *Int J Radiat Oncol Biol Phys* 1996;35:463.

Kam MK, Teo PM, Chau RM, et al. Treatment of nasopharyngeal carcinoma with intensity-modulated radiotherapy: the Hong Kong experience. *Int J Radiat Oncol Biol Phys* 2004;60:1440.

Kwong DL, Pow EH, Sham JS, et al. Intensity-modulated radiotherapy for early-stage nasopharyngeal carcinoma: a prospective study on disease control and preservation of salivary function. *Cancer* 2004;101:1584.

Le QT, Tate D, Koong A, et al. Improved local control with stereotactic radiosurgical boost in patients with nasopharyngeal carcinoma. *Int J Radiat Oncol Biol Phys* 2003;56:1046.

Lee AWM, Law SC, Foo W, et al. Nasopharyngeal carcinoma: local control by megavoltage irradiation. *Br J Radiol* 1993;66:528.

Lee AWM, Poon YF, Foo W, et al. Retrospective analysis of 5037 patients with nasopharyngeal carcinoma treated during 1976–1985. Overall survival and patterns of failure. *Int J Radiat Oncol Biol Phys* 1992;23:261.

Lee N, Xia P, Quivey JM, et al. Intensity-modulated radiotherapy in the treatment of nasopharyngeal carcinoma: an update of the UCSF experience. *Int J Radiat Oncol Biol Phys* 2002;53:12.

Levendag PC, Lagerwaard FJ, Noever I, et al. Role of endocavitary brachytherapy with or without chemotherapy in cancer of the nasopharynx. *Int J Radiat Oncol Biol Phys* 2002;52:755.

Peters LJ, Batsakis JG, Goepfert H, et al. The diagnosis and management of nasopharyngeal cancer in Caucasians. In: Williams CJ, Krikorian JG, Green MR et al., eds. *Textbook of uncommon cancer*. Chichester: John Wiley & Sons, 1988.

Pryzant RM, Wendt CD, Delclos L, et al. Re-treatment of nasopharyngeal carcinoma in 53 patients. *Int J Radiat Oncol Biol Phys* 1992;22:941.

Sanguineti G, Geara FB, Garden AS, et al. Carcinoma of the nasopharynx treated by radiotherapy alone: determinants of local and regional control. *Int J Radiat Oncol Biol Phys* 1997;37:985.

Slevin NJ, Wilkinson JM, Filby HM, et al. Intracavitary radiotherapy boosting for nasopharynx cancer. *Br J Radiol* 1997;70:412.

Teo PML, Kwan WH, Chan AT, et al. How successful is high-dose (60 Gy) reirradiation using mainly external beams in salvaging local failures of nasopharyngeal carcinoma? *Int J Radiat Oncol Biol Phys* 1998;40:897.

Teo P, Shiu W, Leung SF, et al. Prognostic factors in nasopharyngeal carcinoma investigated by computer tomography—an analysis of 659 patients. *Radiother Oncol* 1992;23:79.

Teo P, Tsao SY, Shiu W, et al. A clinical study of 407 cases of nasopharyngeal carcinoma in Hong Kong. *Int J Radiat Oncol Biol Phys* 1989;17:515.

Oropharynx

9

SOFT PALATE

Treatment Strategy

Primary radiotherapy is preferred for T1, T2, and exophytic T3, N0 to N1 carcinomas. Superficial T1 lesions without lymphadenopathy may be amenable to local excision only. Neck dissection is indicated in a few patients with N1 disease who have residual neck mass 6 weeks after completion of radiotherapy.

Combination of radiation with chemotherapy is the treatment of choice for infiltrative T3 and selected T4 or N2 to N3 tumors. Outside the protocol study setting, the combination of conventional radiation fractionation (70 Gy in 35 fractions over 7 weeks) with cisplatin (100 mg per m^2 given on days, 1, 22, and 43 of radiotherapy) is recommended because the benefit of this regimen has been demonstrated in several phase III trials. Neck dissection is indicated in patients who have residual neck mass 6 weeks after completion of therapy.

T4 tumors with bone invasion or extensive normal tissue destruction resulting in deformation and/or impaired functions are best treated with surgery and postoperative radiotherapy.

Primary Radiotherapy

Target Volume

The initial target volume is primary tumor with at least 2-cm margins and bilateral neck nodes, including the retropharyngeal nodes, and levels II, III, and IV nodes. The target volume also includes ipsilateral level IB in the presence of level II node. For lateralized tumors, the target volume includes the ipsilateral tonsillar pillars, parapharyngeal space, and lateral aspect of the pterygoid muscle.

The boost volume encompasses the primary tumor and involved node(s) with 1- to 2-cm margins.

Setup and Field Arrangement

Insertion of metal seeds at the borders of the tumor, when feasible, and marking of oral commissures and palpable nodes facilitate portal shaping. The patient is immobilized in a supine position with thermoplastic mask. An extended head and shoulder mask is used for conformal radiotherapy. With conventional technique, lateral parallel–opposed photon fields are used to treat the primary tumor and upper neck nodes.

- *Anterior border:* at least 2 cm anterior to the tumor.
- *Superior border:* at least 1.5 cm above the soft palate. If the primary tumor spreads into the tonsillar fossa, this border is extended superiorly to encompass the medial pterygoid muscle to the pterygoid plate.
- *Posterior border:* behind the mastoid tip when N0, behind the spinous processes when N+ or more posteriorly in the presence of large nodal mass.
- *Inferior border:* just above the arytenoids except when the extent of nodal disease requires a lower inferior border.

A matching anterior appositional photon field is used to treat the mid and lower neck nodes when indicated.

For the boost volume:

- T1 and small, superficial T2 tumors: it is preferable to administer the boost dose with an intraoral cone whenever feasible (i.e., the lesion is accessible and the patient can tolerate an intraoral cone without gagging) to reduce treatment morbidity by limiting the dose to the mandible and soft tissues. In such cases, it is desirable to administer the boost dose first while the tumor is clearly visible and palpable (see Fig. 9.1).

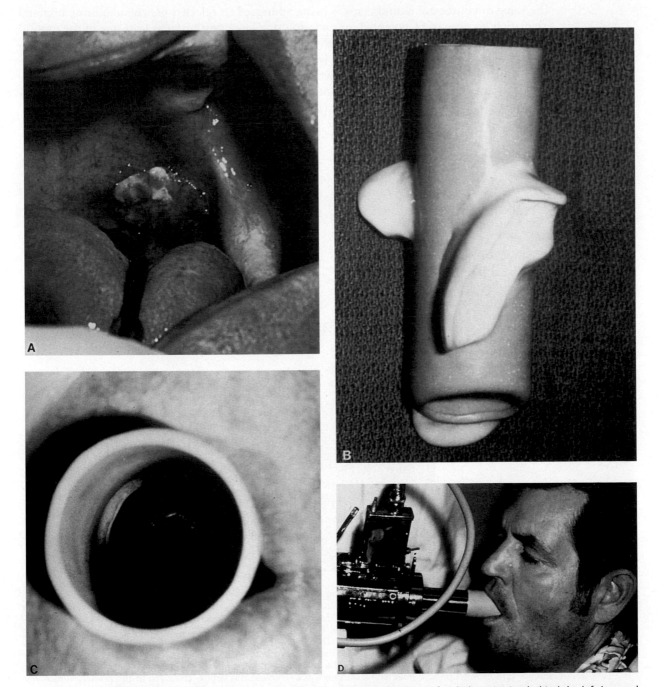

Figure 9.1 A 38-year-old man consulted his physician because of a slight irritation behind the left jaw and blood-streaked saliva. Physical examination revealed a 2.5-cm tumor at the junction of the soft palate and anterior faucial pillar on the left side **(A).** There was no palpable lymphadenopathy. Further examination was unremarkable. Biopsy of this lesion showed poorly-differentiated carcinoma. Stage T2 N0 M0. He received treatment with an intraoral cone followed by external beam irradiation. A customized device was made to ensure reproducible cone positioning **(B,C).** A 3-cm cone was used to deliver irradiations with 125 KVp x-rays to a dose of 15 Gy in five fractions **(D).** The remaining therapy was given through an ipsilateral external beam portal. A combination of electrons and photons, as described in Figure 6.2, was used to administer 50 Gy in 25 fractions over 5 weeks. This patient was alive and well 6 years after completion of therapy.

- Larger tumors: the boost dose is given by external beam. Lateral fields are reduced to cover the primary tumor with 1- to 2-cm margins (see Fig. 9.2).
- Nodal metastases in the upper neck are encompassed in the lateral portals. Nodes in the mid or lower neck can receive boost dose with an appositional glancing photon field or electron portal.

Intensity-Modulated Radiation Therapy

The value of conformal radiotherapy is being addressed in selected patients requiring bilateral irradiation because of its potential for exclusion of a large portion of at least one of the parotid glands from the high-dose volume, thereby reducing xerostomia without compromising the coverage of the primary tumor and draining lymphatics. The patient is immobilized in a supine position with an extended head and shoulder thermoplastic mask. Thin-cut computed tomography (CT) scans are obtained in treatment position. The gross target volume (GTV), clinical target volume (CTV), and planning target volume (PTV) are outlined for dosimetric planning.

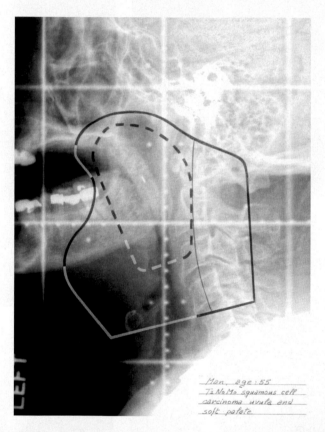

Figure 9.2   A 55-year-old man sought medical attention for a 6-month history of sore throat. Physical examination revealed a 3.5-cm exophytic tumor of the uvula and soft palate with minimal extension to the right anterior tonsillar pillar. The hard palate was uninvolved. There were no palpable neck nodes. Biopsy showed a moderately-differentiated squamous cell carcinoma. Stage: T2 N0 M0. This patient was treated with primary radiotherapy according to the concomitant boost regimen. The fields were designed to encompass the primary tumor and upper neck nodes. The boost volume covered the primary tumor with generous margins. The seed indicated the superior and anterior border of the tumor on the palate. The mid and lower neck nodes were treated through an anterior appositional photon field with a midline block to shield the larynx. The dose to the primary tumor was 70.5 Gy in 41 fractions over 6 weeks. Areas of subclinical disease in the upper neck received 54 Gy in 30 fractions over 6 weeks. The mid and lower neck received 50 Gy in 25 fractions over 5 weeks. He had no evidence of disease 5 years after therapy. However, there was a slight retraction of the soft palate without functional repercussion.

Dose

For T1 N0 and superficial T2 N0 tumors, therapy consists of conventional fractionation delivering 50 Gy in 25 fractions to the initial target volume followed by a boost dose of 15 Gy in five to six fractions given by intraoral cone or 16 Gy in eight fractions by external beam.

For T2 and exophytic T3 N0-1 tumors, therapy consists of concomitant boost schedule to total doses of 69 to 72 Gy in 40 to 42 fractions. The initial volume receives 1.8-Gy fractions to 54 Gy in 6 weeks. The boost volume receives an additional 1.5 Gy to a dose of 15 to 18 Gy given as second daily fractions during the last 2 to 2.5 weeks of the wide-field irradiations. The spinal cord dose is limited to 45 Gy or less.

Patients with T1 to T2, N0 to N1 tumors have been enrolled into a protocol study addressing the role of conformal radiotherapy in reducing the morbidity without compromising the tumor control probability. Currently recommended dose is 66 Gy to PTV of the primary tumor and involved node(s) and 54 Gy to the subclinical disease PTV administered in 30 fractions over 6 weeks.

For exophytic T3 and T4 or N2 to N3 tumors, radiation delivered in the conventional 2-Gy fractions to a dose of 50 Gy to the initial target volume and 70 Gy to the boost volume is given in combination with three cycles of concurrent cisplatin outside the protocol study setting. The spinal cord dose is limited to 45 Gy or less. This group of patients has been enrolled on a study randomizing patients to either conventional 2-Gy fractions to 70 Gy or concomitant boost fractionation (72 Gy in 42 fractions) with concurrent cisplatin.

New protocols are being developed to address the role of integrating biologic therapy (such as antiepidermal growth factor receptor antibody, cetuximab; see Chapter 1) or of adding induction adjuvant chemotherapy to the concurrent radiation therapy–chemotherapy regimen. Some new protocols allow the use of intensity-modulated radiation therapy (IMRT). The recommended doses are mostly 70 Gy to the CTV1 and approximately 56 Gy to regions of elective irradiation delivered in 32 to 35 fractions.

Dose Specification: See "General Principles"

Postoperative Radiotherapy

Target Volume

The initial target volume encompasses the entire surgical bed and all nodal areas of the neck. The boost volume encompasses areas of known disease location with 1- to 2-cm margins.

Setup and Field Arrangement

The general technique is the same as that described under "Primary Radiotherapy." Marking of the external surgical scar facilitates portal design. The *anterior* and *superior field borders* are mainly determined by the local spread of the primary tumor and the extent of surgery (scar/flap). The field borders are placed 2 cm beyond the mucosal scar.

Dose

- A dose of 60 Gy in 30 fractions to areas with high-risk features; that is, close or microscopically positive margins, perineural extension, vascular invasion, positive nodes, or extranodal extension. An additional boost dose of 6 Gy in three fractions may be given when indicated, such as when multiple adverse features are present or when the interval between surgery and radiation is much longer than 6 weeks.
- A dose of 56 Gy in 28 fractions to the surgical bed.
- A dose of 50 Gy in 25 fractions to undissected regions to receive elective irradiation.

Timing of Postoperative Radiotherapy

It is desirable to commence postoperative radiotherapy as soon as possible after healing of the surgical wounds. With good communication between surgical, radiation, and dental oncologists, generally simulation can take place 3 to 4 weeks after surgery and radiotherapy can start a few days later in most patients. When delayed wound healing postpones commencement of postoperative radiation to beyond 5 to 6 weeks, we prescribe accelerated fractionation, such as concomitant boost, by delivering twice-a-day irradiations for 1 week, usually at the end of the radiation course, to reduce the potential hazard of prolonged cumulative treatment time.

Dose Specification: See "General Principles"

Background Data

TABLE 9.1

SITES OF PRIMARY TUMOR[a] IN 188 PATIENTS TREATED AT M.D. ANDERSON CANCER CENTER BETWEEN 1970 AND 1983

Site	No. of Patients	%
Uvula	5	2.7
SP	20	10.6
SP + uvula	14	7.4
AFP	43	22.9
AFP + SP	73	38.8
AFP + SP + uvula	33	17.6
Total	188	100.0

SP, soft palate; AFP, anterior faucial pillar.
[a]Unilateral: 151; midline/bilateral: 37.
Modified from Weber RS, Peters LJ, Wolf P, et al. Squamous cell carcinoma of the soft palate, uvula, and anterior faucial pillar. *Otolaryngol Head Neck Surg* 1988;99(1):16–23, with permission.

TABLE 9.2

LOCAL CONTROL OF SOFT PALATE TUMORS BY T STAGE

Stage	No. of Patients	Local Control (%)	
		3 yr	5 yr
T1	26	92	92
T2	50	70	67
T3	49	58	58
T4	21	49	37

From Keus RB, Pontvert D, Brunin F, et al. Results of irradiation in squamous cell carcinoma of the soft palate and uvula. *Radiother Oncol* 1988;11:311–317, with permission.

TABLE 9.3
THERAPY MODALITY AND OUTCOME BY T STAGE

Primary Treatment	Stage					
	Tx	T1	T2	T3	T4	Total
	No. of Patients (No. Controlled)					
Surgery	2 (2)	9 (9)	12 (11)	4 (4)	1 (0)	28 (26)
Radiation	4 (3)	24 (21)	79 (60)	30 (23)	13 (4)	150 (111)
Surgery + radiation	—	1 (1)	1 (0)	5 (3)	3 (2)	10 (6)
Total	6 (5)	34 (31)	92 (71)	39 (30)	17 (6)	183 (143)

Modified from Weber RS , Peters LJ , Wolf P, et al. Squamous cell carcinoma of the soft palate, uvula, and anterior faucial pillar. *Otolaryngol Head Neck Surg* 1988; 99(1):16–23, with permission.

TABLE 9.4
THERAPEUTIC MODALITY AND INCIDENCE OF NECK RECURRENCE BY N STAGE

Neck Treatment	N0	N1	N2	N3A	N3B	Total
	No. of Patients (No. Controlled)					
Surgery	8 (6)	2 (2)	—	—	—	10 (8)
Radiation	95 (87)	12 (10)	13 (10)	3 (1)	3 (2)	126 (110)
Radiation + surgery	—	1 (1)	13 (10)	3 (3)	2 (1)	19 (15)
Surgery + radiation	2 (2)	5 (4)	1 (1)	—	2 (1)	10 (8)
None	23 (17)	—	—	—	—	23 (17)
Total[a]	128 (112)	20 (17)	27 (21)	6 (4)	7 (4)	188 (158)

[a]Total recurrences, regardless of primary control.
Modified from Weber RS , Peters LJ , Wolf P, et al. Squamous cell carcinoma of the soft palate, uvula, and anterior faucial pillar. *Otolaryngol Head Neck Surg* 1988;99(1):16–23, with permission.

TONSILLAR FOSSA

Treatment Strategy

Primary radiotherapy is preferred for T1, T2, and exophytic T3 N0 to N1 carcinomas. Neck dissection is indicated in a very small number of patients with N1 disease who have residual neck mass 6 weeks after completion of radiotherapy.

Combination of radiation with chemotherapy is the treatment of choice for infiltrative T3 and selected T4 or N2 to N3 tumors. Outside the protocol study setting, the combination of conventional radiation fractionation (70 Gy in 35 fractions over 7 weeks) with cisplatin (100 mg per m^2 given on days, 1, 22, and 43 of radiotherapy) is recommended because the benefit of this regimen has been demonstrated in several phase III trials. Neck dissection is indicated in patients who have residual neck mass 6 weeks after completion of therapy.

T4 tumors with bone invasion or extensive normal tissue destruction, resulting in deformation and/or impaired functions are best treated with surgery and postoperative radiotherapy.

Primary Radiotherapy

Target Volume

For the initial target volume:

- T1 and T2 (with limited extension to the soft palate, and no base of tongue involvement), N0 to N1 tumors: primary lesion with at least 2-cm margins and ipsilateral retropharyngeal and level II–IV nodes. The target volume also includes ipsilateral level IB in the presence of level II node (see Fig. 9.3).
- T2 (with base of tongue or significant soft palate involvement), T3 and selected T4 or N2 to N3 tumors: tonsillar fossa, faucial pillars, soft palate, base of tongue, medial pterygoid muscle, and bilateral neck nodes (parapharyngeal-retropharyngeal, level II–IV, and level IB of the involved neck side).

For the boost volume: primary tumor and involved node(s) with 1- to 2-cm margins.

Setup and Field Arrangement for Ipsilateral Treatment (for T1–T2, N0–N1 Tumors)

Insertion of metal seeds at the borders of the tumor, when feasible, and marking of oral commissures and palpable nodes facilitate portal shaping. The patient is immobilized in a supine position with thermoplastic mask for irradiation of the primary tumor and upper neck nodes with wedge-pair photon portals or IMRT.

Field borders for the initial target volume:

- *Anterior border:* at least 2 cm anterior to the tumor.
- *Superior border:* encompasses the insertion of the medial pterygoid muscle at the pterygoid plate.

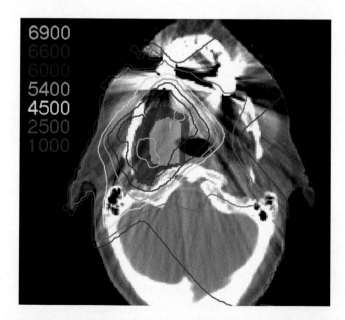

Figure 9.3   A 47-year-old woman presented with a swollen right tonsil and, after some delay, underwent tonsillectomy. Histologic examination revealed invasive poorly-differentiated squamous cell carcinoma with lymphatic and perineural invasion. The final margins after additional resection were free. On presentation to our center, she had postsurgical changes without evidence of residual disease and was, therefore, staged as having a Tx (pT1) N0 tonsil carcinoma. We elected to treat this patient ipsilaterally with a wedged-pair technique, using "field-in-field" compensation (see Fig. 3.17). The total dose was 66 Gy in 33 fractions. The initial volume encompassed the tonsillar bed and upper neck, and was reduced after 50 Gy. This target (*red*) included the pterygoid muscle, parapharyngeal space, the lateral base of tongue, the lateral soft palate and the ipsilateral retropharyngeal nodes. The boost volume encompassed the tonsillar bed only (*green*). An axial isodose distribution through the superior tonsillar region is shown. The initial wedged-pair fields were matched above the arytenoids to an anterior field that covered levels 3 and 4 of the right neck to 50 Gy. She had no evidence of disease and had no sequelae 2 years after therapy.

- *Posterior border:* 2 cm behind the mastoid tip and behind the edge of the sternocleidomastoid muscle.
- *Inferior border:* just above the arytenoids.

A matching anterior photon portal is used to irradiate the mid and lower neck nodes.
For the boost volume, the field is reduced to cover initial gross disease with 1- to 2-cm margins.

Intensity-Modulated Radiation Therapy Planning for Ipsilateral Treatment (for T1–T2, N0–N1 Tumors)

When IMRT is used, the parapharyngeal space, pterygoid muscle to its insertion onto the ptery-goid plates, lateral base of tongue, and soft palate, retropharyngeal, and level II–IV node (also level IB in N1 patients) are included in the CTV (see Fig. 9.4). The primary tumor and nodal regions above the arytenoids are irradiated with IMRT and the lower neck nodes are irradiated with a matching anterior portal.

Setup and Field Arrangement for Bilateral Treatment

Insertion of metal seeds at the borders of the tumor, when feasible, and marking of oral commis-sures and palpable nodes facilitate portal shaping (see Figs. 9.5 and 9.6). Patient is immobilized in a supine position.

Field borders for the initial target volume:

- *Anterior border:* at least 2 cm anterior to the tumor or more anteriorly if necessary to encompass level IB (submandibular) node.

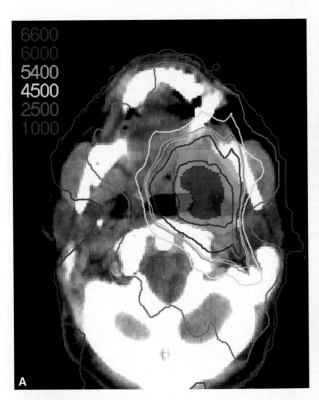 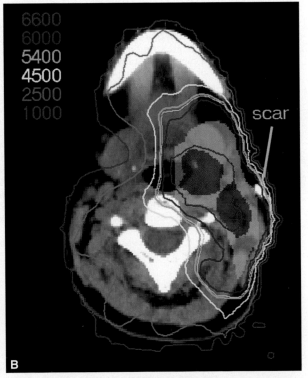

Figure 9.4 A 40- year-old woman presented after an excisional biopsy of an asymptomatic left neck mass. Histologic examination revealed squamous cell carcinoma in a 2.3 cm lymph node. Her workup did not reveal any residual nodal disease, but the left tonsil was firm. A biopsy of the tonsil done during examination under anesthesia revealed squamous cell carcinoma. Stage was T1Nx (pN1). It was elected to treat her ipsilaterally using intensity-modulated radiation therapy (IMRT). Axial isodose distributions are shown. The tonsillar region (*red*) received 66 Gy **(A)** and an additional rim of surrounding tissues (*green*) along with ipsilateral lev-els IB and II nodes received 60 Gy. The involved nodal bed defined from the pre-biopsy imaging (*blue*) was prescribed a minimum dose of 63 Gy **(B)**. The excision scar was wired for planning, and a 2 mm bolus was applied over the scar. The left low neck was treated with an appositional anterior field to 50 Gy, matched with a monoisocentric technique to the IMRT fields. She had no evidence of disease and had no sequelae 2 years after therapy.

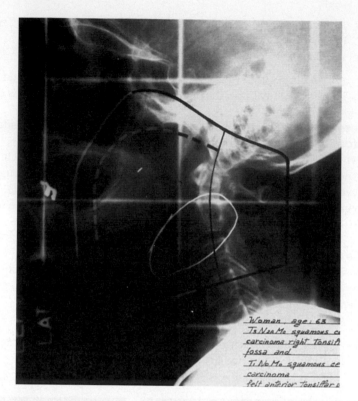

Woman age: 63
Ts Naa Mo squamous ce
carcinoma right Tonsill
fossa and
Tı No Mo squamous ce
carcinoma
left anterior tonsillar p

Figure 9.5 A 63-year-old woman had a 1-month history of sore throat and swelling of the right tonsil. Physical examination revealed a large exophytic and ulcerative tumor filling the right tonsillar fossa, extending across the glossopalatine sulcus to approximately 1.5 cm into the base of tongue. There was also extension to the anterior tonsillar pillar and soft palate, and posteriorly to the lateral pharyngeal wall. The inferior border of the tumor was at the level of the tip of the epiglottis. The largest dimension of the tumor was 4.5 cm. Tongue mobility was normal and there was no trismus. There was also an area at the lower part of the contralateral anterior tonsillar pillar with some nodularity and superficial ulceration that raised suspicion. A 4.5 × 2.5-cm mobile node was palpable in the right subdigastric area. Biopsies from the right tonsillar area as well as from the left anterior tonsillar pillar showed squamous cell carcinoma. The tumor in the right tonsillar fossa was staged as T3 N2 AM0 and the tumor on the left tonsillar pillar was staged as T1 N0 M0. The patient received primary radiotherapy for both lesions. The primary tumors and upper neck nodes were treated with lateral–opposed fields. A seed was inserted to indicate the anterior and superior border of the tonsillar fossa tumor. The palpable lymph node was wired. The part of the node overlying the spinal cord was relatively superficial and it was felt that this could be supplemented with 9 MeV electrons after off-cord reduction. The mid and lower neck nodes were treated electively through an anterior appositional portal. Because the inferior border of the boost field was relatively close to the edge of the node, the right midcervical region was boosted with a lateral appositional 9 MeV electron field matched to the inferior border of the photon field. The dose to the larger primary tumor and involved neck nodes was taken to 72 Gy in 42 fractions over 6 weeks. The right midcervical nodal group, adjacent to the big nodal mass, received 63 Gy in 36 fractions over 6 weeks. Areas of subclinical disease received 54 Gy in 30 fractions over 6 weeks. She had no evidence of disease 4 years after completion of therapy.

Figure 9.6 A 49-year-old man presented with several months of otalgia and sore throat. Examination revealed a right neck mass. A fine needle aspirate specimen of this mass was positive for poorly differentiated squamous cell carcinoma. Physical examination revealed a 3-cm primary tumor located in the superior aspect of the right tonsil and extending onto the soft palate. There was no trismus. The neck examination revealed a 5-cm mass of matted lymph nodes Stage T2 N2b M0. He was treated with radiation alone using concomitant boost regimen. Treatment started with two lateral **(A)** and an anterior **(B)** portals matched at a single isocenter above the arytenoids. The large lateral portals received 41.4 Gy. To encompass the gross disease in the photon fields, for the off–spinal cord reduction and boost fields, parallel–opposed oblique fields were used. The posterior cervical strips were treated with 9 MeV electrons to 54 Gy. The boost was delivered concomitantly, 18 Gy in 12 fractions. The anterior field continued to 54 Gy with a full midline block inserted at 45 Gy to shield the spinal cord. The gross nodal disease in the mid neck was boosted with a posterior photon beam, matched at the single isocenter. **C,D:** Digital reconstructions of the blocks for the boost fields with the gross disease contoured. Axial views of the isodoses through the primary target (*T*) and through the mid neck are shown in **(E,F)**. A selective right neck dissection was performed because a residual neck mass remained 6 weeks after completion of radiotherapy. Ten lymph nodes were removed from levels two and three, but none contained viable tumor.

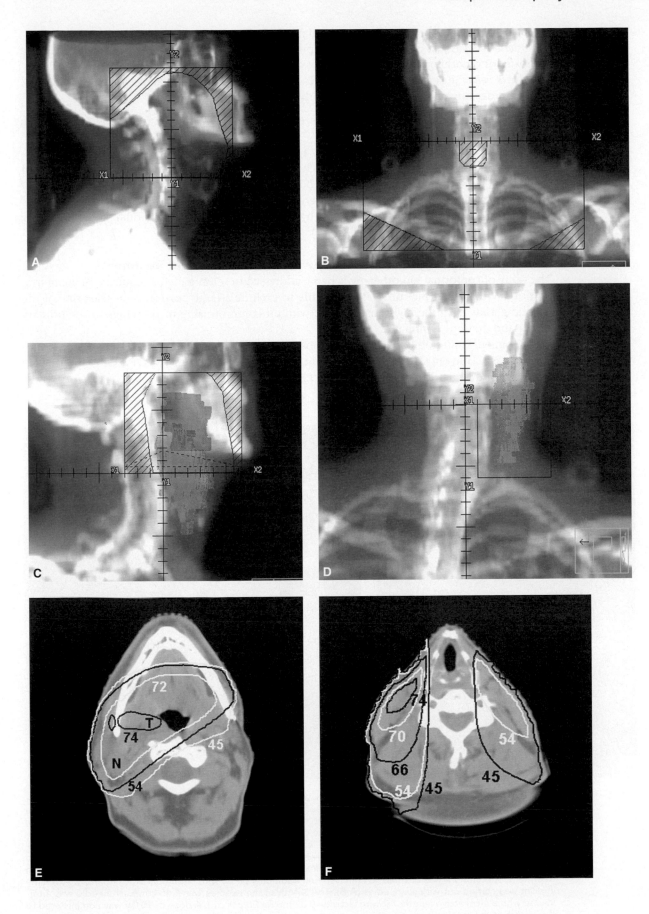

- *Superior border:* encompasses pterygoid plates and retropharyngeal nodes.
- *Posterior border:* just behind the spinous processes or more posteriorly in the presence of large posterior cervical nodal masses.
- *Inferior border:* just above the arytenoids. In the presence of large nodal disease below this level, the border can be extended more inferiorly.

An anterior appositional photon field is used for elective treatment of the mid and lower neck nodes bilaterally.

For the boost volume, the lateral portals are reduced to include the primary tumor with 1- to 2-cm margins and the involved upper neck nodes. In the presence of trismus, the ipsilateral medial pterygoid muscle is included in the boost fields. Nodal disease outside the primary boost field is generally treated with anterior–posterior glancing photon fields.

An additional boost with interstitial brachytherapy is given if there is residual palpable disease, particularly in the tongue base (see Fig. 9.7).

Intensity-Modulated Radiation Therapy Planning for Bilateral Treatment

The value of conformal radiotherapy is being addressed in select patients requiring bilateral irradiation. With careful planning, it is possible to exclude a large portion of at least one of the parotid glands from the high-dose volume without compromising the coverage of the primary tumor and draining lymphatics.

The patient is immobilized in a supine position with an extended head and shoulder thermoplastic mask. Thin-cut CT images are obtained in treatment position. The GTV, CTV, and PTV are outlined for dosimetric planning (see Figs. 9.8 and 9.9).

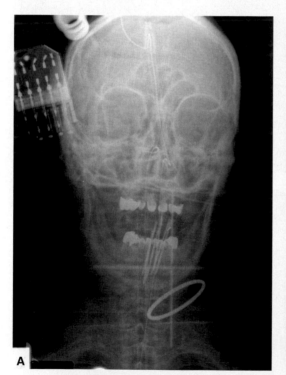
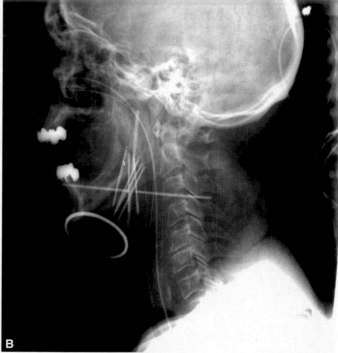

A

B

Figure 9.7 A 62-year-old man presented to a physician because of a burning sensation in his throat. A left tonsillar tumor was found and he was referred to our center for workup and treatment. Physical examination revealed a 5-cm tumor of the left tonsil extending to the anterior faucial pillar, soft palate, lateral pharyngeal wall, and through the glossopalatine sulcus into the base of tongue (2 cm). There was a 4 × 2-cm matted mass palpable at the left subdigastric area. The biopsy of the left tonsillar lesion showed a moderately differentiated squamous cell carcinoma; Stage T3 N2b M0. He received external beam irradiation using a setup as described in Figures 9.5–9.6. A small base of tongue residual lesion was palpable at the completion of the external beam treatment. Therefore, it was decided to administer an additional boost with interstitial brachytherapy. A volume implant was carried out with six needles **(A,B).** The length of the needles was 4.45 cm. Each needle was afterloaded with a 4-cm active-length ^{192}Ir wire (activity: 0.32 mg Ra Eq per cm). A dose of 10 Gy was administered to the border of the residual tumor in 20 hours.

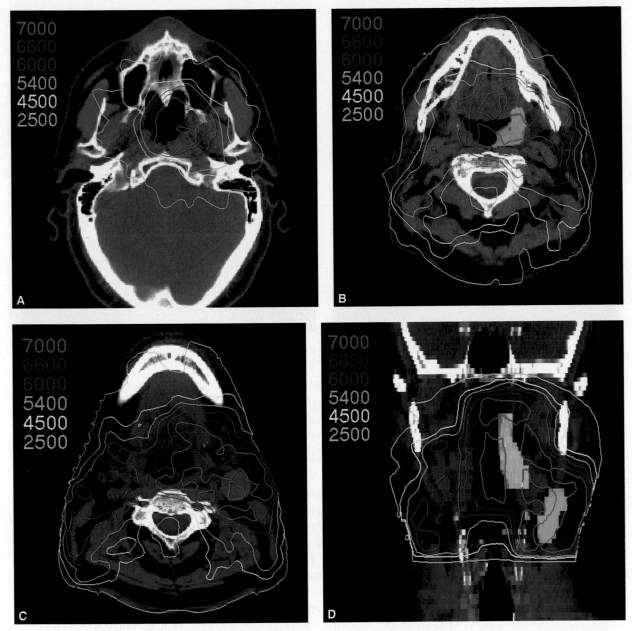

Figure 9.8 A 60-year-old man presented with an asymptomatic left neck mass. A fine needle aspiration showed metastatic squamous cell carcinoma. Physical examination revealed a 3-cm exophytic left tonsillar mass and a 3-cm mobile left level II node. He received treatment with intensity-modulated radiation therapy (IMRT) to a dose of 66 Gy in 30 fractions. The gross target volumes (primary tonsillar tumor and solitary lymph node) were contoured and shown in the figures. Three representative axial distributions are shown at the levels of the pterygoids **(A)**, midtonsil **(B)**, and inferior oropharyngeal wall and midlevel II **(C)** regions. A coronal isodose distribution through the gross tonsil tumor and lymph node is also shown **(D)**. The IMRT fields were matched above the arytenoids to an anterior supraclavicular field, which delivered 50 Gy in 25 fractions. Left level III received additional irradiation to a total of 58 Gy. A selective neck dissection performed after radiotherapy revealed no residual disease. He had no evidence of disease at the last follow-up over 2 years after treatment. He has been able to eat all types of foods including bread.

Dose

For T1 and superficial T2, N0: conventional fractionation delivering 50 Gy in 25 fractions to the initial target volume followed by 16 Gy in eight fractions to the boost volume.

For large T2 and T3, N0 to N1: concomitant boost schedule to total doses of 69 to 72 Gy in 40 to 42 fractions. The initial volume receives 1.8-Gy fractions to 54 Gy in 6 weeks. The boost volume receives an additional 1.5 Gy to a dose of 15 to 18 Gy given as second daily fractions during the last 2 to 2.5 weeks of the wide-field irradiations.

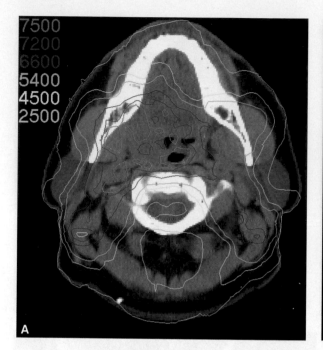 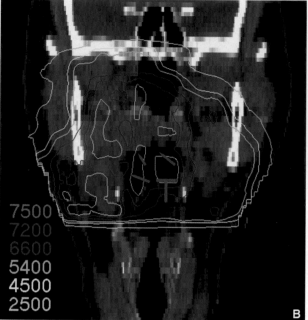

Figure 9.9 A 60-year-old man presented with right otalgia and underwent biopsy of the right tonsil showing a poorly-differentiated squamous cell carcinoma. Staging workup showed a T2 N1 tonsil carcinoma. The primary tumor involved the superior tonsil and extended onto the lateral aspect of the soft palate. He was treated with intensity-modulated radiation therapy (IMRT), using a concomitant boost fractionation regimen. The primary tumor and ipsilateral level II node with margin received 57 Gy in 30 fractions. The primary tumor and gross lymph node with 5-10 mm margins received a concomitant IMRT boost of 15 Gy in 10 fractions for a cumulative prescribed dose of 72 Gy. A representative axial isodose through the tonsillar tumor is shown **(A)**. Note that the tumor causes loss of the fat space between the fossa and pterygoid muscle. These changes can also be appreciated on the coronal isodose **(B)** with the tumor *(T)* labeled. He had a complete response, so a neck dissection was not performed. At last follow-up visit, he was free of disease, although he had grade 1 xerostomia and mild trismus.

Patients with T2 tumor, N0 to N2 (small-node) tumors recommended to receive bilateral irradiation, particularly those with extension to the soft palate, have been more frequently treated with conformal therapy to reduce the morbidity without compromising the tumor control probability. The currently evaluated dose is 66 Gy to PTV of the primary tumor and involved node(s) and 54 Gy to the subclinical disease PTV administered in 30 fractions over 6 weeks (Fig. 9.8).

For exophytic T3 and T4 or N2 to N3 tumors, radiation delivered in the conventional 2-Gy fractions to a dose of 50 Gy to the initial target volume and 70 Gy to the boost volume is given in combination with three cycles of concurrent cisplatin outside the protocol study setting. The spinal cord dose is limited to 45 Gy or less. An additional boost with interstitial brachytherapy is given if there is residual palpable disease in the tongue base (Fig. 9.7). This group of patients has been enrolled on a study randomizing patients to either conventional 2-Gy fractions to 70 Gy or concomitant boost fractionation (72 Gy in 42 fractions) with concurrent cisplatin.

New protocols are being developed to address the role of integrating biologic therapy (such as anti-epidermal growth factor receptor antibody, cetuximab; see Chapter 1) or adding induction adjuvant chemotherapy to concurrent radiation therapy–chemotherapy regimen. Some new protocols allow the use of IMRT. The recommended doses are mostly 70 Gy to the CTV1, 60 to 63 Gy to the region of intermediate risk, and approximately 56 Gy to regions of elective irradiation, all delivered in 32 to 35 fractions.

Dose Specification: See "General Principles"

Postoperative Radiotherapy

Target Volume

The initial target volume encompasses the entire surgical bed and all nodal areas of the neck.

The boost volume encompasses areas of known disease location with 1- to 2-cm margins.

Setup and Field Arrangement

Marking of external surgical scar facilitates portal design. The patient is immobilized in a supine position with a thermoplastic mask. The general technique is the same as that described under "Primary Radiotherapy." The anterior field border is mainly determined by the contiguous primary tumor spread and the extent of the surgery (scar/flap). The field borders are placed 2 cm beyond the scar when possible.

Dose

- A dose of 60 Gy in 30 fractions to areas with high-risk features, i.e., close or microscopically positive margins, perineural extension, vascular invasion, positive nodes, or extranodal extension. An additional boost dose of 6 Gy in three fractions may be given when indicated, such as when multiple adverse features are present or when the interval between surgery and radiation is much longer than 6 weeks.
- A dose of 56 Gy in 28 fractions to the surgical bed.
- A dose of 50 Gy in 25 fractions to undissected regions to receive elective irradiation.

Timing of Postoperative Radiotherapy

It is desirable to commence postoperative radiotherapy as soon as possible after healing of the surgical wounds. With good communication between surgical, radiation, and dental oncologists, generally simulation can take place 3 to 4 weeks after surgery, and radiotherapy can start a few days later in most patients. When delayed wound healing postpones commencement of postoperative radiation to beyond 5 to 6 weeks, we prescribe accelerated fractionation, such as concomitant boost, by delivering twice-a-day irradiations for 1 week, usually at the end of the radiation course, to reduce the potential hazard of prolonged cumulative treatment time.

Dose Specification: See "General Principles"

Background Data

TABLE 9.5

LOCAL CONTROL ANALYSIS IN 150 PATIENTS WITH TONSIL CARCINOMA TREATED AT THE M.D. ANDERSON CANCER CENTER

Tumor Stage	All Patients Local Control After XRT (%)	Evaluable Patients[a] Local Control After XRT (%)	Salvage Surgery	Local Control After Surgery	Ultimate Local Control (%)
T1	16/17 (94%)	15/16 (94%)	1	1/1	16/16 (100%)
T2	48/59 (81%)	41/52 (79%)	6	3/6	44/52 (85%)
T3	44/66 (67%)	30/52 (58%)	10	1/10	31/52 (60%)
T4	5/8 (63%)	3/6 (50%)	1	0/1	3/6 (50%)
Total	113/150 (75%)	89/126 (71%)	18	5/18	94/126 (75%)

Note: July 1968 to December 1983; Analysis, December 1986.
XRT, radiation therapy.
[a]Twenty-four patients who died within 2 years from date of irradiation without local failure are excluded from analysis of local control. Length of follow-up after salvage ranges from 26 to 162 months.
From Wong CS, Ang KK, Fletcher GH, et al. Primary radiotherapy for squamous cell carcinoma of the tonsillar fossa. *Int J Radiat Oncol Biol Phys* 1989;16:657–662, with permission.

TABLE 9.6

REGIONAL CONTROL ANALYSIS ACCORDING TO N-STAGE AND NECK TREATMENT

N Stage	XRT Only	Combined XRT and Surgery	Total
N0	36/36	1/1	37/37
N1	20/20	6/6	26/26
N2A	15/16	5/5	20/21
N2B	10/11	6/7	16/18
N3A	—	0/1	0/1
N3B	1/1	1/1	2/2
Total	82/84	19/21	101/105

Note: Alive minimum 1 year with neck and primary controlled. July 1968 to December 1983; Analysis, December 1986.
XRT, radiation therapy.
From Wong CS, Ang KK, Fletcher GH, et al. Primary radiotherapy for squamous cell carcinoma of the tonsillar fossa. *Int J Radiat Oncol Biol Phys* 1989;16:657–662, with permission.

TABLE 9.7

LATE COMPLICATIONS BY DOSE AND T-STAGE IN 137 PATIENTS TREATED BY CONVENTIONAL FRACTIONATION

	Dose to Primary: T-Stage			
	<67.5 Gy		>67.5 Gy	
Type of Late Complications	T1 and T2 ($n = 39$)	T3 and T4 ($n = 12$)	T1 and T2 ($n = 31$)	T3 and T4 ($n = 55$)
Bone necrosis requiring mandibular resection	0	1	2	4
Soft tissue necrosis	0	0	0	4
Trismus	0	0	3	2
Cranial nerve palsy	0	0	0	1
Total no. of complications	0	1	5	11
Total no. of patients with complications	0	1	5	8
5-yr actuarial incidence of patients developing complications	0	14%	13%	29%

From Wong CS, Ang KK, Fletcher GH, et al. Primary radiotherapy for squamous cell carcinoma of the tonsillar fossa. *Int J Radiat Oncol Biol Phys* 1989;16:657–662, with permission.

TABLE 9.8

COMPARISON OF ALTERED FRACTIONATION SCHEDULES FOR TREATMENT OF CARCINOMA OF THE TONSIL (LITERATURE REVIEW): 5-YR ACTUARIAL LOCAL CONTROL

Institution	Fractionation	T1 No. of Patients (% Control)	T2 No. of Patients (% Control)	T3 No. of Patients (% Control)	T4 No. of Patients (% Control)
MDACC	Concomitant boost	5 (100%)	29 (96%)	41 (78%)	4 (50%)
U of FL[a]	Twice-a-day (1.2 Gy)	5 (100%)	37 (78%)	35 (74%)	14 (57%)
MGH	Split course bid (1.6 Gy)		53[b] (91%)	49 (80%)	ND

[a]Control calculated by direct method.
[b]T1 and T2 combined.
MDACC, M.D. Anderson Cancer Center (Gwozdz[aq 09] et al., 1997); U of FL, University of Florida (Fein et al., 1996); MGH, Massachussetts General Hospital (Wang et al., 1995); ND, not described.

TABLE 9.9

OUTCOMES OF 1042 PATIENTS WITH SQUAMOUS CARCINOMA OF THE OROPHARYNX IRRADIATED AT THE M.D. ANDERSON CANCER CENTER 1975–1998 (ANALYSIS, 2005)

Primary Site	No. of Patients	5-yr Local Control	5-yr Overall Survival[a]
Soft palate	138	70%	44%
Tonsillar fossa	324	76%	56%
Base of tongue	383	77%	49%
Pharyngeal wall	168	68%	39%
T stage[b]			
T1	123	98%	69%
T2	324	84%	63%
T3	383	69%	41%
T4	168	45%	23%
Tx[c]	44	95%	80%
Total	1042	75%	50%

[a]95% of surviving patients alive >5 yr.
[b]Fifth edition AJCC staging manual.
[c]Most common presentation—tonsillectomy done prior to evaluation.
Unpublished data, from the M.D. Anderson Cancer Center.

TABLE 9.10

PRIMARY CONTROL OF 200 PATIENTS WITH OROPHARYNGEAL CARCINOMA IRRADIATED WITH THE CONCOMITANT BOOST TECHNIQUE AT THE M.D. ANDERSON CANCER CENTER BETWEEN 1984 AND 1994 (ANALYSIS, 1999)

T Stage	No. of Patients	5-yr Actuarial 5-yr Control
T1	13	92%
T2	84	94%
T3	91	73%
T4	8	50%

Unpublished data, from the M.D. Anderson Cancer Center.

TABLE 9.11

FIRST SITE OF FAILURE DISTRIBUTION FOR STAGE I AND II OROPHARYNX CANCER TREATED WITH RADIATION AT THE M.D. ANDERSON CANCER CENTER (1970–1998)

		None	L	R	LR	DM	L and DM	R and DM	Total
T stage	T1 and Tx	45	3	1	1	1	0	0	51
	T2	87	21	5	1	8	1	1	124
Total		132	24	6	2	9	1	1	175

L, local recurrence; R, regional recurrence; LR, loco-regional recurrence; DM, distant metastases; L and DM, synchronous local recurrence and distant metastases; R and DM, synchronous regional recurrence and distant metastases. Modified from Selek U, Garden AS, Morrison WH, et al. Radiation therapy for early-stage carcinoma of the oropharynx. *Int J Radiat Oncol Biol Phys* 2004;59:743–775, with permission.

TABLE 9.12

FIRST SITE OF FAILURE DISTRIBUTION FOR STAGE I AND II OROPHARYNX CANCER TREATED WITH IMRT AT THE M.D. ANDERSON CANCER CENTER 2000–2002 (ANALYSIS, 2004)

		First Site of Failure							
		None	L	R	LR	DM	L and DM	R and DM	Total
T stage	T1 and Tx	31	0	2	0	2	0	0	35
	T2	15	2	0	1	1	0	0	19
Total		46	2	2	1	3	0	0	54

L, local recurrence; R, regional recurrence; LR, loco-regional recurrence; DM, distant metastases; L and DM, synchronous local recurrence and distant metastases; R and DM, synchronous regional recurrence and distant metastases. Unpublished data, from the M.D. Anderson Cancer Center.

BASE OF TONGUE

Treatment Strategy

Primary radiotherapy is preferred for T1, T2, and exophytic T3, N0 to N1 carcinomas. Neck dissection is indicated in a very small number of patients with N1 disease who have residual neck mass 6 weeks after completion of radiotherapy.

Combination of radiation with chemotherapy is the treatment of choice for infiltrative T3 and selected T4 or N2 to N3 tumors. Outside the protocol study setting, the combination of conventional radiation fractionation (70 Gy in 35 fractions over 7 weeks) with cisplatin (100 mg per m^2 given on days, 1, 22, and 43 of radiotherapy) is recommended because the benefit of this regimen has been demonstrated in several phase III trials. Neck dissection is indicated in patients who have residual neck mass 6 weeks after completion of therapy.

T4 tumors with bone invasion or extensive normal tissue destruction resulting in deformation and/or impaired functions are best treated with surgery and postoperative radiotherapy.

Primary Radiotherapy

Target Volume

The initial target volume encompasses the base of tongue with a generous margin toward oral tongue, epiglottis, superior pre-epiglottic space, lateral oropharyngeal walls, and bilateral neck nodes, including the retropharyngeal nodes, and levels II, III, and IV nodes. The target volume also includes ipsilateral level IB in the presence of level II node. The margins are more generous in infiltrative lesions.

The boost volume encompasses the primary tumor and involved nodes with 1- to 2-cm margins.

Setup and Field Arrangement

Insertion of metal seeds at the borders of the tumor, when accessible, and marking of oral commissures and palpable nodes facilitate portal shaping (see Figs. 9.10 to 9.12).

An intraoral stent is used to open the mouth and depress the tongue. The patient is immobilized in a supine position with a thermoplastic mask. Lateral parallel–opposed photon fields are used for treatment of the primary tumor and upper neck nodes.

- *Anterior border:* at least 2 cm anterior to the palpable tumor border.
- *Superior border:* to include the retropharyngeal and level II (upper jugular) nodes.
- *Posterior border:* just behind the spinous processes or more posteriorly in the presence of a large nodal mass.
- *Inferior border:* just above the arytenoids or lower in the presence of vallecula or pre-epiglottic space involvement.

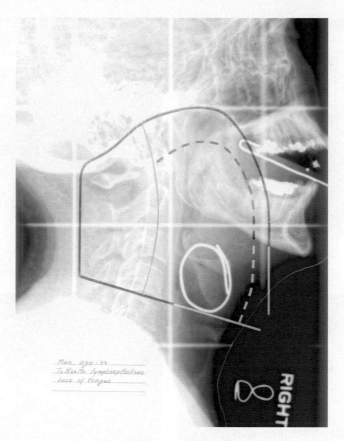

Figure 9.10 A 44-year-old man presented with an asymptomatic right neck mass. Physical examination showed a 5 × 3-cm exophytic tumor of the right base of tongue. The tumor extended anteriorly to the circumvallate papillae and laterally to the glossopharyngeal sulcus and inferiorly the right vallecula. The tumor did not cross the midline. There was a 4 × 3-cm mobile, firm right subdigastric node. Biopsy revealed a poorly differentiated squamous cell carcinoma with features of lymphoepithelioma Stage: T3 N2 AM0. The patient received primary radiotherapy according to the concomitant boost regimen. The primary tumor and upper neck nodes were treated with lateral parallel–opposed photon fields. The seed marked the anterior and superior margin of the tumor. To spare the larynx, the inferior border of the field was placed just at the lower edge of the neck node. The mid and lower neck was treated with an anterior appositional photon field matched to the lateral fields on the skin. Boost to the areas of gross disease was delivered with opposed–lateral fields. An L-shaped electron field was matched to the inferior and posterior borders of the boost field to secure adequate dose to tissues adjacent to the palpable right subdigastric node. The dose to the primary tumor (a lymphoepithelioma) was taken to 69 Gy in 40 fractions over 6 weeks (usually 72 Gy in 42 fractions over 6 weeks for keratinizing squamous cell carcinomas). Areas of subclinical disease received 54 Gy in 30 fractions over 6 weeks. Tissues adjacent to the palpable node received 63 Gy in 35 fractions over 6 weeks.

A matching anterior appositional photon field is used for elective treatment of the mid and lower neck nodes.

For the boost volume, the lateral portals are reduced to include the primary tumor with 1- to 2-cm margin and involved upper neck nodes. Nodal disease outside the primary boost field is treated with appositional electron field or anterior-posterior glancing photon fields.

Intensity-Modulated Radiation Therapy

The value of conformal radiotherapy is being addressed in selected patients requiring bilateral irradiation (see Figs. 9.13 and 9.14). With careful planning, it is possible to exclude a large portion of at least one of the parotid glands from the high-dose volume without compromising the coverage of the primary tumor and draining lymphatics.

The patient is immobilized in a supine position with an extended head and shoulder thermoplastic mask. Thin-cut CT scans are obtained in treatment position. The GTV, CTV, and PTV are outlined for dosimetric planning.

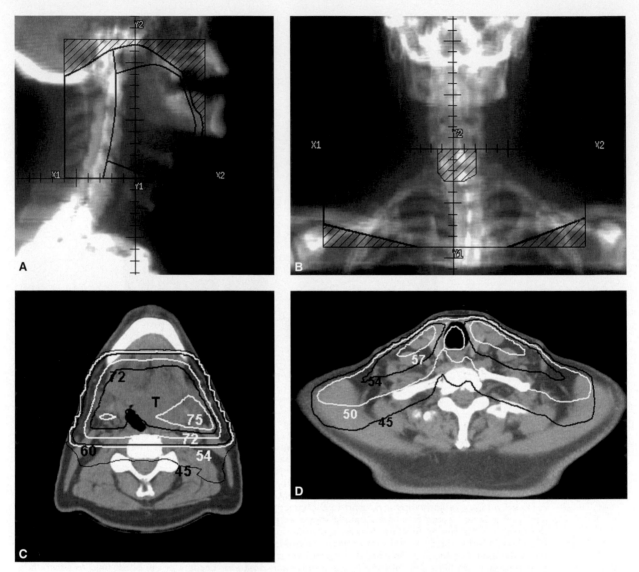

Figure 9.11 A 67-year-old man presented with mild sore throat. Physical examination revealed a 5-cm exophytic mass occupying the left base of tongue with extension to the vallecula and crossing the midline. The tongue mobility was normal and there was no adenopathy. A biopsy was positive for invasive grade-2 squamous cell carcinoma. Stage T3 N0 M0. He was treated with radiation alone using concomitant boost fractionation. Treatment started with two lateral **(A)** and an anterior **(B)** portals matched at a single isocenter localized at the top of the arytenoids. A spinal cord reduction was made at 41.4 Gy, and the boost dose was delivered through parallel–opposed fields. All portals received radiation with 6 MV photons, except that the right lateral boost portal was irradiated with 18 MV photons to minimize hot spot in the right mandible and soft tissues. Representative isodose distribution through the tongue and tumor (*T*) irradiated to 72 Gy is shown in **(C)** and that of the low-neck field to 54 Gy in **(D)**.

Dose

For T1 N0 tumors: conventional fractionation delivering 50 Gy in 25 fractions to the initial target volume. The boost dose by external beam is 16 Gy in eight fractions.

For T2 and exophytic T3, N0 to N1 tumors: concomitant boost schedule to total doses of 69 to 72 Gy in 40 to 42 fractions. The initial volume receives 1.8-Gy fractions to 54 Gy in 6 weeks. The boost volume receives an additional 1.5 Gy to a dose of 15 to 18 Gy given as second daily fractions during the last 2 to 2.5 weeks of the wide-field irradiations.

Patients with T1 to T2, N0 to N1 tumors have been enrolled into a protocol study addressing the role of conformal radiotherapy in reducing the morbidity without compromising the tumor control probability. Currently recommended dose is 66 Gy to PTV of the primary tumor and

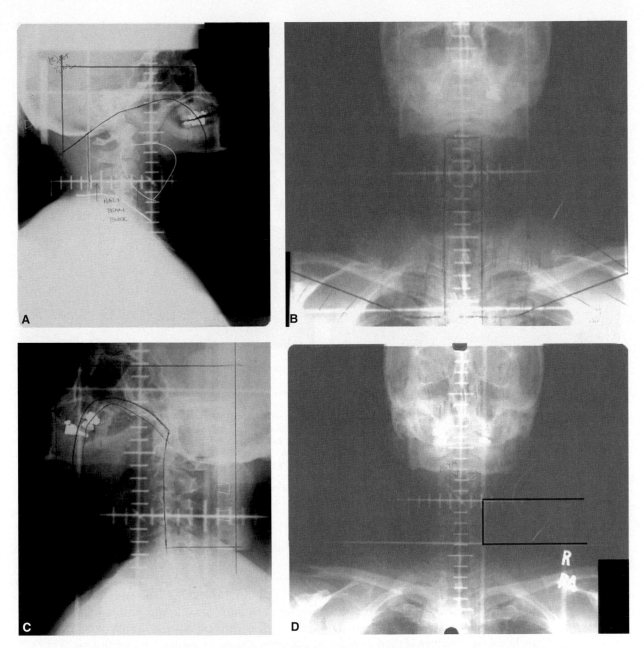

Figure 9.12 A 48-year-old man presented with sore throat and a neck mass. A base-of-tongue mass was found, biopsy of which revealed poorly differentiated squamous cell carcinoma. Physical examination showed a 3-cm exophytic mass confined to the right lateral base of tongue and not extending into the vallecula. The tongue mobility was normal. There was a 4-cm mobile upper jugular lymph node extending into the mid neck palpable. Computed tomography (CT) scan confirmed the physical findings. Stage T2 N2 aM0. He was treated with radiation alone using the concomitant boost regimen. Treatment began with lateral fields covering the primary tumor and upper neck, and an anterior field covering the mid and low neck nodes. The lateral portals **(A)** matched the anterior field **(B)** at a single isocenter just above the arytenoids. The match line transected the palpable node (wired). A larynx and spinal cord block was used in the anterior portal. Planning CT scan verification is obtained to ensure the large nodal disease did not extend medially to fall under the larynx block. Because the lymph node extended posteriorly **(see A)**, the off–spinal cord and boost portals were treated with parallel oblique fields to encompass the node in the photon fields **(C)**. The inferior portion of the lymph node received boost dose with a posterior mid neck photon field **(D)**. A single isocenter was used for these fields as well. The off–spinal cord fields were matched to the low neck supraclavicular field, and the parallel oblique boost fields covering the primary tumor and upper portion of the gross nodal disease matched the posterior boost portal to the lower part of the node. The gross disease received 72 Gy and the low neck 54 Gy. A full midline block was placed after 45 Gy to limit the spinal cord dose. This was verified with planning CT dosimetry. The patient had a complete response in the primary and neck node and, therefore, neck dissection was not performed. The patient remained free of disease 3 years from diagnosis.

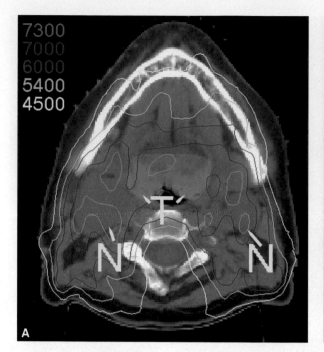
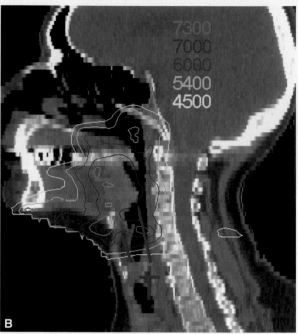

Figure 9.13   A 58-year-old woman presented with an asymptomatic right neck mass. Examination revealed an exophytic mass, over 4 cm, in the middle of base of tongue, involving both sides and extending to the valleculae. Biopsy was positive for squamous cell carcinoma. Neck examination revealed bilateral adenopathy, a 5-cm level II–III right neck mass and a 3-cm left level II node. Stage T3 N2 cM0. She was treated with concurrent cisplatin and conventional radiation (70 Gy in 35 fractions). Intensity-modulated radiation therapy (IMRT) was chosen because it was anticipated to provide a better distribution to the bilateral adenopathy that was located deep in the neck. A representative axial isodose distribution through the base of tongue tumor (T) and bilateral nodes (N) is shown **(A)** along with a sagittal isodose **(B)** through the miplane including the primary (T). The patient had residual bilateral masses 6 weeks after treatment. She underwent bilateral neck dissections and examination under anesthesia. No residual primary tumor was detected. All 29 nodes had fibrosis and treatment effects but contained no detectable viable tumor cells. She remained without disease nearly 4 years from post-treatment.

involved node(s) and 54 Gy to the subclinical disease PTV administered in 30 fractions over 6 weeks (Fig. 9.8).

For exophytic T3 and T4 or N2 to N3 tumors, radiation delivered in the conventional 2-Gy fractions to a dose of 50 Gy to the initial target volume and 70 Gy to the boost volume is given in combination with three cycles of concurrent cisplatin outside the protocol study setting. The spinal cord dose is limited to 45 Gy or less. An additional boost with interstitial brachytherapy is given if there is residual palpable disease at the base of the tongue (Fig. 9.7). This group of patients has been enrolled in a study randomizing patients to either conventional 2-Gy fractions to 70 Gy or concomitant boost fractionation (72 Gy in 42 fractions) with concurrent cisplatin.

New protocols are being developed to address the role of integrating biologic therapy (such as antiepidermal growth factor receptor antibody, cetuximab; see Chapter 1) or adding induction adjuvant chemotherapy to the concurrent radiation–chemotherapy regimen. Some new protocols allow the use of IMRT. The recommended doses are mostly 70 Gy to the CTV1 and approximately 56 Gy to regions of elective irradiation delivered in 32 to 35 fractions.

Dose Specification: See "General Principles"

Postoperative Radiotherapy

Target Volume

The initial target volume encompasses the surgical bed and the entire neck. In patients who have had laryngectomy, the initial target volume includes the tracheal stoma if there is tumor extension

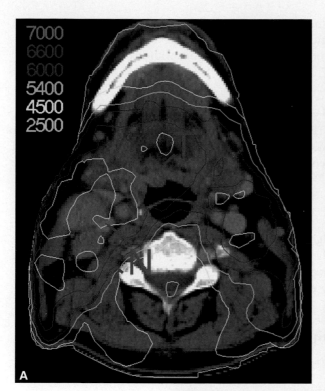

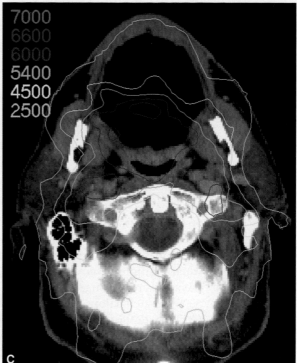

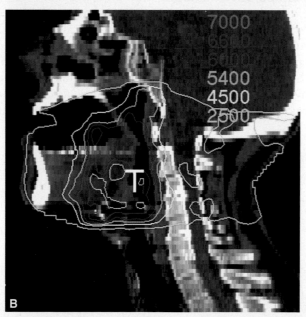

Figure 9.14   A 57-year-old man presented with asymptomatic right neck adenopathy. A right inferior base of tongue tumor was detected. Clinical stage was T1 N2b. He was treated with intensity-modulated radiation therapy (IMRT). A total dose of 66 Gy was delivered in 30 fractions to the primary and gross nodes with margin (CTV1). An axial isodose distribution is shown **(A)** at the level of the primary tumor (T) and nodes (N) in the right neck. A sagittal dose distribution is shown **(B)** with the primary tumor seen just above the vallecula. Note the patient was positioned with a mouth opening stent. An axial isodose distribution through the level of the retropharyngeal nodes is also shown **(C)**. These nodes and the contralateral (left neck) nodes were defined as a clinical target to receive 54 Gy. The patient had a complete response in the primary and dubious node remaining in the right neck. A follow-up ultrasound was performed and demonstrated the node with central fatty replacement. A fine needle aspiration was negative. It was elected not to perform a neck dissection. He was without evidence of disease 2 years later. He had grade I xerostomia and chemical hypothyroidism treated with low dose Synthroid.

into the soft tissues of the neck (including nodes with extracapsular extension), or the patient underwent an emergency tracheostomy prior to resection.

The boost volume encompasses areas of known disease locations with 1- to 2-cm margins.

Setup and Field Arrangement

The patient is immobilized in a supine position. Marking of external surgical scar and stoma, when present, facilitates portal design. The technique used is the same as that described under "Primary Radiotherapy." The *anterior* and *superior field borders* are mainly determined by the local spread of the primary tumor and the extent of surgery. The field borders are placed 2 cm from the mucosal scar.

Dose

- 60 Gy in 30 fractions to areas with high-risk features, that is, close or microscopically positive margins, perineural extension, vascular invasion, positive nodes, or extranodal extension. An additional boost dose of 6 Gy in three fractions may be given when indicated, for example, when multiple adverse features are present or when the interval between surgery and radiotherapy is much longer than 6 weeks.
- 56 Gy in 28 fractions to the surgical bed.
- 50 Gy in 25 fractions to undissected regions to receive elective irradiation.

Timing of Postoperative Radiotherapy

It is desirable to commence postoperative radiotherapy as soon as possible after healing of surgical wounds. With good communication between surgical, radiation, and dental oncologists, generally simulation can take place 3 to 4 weeks after surgery and radiotherapy can start a few days later in most patients. When delayed wound healing postpones commencement of postoperative radiation to beyond 5 to 6 weeks, we prescribe accelerated fractionation, such as concomitant boost, by delivering twice-a-day irradiations for 1 week, usually at the end of the radiation course, to reduce the potential hazard of prolonged cumulative treatment time.

Dose Specification: See "General Principles"

Background Data

TABLE 9.13
CONTROL OF BASE OF TONGUE CARCINOMA CORRELATED WITH T STAGE

Stage	No. of Patients	NED at Primary (Survival >2 yr)	Failure at Primary	Died <2 yr, Other Causes (N, DM, ID)
T1	32	23	9% (3)	6
T2	49	23	29% (14)	12
T3	64	33	22% (14)	17
T4	29	6	48% (14)	9

NED, no evidence of disease; N, neck recurrence; DM, distant metastases; ID, intercurrent disease.
From Spanos WJ Jr, Shukovsky LJ, Fletcher GH. Time dose and tumor volume relationships in irradiation of squamous cell carcinomas of the base of the tongue. *Cancer* 1976;37:2591–2599, with permission.

TABLE 9.14

LOCAL CONTROL ("LOCAL NON-FAILURE") AND COMPLICATIONS FOLLOWING CURATIVE IRRADIATION FOR BASE OF TONGUE CARCINOMA: LITERATURE REVIEW

Author, Year, Institution	Boost Technique	Local Control[a] by T Stage				Incidence of Soft Tissue ± Bone Necrosis[b]
		T1	T2	T3	T4	
Housset et al, 1987 Hopital Necker, Paris, France	Implant	6/6	17/23 (74%)	—	—	3/29 (10%)
Puthawala et al, 1988 Memorial Med. Center, Long Beach, Calif.	Implant	2/2	14/16 (88%)	30/40 (75%)	8/12 (67%)	10/70 (14%)
Crook et al, 1988 Hopital Henri Mondor, Creteil, France	Implant	11/13 (85%)	25/35 (71%)	—	—	12/48 (25%)
Lusinchi et al, 1988 Inst. Gustave Roussy, Paris, France	Implant	15/18 (83%)	20/39 (51%)	35/51 (69%)	—	29/108 (27%)
Sessions et al, 1988 Memorial-Sloan Kettering, New York	Implant	4/4	5/6	5/6	1/1	6/17 (35%)
Goffinet et al, 1988 Stanford Univ., Stanford, Calif.	Implant	4/5	7/7	9/10	5/7	8/29 (28%)[c]
Spanos et al, 1976 M. D. Anderson, Houston, Texas	External beam	29/32 (91%)	35/49 (71%)	50/64 (78%)	15/29 (52%)	15/91 (16%)[d]
Jaulerry et al, 1991	External beam	21/22 (95%)	25/45 (56%)	26/64 (41%)	4/31 (13%)	ND
Mendenhall et al, 2000 Univ. of Florida, Gainesville, Florida	External beam	29[e] (96%)	76 (91%)	70 (81%)	42 (38%)	8/217 (4%)[f]

ND, not described.
[a]No. continuously free of disease at the primary site/total no. treated.
[b]All degrees of severity.
[c]Three patients with development of hemorrhage are included.
[d]Bone only.
[e]Total patients and 5-year actuarial control.
[f]Severe late complications.
Modified from Foote RL, Parsons JT, Mendenhall WM, et al. Is interstitial implantation essential for successful radiotherapeutic treatment of base of tongue carcinoma? *Int J Radiat Oncol Biol Phys* 1990;18:1293 and Mendenhall WM, Amdur RJ, Stringer SP, et al. Radiation therapy for squamous cell carcinoma of the base of tongue: a preferred alternative to surgery? *J Clin Oncol* 2000;18:35 with permission.

TABLE 9.15

COMPARISON OF ALTERED FRACTIONATION SCHEDULES FOR TREATMENT OF BASE OF TONGUE CARCINOMA (LITERATURE REVIEW): 5-YEAR ACTUARIAL LOCAL CONTROL

Institution	Fractionation	T1 No. of Patients (% Control)	T2 No. of Patient (% Control)	T3 No. of Patient (% Control)	T4 No. of Patient (% Control)
MDACC	Concomitant boost	4 (100%)	27 (96%)	22 (67%)	1 (NE)
U of FL[a]	Twice-a-day (1.2 Gy)	4 (100%)	17 (94%)	23 (78%)	14 (43%)
MGH	Split course bid (1.6 Gy)		47[b] (85%)	43 (54%)	ND

[a]Control calculated by direct method.
[b]T1 and T2 combined.
MDACC, M.D. Anderson Cancer Center (Mak et al, 1997); U of FL, University of Florida (Fein et al, 1996); MGH, Massachussetts General Hospital (Wang et al, 1995); ND, not described; NE, not evaluated.

POSTERIOR OROPHARYNGEAL WALL

Treatment Strategy

Primary radiotherapy is preferred for T1, T2, and exophytic T3, N0 to N1 carcinomas. Neck dissection is indicated in a very small number of patients with N1 disease who have residual neck mass 6 weeks after completion of radiotherapy.

Combination of radiation with chemotherapy is the treatment of choice for T3 and T4 or N2 to N3 tumors. Outside the protocol study setting, the combination of conventional radiation fractionation (70 Gy in 35 fractions over 7 weeks) with cisplatin (100 mg per m^2 given on days 1, 22, and 43 of radiotherapy) is recommended because the benefit of this regimen has been demonstrated in several phase III trials. Neck dissection is indicated in patients who have residual neck mass 6 weeks after completion of therapy.

Occasionally, advanced tumors are treated with surgery and postoperative radiotherapy.

Primary Radiotherapy

Target Volume

The initial target volume encompasses the primary tumor with at least 2- to 3-cm margins (submucosal spread can be extensive) and retropharyngeal and level II–IV nodes. The target volume also includes ipsilateral level IB in the presence of level II node.

The boost volume encompasses the primary tumor and involved nodes with 1- to 2-cm margins.

Setup and Field Arrangement

Marking of palpable nodes and shoulders facilitates portal design (see posterior hypopharyngeal wall). The patient is immobilized in a supine position with a thermoplastic mask. Lateral parallel–opposed photon fields are used for treatment of the primary tumor and upper neck nodes (see Fig. 9.15).

- *Anterior border:* at least 2 cm anterior to the known extent of the tumor, but when feasible, short of fall-off anteriorly.
- *Superior border:* at the base of skull to cover parapharyngeal lymphatics and level II nodes.
- *Posterior border:* just behind the spinous processes or more posteriorly in the presence of large nodal masses. After off cord reduction, the posterior portal margin is at the posterior one third of vertebral bodies to include the retropharyngeal nodes and provide the margin for the posterior pharyngeal wall.
- *Inferior border:* because the caudal extent of these tumors is often poorly defined, and submucosal extension beyond gross disease is frequent, a generous inferior margin (3 cm or more) is used to include the whole pharynx in the initial target volume.

An anterior appositional portal is used for treating lower neck nodes.

For the boost volume, the lateral fields are reduced to include the primary tumor with 1.5- to 2-cm margins; involved lymph nodes are either encompassed by lateral fields or, when overlying the spinal cord or low in the neck, by an appositional electron field or glancing photon portals.

Intensity-Modulated Radiation Therapy

Conformal radiotherapy is best suited for treating tumors extending to the paravertebral region without overdosing the spinal cord because this technique can produce a horseshoe shape isodose distribution. The patient is immobilized in a supine position with an extended head and shoulder thermoplastic mask. Thin-cut CT scans are obtained in treatment position. The GTV, CTV, and PTV are outlined for dosimetric planning. The high dose CTV encompasses the GTV with 1- to 1.5-cm cranial and caudal margins. An additional 1 cm is used to define the subclinical CTV of the primary tumor. The role of image-guided therapy, and positron emission tomography (PET) scanning to identify tumor borders is under investigation. These investigations will be beneficial to define borders especially in posterior pharyngeal tumors where there is difficulty in border definition.

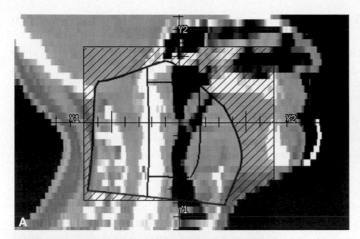

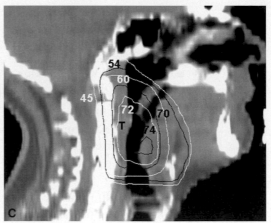

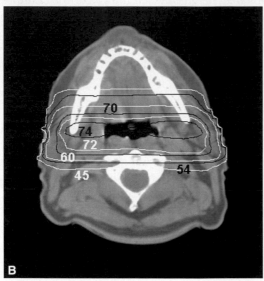

Figure 9.15 A 55-year-old man presented with a globus sensation on swallowing. A tumor was detected on the posterior oropharyngeal wall and biopsy was positive for squamous cell carcinoma. The tumor was approximately 5 mm in thickness and extended from the level of the soft palate superiorly to the level of mid tongue base inferiorly. There was no clinical adenopathy. Stage T2 N0 M0. He was treated with primary radiotherapy with concomitant boost regimen to a total dose of 72 Gy in 42 fractions. The lateral portals are shown on a sagittal digital reconstruction **(A)**. Initial fields received 41.4 Gy in 23 fractions with 6 MV photons. A supraclavicular field with a larynx block was matched on skin. This anterior field received 50 Gy in 25 fractions prescribed at D_{max}. The lateral fields were reduced off the spinal cord and continued to 54 Gy. The posterior cervical strips excluded from the off–spinal cord photon fields were supplemented with 9 MeV electrons, 12.6 Gy at D_{max} in seven fractions. The boost was delivered as second daily fractions, 18 Gy in 12 fractions, with 18 MV photons. An axial and sagittal isodose distribution through the middle of the tumor (T) is shown **(B, C)**.

Dose

The dose is the same as that for tonsillar fossa primary lesion.

Dose Specification: See "General Principles"

Postoperative Radiotherapy

Target Volume

The initial target volume encompasses the entire surgical bed and retropharyngeal and level II–IV nodes. The target volume also includes ipsilateral level IB in the presence of level II node. When a laryngectomy is performed, indications for treatment of the tracheal stoma are as outlined for a base of tongue tumor.

The boost volume encompasses areas of known disease locations with 1- to 2-cm margins.

Setup and Field Arrangement

The patient is immobilized in a supine position. Marking of the external surgical scar, tracheal stoma (when present), and shoulders facilitate portal design. Lateral parallel–opposed photon fields are used for treatment of the primary tumor bed and upper neck node areas.

■ *Anterior border:* depends on the extent of local spread of the primary tumor and surgery. If possible, the field border is placed at least 2 cm beyond the scar. It is generally not possible to spare a strip of anterior neck skin due to the location of the external surgical scar.

- *Superior border:* at the base of skull to cover the parapharyngeal lymphatics and upper jugular nodes.
- *Posterior border:* just behind the spinous processes or more posteriorly, depending on the extent of resection.
- *Inferior border:* depends on the extent of local spread of the primary tumor and surgery; usually just above the stoma or shoulders (if laryngectomy was not performed).

An anterior portal is used to treat the lower neck nodes and, when indicated, tracheal stoma.

For the boost volume, lateral portals are reduced to encompass the areas of known tumor locations. Electrons are used to boost the nodal areas overlying the spinal cord.

Dose

- 60 Gy in 30 fractions to areas with high-risk features, i.e., close or microscopically positive margins, perineural extension, vascular invasion, positive nodes, or extranodal extension. An additional boost dose of 6 Gy in three fractions may be given when indicated, for example, when multiple adverse features are present or when the interval between surgery and radiation is much longer than 6 weeks.
- 56 Gy in 28 fractions to the surgical bed.
- 50 Gy in 25 fractions to undissected regions to receive elective irradiation.

Timing of Postoperative Radiotherapy

It is desirable to commence postoperative radiotherapy as soon as possible after healing of surgical wounds. With good communication between surgical, radiation, and dental oncologists, generally simulation can take place 3 to 4 weeks after surgery and radiotherapy can start a few days later in most patients. When delayed wound healing postpones commencement of postoperative radiation to beyond 5 to 6 weeks, we prescribe accelerated fractionation, such as concomitant boost, by delivering twice-a-day irradiations for 1 week, usually at the end of the radiation course, to reduce the potential hazard of prolonged cumulative treatment time.

Dose Specification: See "General Principles"

Background Data

TABLE 9.16

SQUAMOUS CELL CARCINOMAS OF THE PHARYNGEAL WALLS TREATED WITH IRRADIATION ALONE: FAILURE RATES FOR TREATMENT OF PRIMARY TUMOR IN PATIENTS TREATED AT THE M.D. ANDERSON CANCER CENTER BETWEEN 1954 AND 1974 (ANALYSIS IN OCTOBER 1976)

Stage	Primary Tumor Control	No. Salvaged by Surgery	Ultimate Primary Control	No. Complications[a]
T1	10/11 (91%)	1	11/11 (100%)	0 (0%)
T2	33/45 (73%)	2	35/45 (78%)	3 (7%)
T3	38/62 (61%)	6	44/62 (71%)	9 (15%)
T4	17/46 (37%)	2	19/46 (41%)	8 (17%)

[a]Pharyngeal wall necrosis: 3; carotid rupture: 8 (5 associated with salvage surgery); osteonecrosis: 3; radiation myelitis: 2; severe larynx edema: 2; and severe neck fibrosis: 2.
Modified from Meoz-Mendez RT, Fletcher GH, Guillamondegui OM, et al. Analysis of the results of irradiation in the treatment of squamous cell carcinomas of the pharyngeal walls. *Int J Radiat Oncol Biol Phys* 1978;4:579–585, with permission.

TABLE 9.17

SQUAMOUS CELL CARCINOMAS OF THE PHARYNGEAL WALLS TREATED WITH IRRADIATION ALONE: RESULTS OF TREATMENT OF NECK DISEASE IN PATIENTS WITH PRIMARY CONTROL (JANUARY 1954–DECEMBER 1974; ANALYSIS OCTOBER 1976) (1 YEAR MINIMUM TO UNLIMITED FOLLOW-UP)

| Stage | No. of Patients | No. Control | No. of Patients Salvaged | | Ultimate Control |
			Neck Dissection	Irradiation	
N0	40	35 (88%)	3	1	39/40 (98%)
N1	15	12 (80%)	3	0	15/15 (100%)
N2A–N3B	27	18 (67%)	3	0	21/27 (78%)

Modified from Meoz-Mendez RT, Fletcher GH, Guillamondegui OM, et al. Analysis of the results of irradiation in the treatment of squamous cell carcinomas of the pharyngeal walls. *Int J Radiat Oncol Biol Phys* 1978;4:579–585, with permission.

TABLE 9.18

SQUAMOUS CELL CARCINOMA OF THE PHARYNGEAL WALLS TREATED WITH COMBINATION OF SURGERY AND PREOPERATIVE OR POSTOPERATIVE IRRADIATION: PRIMARY CONTROL BY STAGE

Stage	No. of Patients	Primary Control	Alive and NED at 1 yr	Died of Intercurrent Diseases <1 yr
T2	5	5/5 (100%)	4	1
T3 + T4	20	15/20 (75%)	10	5

NED, no evidence of disease.
Modified from Meoz-Mendez RT, Fletcher GH, Guillamondegui OM, et al. Analysis of the results of irradiation in the treatment of squamous cell carcinomas of the pharyngeal walls. *Int J Radiat Oncol Biol Phys* 1978;4:579–585, with permission.

TABLE 9.19

SQUAMOUS CELL CARCINOMA OF THE OROPHARYNGEAL WALL TREATED WITH RADICAL IRRADIATION: LOCAL CONTROL (NO. CONTROLLED/NO. TREATED)

T Stage[a]	T1	T2	T3	T4
Patient number	3	9	11	1
2-yr actuarial control	100%	89%	82%	100%

[a]Oropharyngeal T stage using the AJCC system (1983).
Modified from Fein DA, Lee WR, Amos WR, et al.Oropharyngeal carcinoma treated with radiotherapy: a 30-year experience. *Int J Radiat Oncol Biol Phys* 1996;34:289–296, with permission.

SUGGESTED READINGS

Amdur RJ, Mendenhall WM, Parsons JT, et al. Carcinoma of the soft palate treated with irradiation: analysis of results and complications. *Radiother Oncol* 1987;9:185.

Ang KK, Peters LJ, Weber RS, et al. Concomitant boost radiotherapy schedules in the treatment of carcinoma of the oropharynx and nasopharynx. *Int J Radiat Oncol Biol Phys* 1990;19:1339.

Bataini JP, Asselain B, Jaulerry C, et al. A multivariate primary tumour control analysis in 465 patients treated by radical radiotherapy for cancer of the tonsillar region: clinical and treatment parameters as prognostic factors. *Radiother Oncol* 1989;14:265.

Calais G, Alfonsi M, Bardet E, et al. Randomized trial of radiation therapy versus concomitant chemotherapy and radiation therapy for advanced-stage oropharynx carcinoma. *J Natl Cancer Inst* 1999;91:2081.

Chao KS, Ozyigit G, Blanco AI, et al. Intensity-modulated radiation therapy for oropharyngeal carcinoma: impact of tumor volume. *Int J Radiat Oncol Biol Phys* 2004;59:43.

Cooper RA, Slevin NJ, Carrington BM, et al. Radiotherapy for carcinoma of the posterior pharyngeal wall. *Int J Radiat Oncol Biol Phys* 2000;16:611.

Denis F, Garaud P, Bardet E, et al. Final results of the 94-01 French Head and Neck Oncology and Radiotherapy Group randomized trial comparing radiotherapy alone with concomitant radiochemotherapy in advanced-stage oropharynx carcinoma. *J Clin Oncol* 2004;22:69.

Fein DA, Lee WR, Amos WR, et al. Oropharyngeal carcinoma treated with radiotherapy: a 30-year experience. *Int J Radiat Oncol Biol Phys* 1996;34:289.

Fein DA, Mendenhall WM, Parsons JT, et al. Pharyngeal wall carcinoma treated with radiotherapy: impact of treatment technique and fractionation. *Int J Radiat Oncol Biol Phys* 1993;26:751.

Fletcher GH. Oral cavity and oropharynx. In: Fletcher GH, ed. *Textbook of radiotherapy*, 3rd ed. Philadelphia, PA: Lea & Febiger, 1980.

Foote RL, Parsons JT, Mendenhall WM, et al. Is interstitial implantation essential for successful radiotherapeutic treatment of base of tongue carcinoma? *Int J Radiat Oncol Biol Phys* 1990;18:1293.

Garden AS, Asper JA, Morrison WH, et al. Is concurrent chemoradiation the treatment of choice for all patients with Stage III or IV head and neck carcinoma? *Cancer* 2004;100:1171.

Gelinas M, Fletcher GH. Incidence and causes of local failure of irradiation in squamous cell carcinoma of the faucial arch, tonsillar fossa and base of the tongue. *Radiology* 1973;108:383.

Gwozdz JT, Morrison WH, Garden AS, et al. Concomitant boost radiotherapy for squamous carcinoma of the tonsillar fossa. *Int J Radiat Oncol Biol Phys* 1997;39:127.

Hansen E, Panwala K, Holland J. Post-operative radiation therapy for advanced-stage oropharyngeal cancer. *J Laryngol Otol* 2002;116:920.

Hicks WL Jr, Kuriakose MA, Loree TR, et al. Surgery versus radiation therapy as single-modality treatment of tonsillar fossa carcinoma: the Roswell Park Cancer Institute experience (1971–1991). *Laryngoscope* 1998;108:1014.

Horiot JC, Le Fur R, Nguyen T, et al. Hyperfractionation versus conventional fractionation in oropharyngeal carcinoma: final analysis of a randomized trial of the EORTC cooperative group of radiotherapy. *Radiother Oncol* 1992;25:23.

Housset M, Baillet F, Dessard-Diana B, et al. A retrospective study of three treatment techniques for T1–T2 base of tongue lesions: surgery plus postoperative radiation, external radiation plus interstitial implantation and external radiation alone. *Int J Radiat Oncol Biol Phys* 1987;13:511.

Jaulerry C, Rodriguez J, Brunin F, et al. Results of radiation therapy in carcinoma of the base of the tongue: the Curie Institute experience with about 166 cases. *Cancer* 1991;67:1532.

Jesse RH, Lindberg RD. The efficacy of combining radiation therapy with a surgical procedure in patients with cervical metastasis from squamous cancer of the oropharynx and hypopharynx. *Cancer* 1975;35:1163.

Keus RB, Pontvert D, Brunin F, et al. Results of irradiation in squamous cell carcinoma of the soft palate and uvula. *Radiother Oncol* 1988;11:311.

Langlois D, Hoffstetter S, Pernot M. Selection of patients for re-irradiation with local implants in carcinomas of oropharynx and tongue. *Acta Oncol* 1988;27:571.

Lee HJ, Zelefsky MJ, Kraus DH, et al. Long-term regional control after radiation therapy and neck dissection for base of tongue carcinoma. *Int J Radiat Oncol Biol Phys* 1997;38:995.

Lusinchi A, Eskandari J, Son Y, et al. External irradiation plus curietherapy boost in 108 base of tongue carcinomas. *Int J Radiat Oncol Biol Phys* 1989;17:1191.

Lusinchi A, Wibault P, Marandas P, et al. Exclusive radiation therapy: the treatment of early tonsillar tumors. *Int J Radiat Oncol Biol Phys* 1989;17:273.

Mak AC, Morrison WH, Garden AS, et al. Base-of-tongue carcinoma: treatment results using concomitant boost radiotherapy. *Int J Radiat Oncol Biol Phys* 1995;33:289.

Mak-Kregar S, Baris G, Lebesque JV, et al. Radiotherapy of tonsillar and base of the tongue carcinoma. Prediction of local control. *Eur J Cancer B Oral Oncol* 1993;29B:119.

Mendenhall WM, Amdur RJ, Stringer SP, et al. Radiation therapy for squamous cell carcinoma of the tonsillar region: a preferred alternative to surgery? *J Clin Oncol* 2000;18:2219.

Mendenhall WM, Stringer SP, Amdur RJ, et al. Is radiation therapy a preferred alternative to surgery for squamous cell carcinoma of the base of tongue? *J Clin Oncol* 2000;18:35.

Meoz-Mendez RT, Fletcher GH, Guillamondegui OM, et al. Analysis of the results of irradiation in the treatment of squamous cell carcinomas of the pharyngeal walls. *Int J Radiat Oncol Biol Phys* 1978;4:579.

Nathu RM, Mancuso AA, Zhu TC, et al. The impact of primary tumor volume on local control for oropharyngeal squamous cell carcinoma treated with radiotherapy. *Head Neck* 2000;22:1.

Olmi P, et al. Locoregionally advanced carcinoma of the oropharynx: conventional radiotherapy vs. accelerated hyperfractionated radiotherapy vs. concomitant radiotherapy and chemotherapy—a multicenter randomized trial. *Int J Radiat Oncol Biol Phys* 2003;55:78.

O'Sullivan B, Warde P, Grice B, et al. The benefits and pitfalls of ipsilateral radiotherapy in carcinoma of the tonsillar region. *Int J Radiat Oncol Biol Phys* 2001;51:332.

Parsons JT, Mendenhall WM, Stringer SP, et al. Squamous cell carcinoma of the oropharynx: surgery, radiation therapy or both. *Cancer* 2002;94:2967.

Perez CA, Carmichael T, Devineni VR, et al. Carcinoma of the tonsillar fossa: a nonrandomized comparison of irradiation alone or combined with surgery: long-term results. *Head Neck* 1991;13:282.

Pierquin B, Wilson JF, Chassagne D, eds. *Modern brachytherapy*. New York: Masson Publishers, 1987.

Puthawala AA, Syed AM, Gates TC. Iridium-192 implants in the treatment of tonsillar region malignancies. *Arch Otolaryngol* 1985;111:812.

Remmler D, et al. Treatment of choice for squamous carcinoma of the tonsillar fossa. *Head Neck Surg* 1985;7:206.

Selek U, Garden AS, Morrison WH, et al. Radiation therapy for early-stage carcinoma of the oropharynx. *Int J Radiat Oncol Biol Phys* 2004;59:743.

Shukovsky LJ, Fletcher GH. Time-dose and tumor volume relationships in the irradiation of squamous cell carcinoma of the tonsillar fossa. *Radiology* 1973;107:621.

Spanos WJ Jr, Shukovsky LJ, Fletcher GH. Time dose and tumor volume relationships in irradiation of squamous cell carcinomas of the base of the tongue. *Cancer* 1976;37:2591.

Thomas F, Ozanne F, Mamelle G, et al. Radiotherapy alone for oropharyngeal carcinomas: the role of fraction size (2 Gy vs 2.5 Gy) on local control and early and late complications. *Int J Radiat Oncol Biol Physiol* 1988;15:1097.

Tiwari RM, et al. Advanced squamous cell carcinoma of the base of the tongue treated with surgery and post-operative radiotherapy. *Eur J Surg Oncol* 2000;26:556.

Wang CC, Montgomery W, Efird J. Local control of oropharyngeal carcinoma by irradiation alone. *Laryngoscope* 1995;105:529.

Weber RS, Gidley P, Morrison WH, et al. Treatment selection for carcinoma of the base of the tongue. *Am J Surg* 1990;160:415.

Weber RS, Peters LJ, Wolf P, et al. Squamous cell carcinoma of the soft palate, uvula, and anterior faucial pillar. *Otolaryngol Head Neck Surg* 1988;99:16,23.

Withers HR, Peters LJ, Taylor JM, et al. Late normal tissue sequelae from radiation therapy for carcinoma of the tonsil: patterns of fractionation study of radiobiology. *Int J Radiat Oncol Biol Phys* 1995a;33(3):563.

Withers HR, Peters LJ, Taylor JM, et al. Local control of carcinoma of the tonsil by radiation therapy: an analysis of patterns of fractionation in nine institutions. *Int J Radiat Oncol Biol Physiol* 1995b;33(3):549.

Wong CS, Ang KK, Fletcher GH, et al. Primary radiotherapy for squamous cell carcinoma of the tonsillar fossa. *Int J Radiat Oncol Biol Phys* 1989;16:657.

Zelefsky MJ, Harrison LB, Armstrong JG. Long-term treatment results of postoperative radiation therapy for advanced stage oropharyngeal carcinoma. *Cancer* 1992;70:2388.

Larynx

10

SUPRAGLOTTIS

Treatment Strategy

Primary radiotherapy is preferred for T1 tumors. The preferred larynx-preserving therapy for T2 to T3 tumors depends on the disease and patient characteristics. For relatively small exophytic T2 lesions, therapy consists of concomitant boost or hyperfractionated radiotherapy regimen.

For T2 lesions, bulky or infiltrating:

- *Good pulmonary function and general condition:* supraglottic laryngectomy or other type of conservative surgery with or without postoperative radiotherapy.
- *Medically unfit or technically not suitable for supraglottic laryngectomy:* concomitant boost or hyperfractionated radiotherapy regimen or concurrent chemotherapy (if medically fit for systemic treatment).

For T3 lesions, mobile vocal cord:

- *Good pulmonary function and general condition:* supraglottic laryngectomy or other type of conservative surgery with or without postoperative radiotherapy.
- *Medically unfit or technically not suitable for supraglottic laryngectomy:* concurrent radiation and chemotherapy or ongoing trial.

For T3 lesions, fixed vocal cords, therapy consists of concurrent radiation and chemotherapy or ongoing clinical trials.

The standard treatment for T4 tumors is total laryngectomy, usually with postoperative radiotherapy and, in the presence of high-risk features such as positive extracapsular nodal extension or positive margin, with concurrent cisplatin. Selected patients may be enrolled in an ongoing trial. In patients with palpable lymphadenopathy receiving primary radiotherapy, neck dissection is carried out if the nodal mass does not regress completely 6 weeks after completion of radiation.

Indications for postoperative radiotherapy are close or positive surgical margins, extension of primary lesion through cartilage into soft tissues of the neck, perineural invasion, extensive subglottic extension, multiple positive nodes, or presence of extracapsular extension (ECE). The need for emergent tracheotomy is also an indication for postoperative radiation.

Primary Radiotherapy

Target Volume

Initial target volume:

- *T1 to T3 N0:* larynx and levels II, III, and IV (subdigastric, mid, and lower jugular) nodes (see Figs. 10.1 and 10.2).
- *T1 to T3 N+:* larynx and levels IB, II, III, and IV nodes. The initial target volume includes level IB and/or level V nodes in the presence of upper neck or bulky node(s).

For boost volume: primary tumor and, when present, involved nodes with 1- to 2-cm margins.

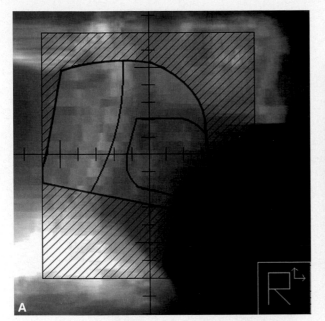

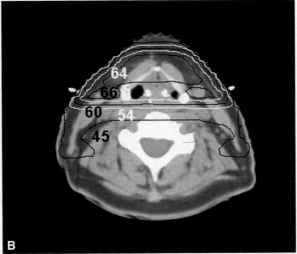

Figure 10.1 A 57-year-old woman presented with hoarseness, right otalgia, and odynophagia. A biopsy of a 1-cm tumor confined to the right false vocal cord was positive for squamous cell carcinoma. The vocal cord mobility was normal and there was no palpable adenopathy. Stage T1 N0 M0. She was treated with primary radiation. Treatment started with parallel–opposed fields covering the upper and midjugular nodes and the primary tumor using ^{60}Co γ-ray. An off–spinal cord reduction was made at 42 Gy and treatment continued to 50 Gy with 6 MV photons. A boost of 16 Gy was delivered to the primary tumor. This figure shows the three pairs of lateral–opposed portals (**A**) and an isodose distribution through the isocenter (**B**). The beams were modified by the use of 30- and 45-degree wedges.

Setup and Field Arrangement

The patient is immobilized in a supine position with a thermoplastic mask. Marking of shoulders and, when present, involved nodes, facilitates portal design. Lateral parallel–opposed photon fields are used to treat the primary tumor and upper neck nodes.

- *Superior border:* approximately 2 cm above the angle of mandible when N0 or approximately 1 cm above the tip of mastoid process when N+.
- *Anterior border:* fall-off anteriorly; when there is extension into the oropharynx, a generous part of the base of tongue is encompassed in the field. In patients with loose skin overlying the larynx, the anterior tip of skin can be spared by pulling it forward out of the field with wooden clothespins.
- *Posterior border:* behind the spinous processes or more posteriorly in the presence of large nodal mass.
- *Inferior border:* depends on the extent of disease—middle or bottom of the cricoid cartilage for tumors of the epiglottis or false cord; upper trachea when there is subglottic extension (at least 2 cm below the inferior tumor extent).
- Except in heavy patients, treatment is usually delivered with low energy photon (4 to 6 MV) beams.

A matching anterior portal is used to treat the lower neck. It may be necessary to use anterior and inferior tilts for patients with a short neck. In this case the supraclavicular fossa is included in the primary portal (see Fig. 10.8).

For boost volume, the lateral fields are reduced to 1- to 2-cm margins around the primary tumor and involved nodes. Nodes overlying the spinal cord can usually receive boost dose through oblique–lateral primary boost portals and those in the lower neck through an appositional electron portal or glancing photon fields.

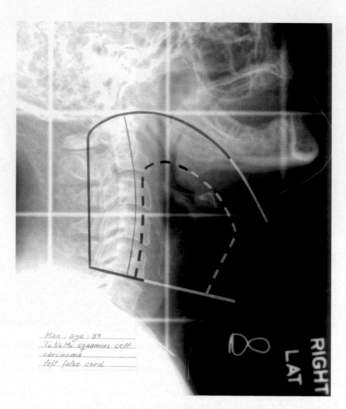

Figure 10.2   A 39-year-old man presented with intermittent hoarseness for 6 months. Mirror examination showed a tumor on the left false cord, extending upward to the left aryepiglottic fold and downward to obliterate the left ventricle. There was no evidence of glottic or pyriform sinus involvement. The mobility of both true vocal cords was normal. There was no palpable neck adenopathy. Biopsy showed moderately differentiated squamous cell carcinoma. Stage: T2 N0 M0. This patient was treated with primary radiotherapy using a hyperfractionation schedule. The primary tumor and upper and middle neck nodes were treated with lateral parallel–opposed ^{60}Co fields. Because the tumor was mainly located in the posterior part of the larynx, it was thought that the anterior skin could be excluded from the boost volume. Lower neck nodes were irradiated through an anterior appositional ^{60}Co field. The primary tumor received 76.6 Gy over 7 weeks (55.2 Gy in 46 fractions for 4.6 weeks + 21.6 Gy in 18 fractions for 2 weeks), uninvolved upper neck nodes 55.2 Gy in 46 fractions over 4.6 weeks, and lower neck nodes 50 Gy in 25 fractions for 5 weeks. He had no evidence of disease and worked full time 3 years after therapy.

Intensity-Modulated Radiation Therapy Planning

Intensity-modulated radiation therapy (IMRT) may offer an advantage in sparing the parotid gland(s) in patients with upper neck nodes or in improving tumor coverage in those with short, muscular necks.

Dose

For T1 N0 tumors: 50 Gy in 25 fractions to the initial target volume followed by 16 Gy in eight fractions to the primary tumor. Neck nodes, when present, can receive higher doses appropriate for the size.

For nonbulky, exophytic T2 to T3 tumors: concomitant boost or hyperfractionated regimen. Concomitant boost delivers 1.8-Gy fractions to 54 Gy in 30 fractions to the initial target volume and 1.5-Gy fractions to 15 to 18 Gy given as second daily fractions during the last 2 to 2.5 weeks; the spinal cord dose is limited to 45 Gy or less. Hyperfractionation delivers 55.2 Gy in 46 fractions to the initial target volume then 21.6 to 24 Gy in 18 to 20 fractions (1.2-Gy fractions, twice daily, at 6-hour interval); the spinal cord dose is limited to 44.4 to 45.6 Gy or less and uninvolved posterior cervical nodes are supplemented with 2 Gy daily to approximately 55 Gy.

For T3, fixed vocal cord, or bulky tumor: in combination with three cycles of concurrent cisplatin, radiation is given in the conventional 2-Gy fractions to a dose of 50 Gy to the initial target volume and 70 Gy to the boost volume. The spinal cord dose is limited to less than 45 Gy.

Positive nodes receive doses appropriate for the size and the fractionation schedule used; e.g., 66 to 70 Gy in 2-Gy fractions, 69 to 72 Gy with concomitant boost, or 74.4 to 79.2 Gy with hyperfractionation.

For uninvolved lower neck nodes: 50 Gy in 25 fractions (treated once a day).

Dose Specification: See "General Principles"

Postoperative Radiotherapy

Target Volume

The initial target volume encompasses the entire surgical bed, levels II–IV nodes and, when indicated, levels IB and V nodes and tracheal stoma (see indications list in the following text) (see Fig. 10.3). The boost volume encompasses areas of known disease locations with 1- to 2-cm margins. Indications for postoperative radiotherapy to the tracheal stoma are subglottic extension, emergency tracheostomy, tumor invasion into the soft tissues of the neck (including ECE), close or positive tracheal margin, or surgical scar crosses the stoma.

Setup and Field Arrangement

The patient is immobilized in a supine position with a thermoplastic mask. Marking of surgical scar, tracheal stoma, and shoulders facilitates portal design. Lateral parallel–opposed fields are used to treat the tumor bed and upper neck lymphatics.

- *Anterior, superior, and posterior borders:* similar to those of primary radiotherapy (ensure an adequate coverage of the entire surgical bed).
- *Inferior border:* just above the tracheal stoma.

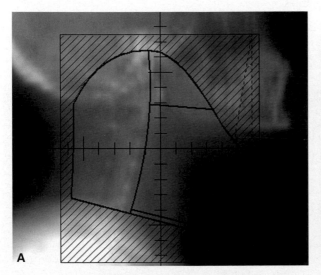
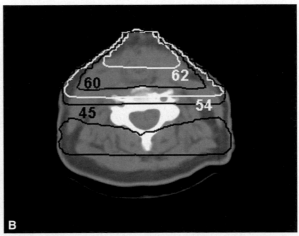

Figure 10.3 This 61-year-old woman underwent a total laryngectomy at another institution for a primary tumor involving the entire epiglottis, right aryepiglottic fold, and medial wall of the pyriform sinus. Pathologic studies revealed a 2.5-cm tumor with a 2-mm mucosal margin. One of 40 lymph nodes in the right neck harbored metastatic disease. Stage: pT2 N1. Treatment began with a pair of lateral-opposed ^{60}Co beams encompassing the neopharynx and draining lymphatics of the upper and mid neck. After 42 Gy, an off–spinal cord reduction was made, with treatment continuing to 56 Gy. The areas considered at highest risk received an additional 4 Gy boost. Digital reconstructions of the initial, off–spinal cord and boost fields are shown in **(A)**. The beams were modified with a combination of 20-degree wedges with the heel placed inferiorly for the ^{60}Co beam and 30-degree wedges heel anterior for the off-spinal cord and boost fields. An isodose distribution through a selected axial image is shown in **(B)**. The posterior cervical strips were supplemented to 56 Gy with 9 MeV electrons to 56 Gy. The tracheal stoma and low neck nodes were treated with an anterior field to 50 Gy.

A matching anterior portal is used for the lower neck nodes and, when indicated, the tracheal stoma.

For the boost volume, lateral portals are reduced to encompass the areas of known tumor bed with 1- to 2-cm margins. Nodes overlying the spinal cord can usually receive boost dose through oblique-lateral primary boost portals and those in the lower neck through an appositional electron portal or glancing photon fields.

Dose

General guidelines after total laryngectomy are:

- 60 Gy in 30 fractions to areas with high-risk features, that is, close or microscopically positive margins, perineural extension, vascular invasion, positive nodes, or extranodal extension. An additional boost dose of 6 Gy in three fractions may be given when indicated, for example, when multiple adverse features are present or when the interval between surgery and radiation is much longer than 6 weeks.
- 56 Gy in 28 fractions to the surgical bed.
- 50 Gy in 25 fractions to undissected regions to receive elective irradiation.
- When delayed wound healing postpones commencement of postoperative radiation to beyond 5 to 6 weeks, we prescribe accelerated fractionation, such as concomitant boost, by delivering twice-a-day irradiations for 1 week, usually at the end of the radiation course, to reduce the potential hazard of prolonged cumulative treatment time.

After supraglottic laryngectomy, the dose is decreased to 55 Gy in 30 fractions over 6 weeks to minimize potential exacerbation of postsurgical edema by irradiation and facilitate rehabilitation of swallowing.

The dose to the tracheal stoma is usually 50 Gy in 25 fractions.

Dose Specification: See "General Principles"

Background Data

TABLE 10.1

SQUAMOUS CELL CARCINOMA OF THE SUPRAGLOTTIC LARYNX: CONTROL OF PRIMARY LESION BY IRRADIATION

| | Stage | | | | | | | |
| | 1954–1963 | | | | 1964–1972 | | | |
Site	T1	T2	T3	T4	T1	T2	T3	T4
Suprahyoid epiglottis	6/6	3/4	9/13	9/15	3/4	7/7	13/15	3/5
Infrahyoid epiglottis	3/5	5/8	0/0	1/4	5/5	11/12	3/4	1/1
Aryepiglottic folds	2/2	9/11	4/7	1/1	5/5	6/7	3/4	3/6
False cords	3/3	5/6	1/1	0/0	2/2	8/10	0/0	1/1
Arytenoids	0/0	2/3	0/1	0/0	2/2	1/1	0/0	0/0
Total	14/16	24/32[a]	14/22[a]	11/20	17/18	33/37[a]	19/23[a]	8/13

Data from the M.D. Anderson Cancer Center.
Note: Approximately 500 rad higher dose in second period.
[a]T2 + T3: 1954–1963, 30% failure rate; 1964–1972, 13% failure rate. $\chi^2 = 4.9386$; $P < 0.05$. Analysis: August 1976.
Modified from Fletcher GH, Goepfert H. Larynx and pyriform sinus. In: Fletcher GH, ed. *Textbook of radiotherapy,* 3rd ed. Philadelphia, PA: Lea & Febiger, 1980:330–363, with permission.

TABLE 10.2

LOCAL CONTROL AND COMPLICATION RATES FOLLOWING RADICAL RADIATION OF T2 TO T3, N0 TO N3 CANCERS OF THE SUPRAGLOTTIC LARYNX

		Local Control		
Radiation Schedules	**No. of Patients**	**2 yr**	**5 yr**	**Severe Complication[a](%)**
Hyperfractionation[b] (1984–1991)	77	87%	80%	2.7
Standard fractionation[b] (1970–1981)	98	78%	70%	3.0

Data from the M.D. Anderson Cancer Center.
Note: Patients treated in 1982 and 1983 were excluded because some received treatment with conventional fractionation and others with hyperfractionation. Analysis, July 1992.
[a]Requiring tracheotomy or laryngectomy.
[b]P = 0.04.

TABLE 10.3

T2 TO T3 SUPRAGLOTTIC LARYNX CARCINOMA: LOCAL CONTROL FOLLOWING RADIOTHERAPY ACCORDING TO MEDICAL AND ANATOMIC SUITABILITY FOR OPERATION IN 83 PATIENTS TREATED AT THE UNIVERSITY OF FLORIDA[a]

	Anatomically Suitable for Supraglottic Laryngectomy			Anatomically Unsuitable
Stage	**Medically Suitable**	**Medically Unsuitable**	**Total**	
T2	35/41 (85%)	14/16 (88%)	49/57 (86%)	44/52 (85%)
T3	9/13 (69%)	8/13 (62%)	17/26 (66%)	17/26 (65%)
Total	44/54 (81%)	22/29 (76%)	66/83 (80%)	61/78 (78%)

[a]Excludes patients who died within 2 years of radiotherapy with primary site continuously disease free.
Modified from Hinerman RW, Mendenhall WM, Amdur RJ, et al. Carcinoma of the supraglottic larynx: treatment results with radiotherapy alone or with planned neck dissection. *Head Neck* 2002;24:456–467, with permission.

TABLE 10.4

RESULTS OF RADIATION AND CHEMOTHERAPY FOR ORGAN PRESERVATION IN LARYNX CANCER: RTOG 91-11

	Radiotherapy Alone	Cisplatin+5-FU followed by Radiotherapy	Radiation+ Concurrent Cisplatin
Patient number	173	173	172
Supraglottic/glottic (%)	72/28	68/32	66/34
T2/T3/T4 (%)	12/79/9	12/78/10	11/78/10
Node positive (%)	50	50	50
2-yr local control (%)	58	64	80
2-yr laryngeal preservation (%)	70	75	88
2-yr distant failure (%)	16	9	8
2-yr overall survival (%)	75	74	75
2-yr difficulty swallowing (%)	14	16	15

Adapted from Forastiere AA, Goepfert H , Maor M, et al. Concurrent chemotherapy and radiotherapy for organ preservation in advanced laryngeal cancer. *N Engl J Med* 2003;349:2091–2098, with permission.

GLOTTIS

Treatment Strategy

Primary radiotherapy is preferred for T1 to T2 tumors. Concurrent radiation and chemotherapy is the preferred larynx-preserving treatment for T3 tumors. Selected patients may be enrolled into ongoing trials.

The standard treatment for T4 tumors is total laryngectomy, usually with postoperative radiotherapy and, in the presence of high-risk features such as positive extracapsular nodal extension or positive margin, with concurrent cisplatin. Selected patients may be enrolled in ongoing trials.

Primary Radiotherapy for T1 to T2 N0 Tumors

The target volume encompasses the larynx proper (sparing suprahyoid epiglottis) (see Figs. 10.4 and 10.5).

Setup and Field Arrangement

The patient is immobilized in a supine position with a short thermoplastic mask. Marking of shoulders facilitates portal design. Lateral parallel–opposed photon fields are used. In patients

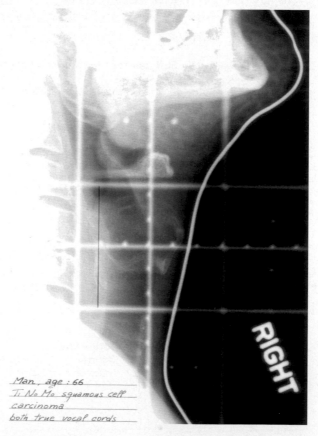

Figure 10.4   A 66-year-old man presented with a 6-month history of progressive hoarseness. Mirror examination showed mild edema and leukoplakia of the anterior commissure and the anterior one third of both true vocal cords. There was no supraglottic or subglottic spread and vocal cord mobility was normal. No lymph nodes were palpated in the neck. Tomography of the larynx was without abnormalities. Biopsies showed microinvasive squamous cell carcinoma on both true vocal cords. Stage: T1 N0 M0. The patient was treated with lateral parallel–opposed ^{60}Co fields. A dose of 64 Gy specified in the isocenter was delivered in 2-Gy fractions. After a dose of 50 Gy, the posterior border was moved 1 cm anteriorly to reduce the dose to the arytenoids. A 15-degree wedge was used to produce a slight dose gradient delivering a higher dose to the thickest part of the lesion at the anterior third of the cords. He had no evidence of disease and had good voice quality 2.5 years after therapy.

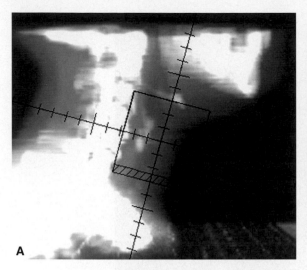
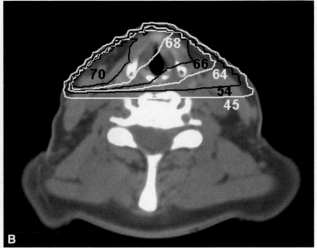

Figure 10.5 A 52-year-old woman who smoked cigarettes presented with hoarseness. Examination revealed a tumor involving the entire length of the right true vocal cord. There was normal vocal cord mobility and the tumor did not extend into the supraglottic or subglottic larynx. A biopsy was positive for invasive squamous cell carcinoma. Stage T1 N0 M0. She was treated with primary radiation to the larynx only. Parallel–opposed fields using ⁶⁰Co were used to deliver a dose of 66 Gy in 33 fractions. The digitally reconstructed radiograph of the portal **(A)** and the isodose distribution through the larynx **(B)** are shown. A combination of 30- and 45-degree wedges was used to modify the beam and the dose was delivered preferentially from the right side.

with a short neck, a 5- to 10-degree inferior tilt may be necessary to avoid irradiation through the wider part of the shoulder.

- *Superior border:* top of thyroid cartilage for T1 or higher for T2 tumor with supraglottic extension.
- *Anterior border:* approximate 1 cm falloff.
- *Posterior border:* anterior margin of the vertebral bodies.
- *Inferior border:* lower edge of the cricoid cartilage for T1, or lower for T2 tumor with subglottic extension.

Dose

T1 tumors: 66 Gy in 33 fractions depending on the size. For microscopic disease (e.g., after "stripping" or excisional biopsy of T1 tumors) the dose can be reduced to 60 Gy in 30 fractions.

T2 tumors: 70 Gy in 35 fractions or 79.2 Gy in 66 fractions (twice daily, 6-hour interval) over 7 or 6.5 weeks, respectively.

T3 tumors: in combination with three cycles of concurrent cisplatin, radiation is given in conventional 2-Gy fractions to a dose of 50 Gy to the initial target volume and 70 Gy to the boost volume. The spinal cord dose is limited to 45 Gy or less.

The dose is specified at an isodose line. Treatment is usually given with 15- or 30-degree wedges. Differential loading (2:1) may be used for one-side lesions.

Primary Radiotherapy for T3 or N+ Tumors

Target Volume

The initial target volume encompasses larynx and levels II, III, and IV (subdigastric, midjugular, and lower neck) nodes in the absence of involved nodes (see Fig. 10.6). The initial target volume includes levels IB and/or V nodes in the presence of upper neck or bulky node(s). The boost volume encompasses primary tumor and involved nodes with 1- to 2-cm margins.

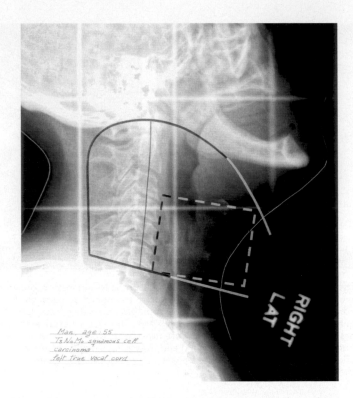

Figure 10.6   A 55-year-old man presented with a long history of persistent hoarseness and recent onset of left ear pain. Mirror examination showed a whitish exophytic lesion over the entire length of the left true vocal cord, which was fixed. The tumor extended into the left ventricle and there was minimal edema of the left false cord. The right true vocal cord showed an area of leukoplakia, but the mobility was normal. There was no palpable lymphadenopathy in the neck. Computed tomography (CT) scan of the larynx confirmed the physical findings. Biopsy showed a well-differentiated squamous cell carcinoma of the left true vocal cord. Stage: T3 N0 M0. The patient declined laryngectomy and elected to have primary radiotherapy. He was treated with a hyperfractionation regimen. The lateral portals were designed to encompass the primary tumor, subdigastric, and midjugular lymph nodes. The lower neck nodes were treated with an anterior appositional field. The boost dose was delivered through small lateral fields as are used for T1 to T2 vocal cord tumors. The primary tumor received 76.8 Gy over 7 weeks (55.2 Gy in 46 fractions for 4.6 weeks + 21.6 Gy in 18 fractions for 2 weeks), uninvolved upper and mid neck nodes 55.2 Gy in 46 fractions over 4.6 weeks, and lower neck nodes 50 Gy in 25 fractions for 5 weeks. This patient continued to smoke during and after treatment. Follow-up examination 2.5 years later revealed no evidence of disease, but the arytenoids were edematous.

Setup and Field Arrangement

The patient is immobilized in a supine position with a thermoplastic mask. Marking of shoulders and palpable lymph nodes, when present, facilitates portal design. Lateral parallel–opposed photon fields are used to treat the primary tumor and upper neck nodes. Field borders are similar to those used for supraglottic carcinoma. A matching anterior portal is used for treatment of the lower neck nodes.

It may be necessary to use anterior and inferior tilts for patients with a short neck. In this case the supraclavicular fossae are included in the primary portal (Fig. 10.8).

For boost volume, lateral portals are reduced to encompass gross disease. Nodes overlying the spinal cord can usually receive boost dose through oblique–lateral primary boost portals and those in the lower neck through an appositional electron portal or glancing photon fields.

Dose

In combination with three cycles of concurrent cisplatin, radiation is given in the conventional 2-Gy fractions to a dose of 50 Gy to the initial target volume and 70 Gy to the boost volume. Positive nodes receive 66 to 70 Gy depending on the size. The spinal cord dose is limited to 45 Gy or less (see "Supraglottis").

Dose Specification: See "General Principles"

Postoperative Radiotherapy

See "Supraglottis" and Figures 10.7 and 10.8.

Treatment of Recurrent Disease

Occasionally, small recurrences from irradiated T1 to T2 glottic cancers can be salvaged by voice-preserving procedures (e.g., laser vaporization or hemilaryngectomy). In most cases, however, laryngectomy is necessary for salvaging the local relapse. Postoperative irradiation to the tracheal stoma and the neck is administered when the recurrent lesion extends to the subglottic region or when the neck dissection reveals multiple nodes or extracapsular nodal disease.

Setup and Field Arrangement

The patient is immobilized in a supine position with a thermoplastic mask. An appositional electron field is used when only the stoma needs additional irradiation. Opposed anterior–posterior

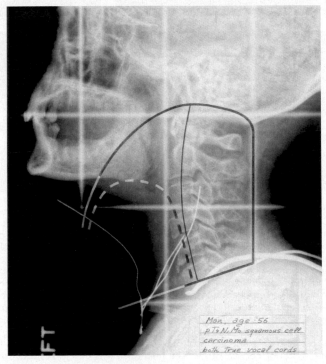

Figure 10.7 A 56-year-old man from Spain presented with a 3-month history of hoarseness and dysphagia. Mirror examination showed a tumor of the infrahyoid epiglottis and both false cords. The true cords could not be visualized because of the swelling of the false cords. The pyriform sinuses appeared free of disease. There were no palpable neck nodes. A computed tomography (CT) scan showed a large tumor of the larynx involving both true cords with upward extension to the false cords and infrahyoid epiglottis and downward extension to the right lateral subglottic area. There was significant destruction of the thyroid cartilage and extension of the tumor into the anterior soft tissues of the neck. A biopsy showed squamous cell carcinoma. Stage: T4 N0 M0. This patient underwent a wide-field laryngectomy. Pathologic examination showed a moderately differentiated squamous cell carcinoma involving both true vocal cords, right false cord, and infrahyoid epiglottis. There was 1.9-cm subglottic extension at the right side. The tumor penetrated through the thyroid cartilage into the anterior soft tissues of the neck. One of 14 recovered lymph nodes contained tumor. This node was located in the left paratracheal area and measured 1 cm in its largest diameter. Stage: pT4 N1 M0. He was enrolled into the postoperative radiotherapy protocol. The surgical scar, tracheal stoma, anterior skin of the neck and shoulders were wired at simulation. The tumor bed and upper and midjugular nodes were irradiated through lateral–opposed fields. The lower neck and tracheal stoma was treated with an anterior field. Primary tumor bed received a total dose of 63 Gy, and dissected nodal areas along with tracheal stoma a dose of 57.6 Gy delivered in 1.8 Gy per fraction. He saw his otolaryngologist 36 months after radiotherapy and was found to have no evidence of disease. Current preference is to treat with 2-Gy fractions to 60 Gy to the tumor bed and 56 Gy to the dissected nodal areas and tracheal stoma.

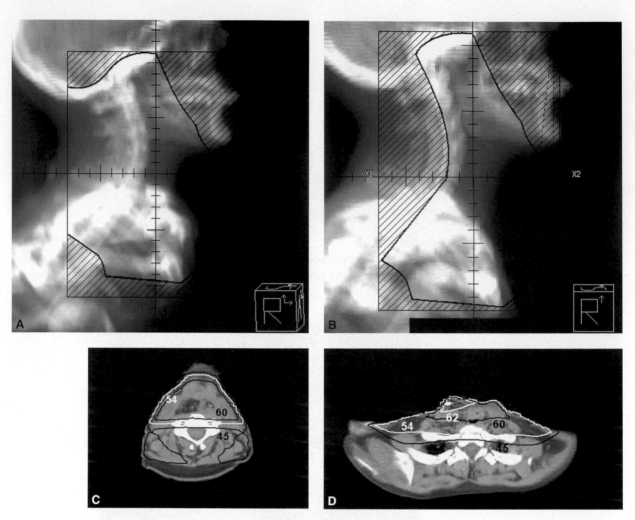

Figure 10.8   A 52-year-old man presented with a transglottic tumor of the larynx and bilateral adenopathy. Computed tomography (CT) scan evaluation of the head and neck revealed the primary tumor invaded the thyroid cartilage. He underwent a total laryngectomy and bilateral neck dissection. Pathology revealed basaloid squamous cell carcinoma of the right hemilarynx and pyriform sinus. The tumor invaded the thyroid cartilage, hyoid bone, and skeletal muscle of the neck. The margins were negative. Nine of 32 lymph nodes in the right neck and two of 32 nodes in the left neck were positive for metastatic regional disease. Stage: T4 N2 M0. Radiation commenced 4 weeks after surgery. It was thought that the initial tumor volume extended inferiorly, and parallel–opposed fields would inadequately cover the volume at risk. It was elected instead to use oblique portals angled caudally and posteriorly **(A)**. These two fields encompassed the primary tumor volume at risk as well as the retropharyngeal nodes and nodal levels II through V. The stoma was covered in these fields, as well. At 42 Gy, the fields were reduced off the spinal cord. The caudal angulation was continued, but the fields were placed in true lateral position **(B)** to facilitate matching the electron fields for delivering supplemental dose to the posterior cervical strips. The final dose was 60 Gy. A reduction was not made off the superior border because the larger tissue diameter in this region resulted in a lower dose per fraction to the retropharyngeal and highest jugular nodes. Thus the high-risk volume received 60 Gy, while the lower risk subclinical volume received 54 Gy (all in 30 fractions). Representative isodose distributions through axial cuts of the mid and low neck are shown in **(C)** and **(D)**.

photon fields are used to irradiate jugular and supraclavicular nodes and the tracheal stoma. A slightly larger midline block is used to shield the previously treated pharynx. Some overlap with the previously irradiated soft tissues of the neck laterally is allowed.

Dose

Stoma only: 50 Gy (at D_{max}) in 25 fractions with 9 to 12 MeV electrons.

Neck and stoma: 50 Gy (at D_{max}) is delivered with the anterior field in 25 fractions; the posterior portal is used to bring the dose at the midline to 50 Gy. Areas of the positive nodes and extranodal extension then receive boost irradiation to a final dose of 60 Gy in 30 fractions.

Background Data

TABLE 10.5

INVASIVE SQUAMOUS CELL CARCINOMA OF THE VOCAL CORDS: 1948–1973

Stage	No. of Patients	Control (%)	Control of Failures by Surgery (%)	Ultimate Control (%)
T1				
No visible lesion	32	29 (91%)	3/3 (100%)	32 (100%)
Post cord stripping	12	11(91%)	0/1 (0%)	11(91%)
Visible-one cord	193	166 (86%)	23/26[a] (88%)	189 (98%)
Bulky lesion	40	39 (97%)	1/1 (100%)	40 (100%)
Anterior comm. involved	55	50 (91%)	4/5 (80%)	54 (98%)
Total	332	295 (89%)	31/36 (86%)	226 (98%)
T2				
Partial mobility	26	21 (81%)	5/5 (100%)	26 (100%)
Extension beyond cord	59	49 (83%)	8/8[b](100%)	57 (97%)
Anterior comm. below cord	49	34 (69%)	14/14[a] (100%)	48/ (98%)
Combinations of features	41	25 (61%)	9/14[c] (64%)	34/ (83%)
Total	175	129 (74%)	36/41 (88%)	165 (94%)

Data from the M.D. Anderson Cancer Center.
[a]One patient refused treatment.
[b]One patient refused treatment, one patient re-treated by irradiation and failed.
[c]One patient refused treatment, one patient not treated.
Modified from Fletcher et al. The place of irradiation in management of the squamous cell carcinomas of the larynx. In: *Otolaryngology*. Vol. 5. Hagerstown, MD: Harper & Row Publishers, 1977:1–45.

TABLE 10.6

LOCAL CONTROL IN 279 PATIENTS TREATED AT THE UNIVERSITY OF FLORIDA

T Stage	Subgroup	Size	Excluded	Local Control (%)	No. Salvaged/No. Attempted Hemilaryn-gectomy	Total Laryngectomy	Ultimate Local Control (%)
T1a	C	<5 mm	1	12/12 (100%)	ND	ND	12/12 (100%)
		5–15 mm	8	73/78 (94%)	3/4	0/1	76/78 (97%)
		>15 mm	2	45/50 (90%)	ND	4/5	49/50 (98%)
T1b	HL	All	0	14/15 (93%)	ND	0/1	14/15 (93%)
	TL	All	2	15/16 (94%)	0/1	ND	15/16 (94%)
T2a	HL	All	5	23/27 (85%)	ND	4/4	27/27 (100%)
	TL	All	2	27/38 (71%)	2/3	7/8	36/38 (95%)
T2b	HL	All	3	13/18 (72%)	1/2	2/3	16/18 (89%)
	TL	All	2	18/25 (72%)	ND	4/6	22/25 (88%)

C, suitable for cordectomy; HL, suitable for hemilaryngectomy; TL, suitable for total laryngectomy; ND, no data.
From Mendenhall WM, Parsons JT, Stringer SP, et al. T1–T2 vocal cord carcinoma: a basis for comparing the results of radiotherapy and surgery. *Head Neck Surg* 1988;10:373–377, with permission.

TABLE 10.7

T2 N0 SQUAMOUS CELL CARCINOMA OF THE TRUE VOCAL CORD: CONTROL OF DISEASE IN THE NECK IN 98 PATIENTS TREATED AT THE UNIVERSITY OF FLORIDA

Primary Site Free of Disease	Surgical Alternative	Initial Control of Neck Disease	No. Salvaged/ No. Attempted	Ultimate Control of Neck Disease
Yes	Hemilaryngectomy	35/36 (97%)	0/1	35/36 (97%)
	Total laryngectomy	38/39 (97%)	0/1	38/39 (97%)
No	Hemilaryngectomy	5/9 (56%)	3/4	8/9 (88%)
	Total laryngectomy	13/14 (93%)	1/1	14/14 (100%)

From Mendenhall WM, Parsons JT, Brant TA, et al. Is elective neck treatment indicated for T2 N0 squamous cell carcinoma of the glottic larynx? *Radiother Oncol* 1989;14:199–202, with permission.

TABLE 10.8

RESULTS OF RADIATION FOR T1 CARCINOMAS OF THE TRUE VOCAL CORDS (REVIEW)

Series	No. of Patients	Local Control
Harwood et al. (1979)	333	86% (5-yr A)
Fletcher and Goepfert (1980)	332	89% (C)
Lustig et al. (1984)	342	90% (3-yr A)
Hendrickson (1985)	364	90% (C)
Wang (1997)	665	93% (5-yr A)
Le et al. (1997)	315	84% (C)
Mendenhall et al. (2004)	291	94% (5-yr A)

A, actuarial; C, crude.

TABLE 10.9

CONTROL PROBABILITY OF T2 GLOTTIC CANCER AS A FUNCTION OF CORD MOBILITY (REVIEW)

Series	No. of Patients		Local Control (%) After Radiotherapy (3 or 5 yr)		Ultimate Control (%) (3 or 5 yr)	
	T2a	T2b	T2a (%)	T2b (%)	T2a (%)	T2b (%)
Martensson et al.	30	19	70	47	—	—
Kun et al.	12	43	75	58	—	—
Fletcher	108	67	77	69	97	90
Harwood et al.	156	80	80	52	—	—
Van den Bogaert et al.	33	28	62	65	81	68
Wang	102	88	79	61	—	—
Karim et al.	111	45	78	80	90	95
Mendenhall et al.	65	43	77	72	97	88
Wiggenraad et al.	50	21	78	71	98	76
Howell-Burke et al.	40	74	73	72	95	97

From Ang KK, Peters LJ. Vocal cord cancer: 2b worse than not 2b? *Radiother Oncol* 1990;18:365–366, with permission.

TABLE 10.10

FIVE-YEAR LOCAL CONTROL RATES IN 230 PATIENTS WITH T2 N0 GLOTTIC CARCINOMA: PROGNOSTIC VARIABLES

	No. of Patients	5-yr Control Rate (%)	P-value
No subglottic extension	111	81	
Subglottic extension	119	63	0.004
T2A	114	74	
T2B	116	70	0.37
Daily dose >2Gy[a]	138	80	
Daily dose ≤ 2 Gy	90	59	<0.001
Once-daily fractionation[a]	147	67	0.06
Twice-daily fractionation	81	79	
Total	230	72	

[a]Two patients with compliance difficulties had fractionation schedule changes during their treatments and are excluded.
Data from M.D. Anderson Cancer Center.
Modified from Garden. AS, Forster.K, Wong. PF, et al. Results of radiotherapy for T2 N0 glottic carcinoma: does the "2" stand for twice-daily treatment? *Int J Radiat Oncol Biol Phys* 2003;55:322–328.

TABLE 10.11

OUTCOME OF TREATMENT OF FIRST RECURRENCES AFTER PRIMARY RADIOTHERAPY IN 37 PATIENTS[a] TREATED AT THE M.D. ANDERSON CANCER CENTER

Site of Recurrence	Local–Regional Control by Treatment Modality					
	Laryngectomy Only	Laryngectomy and Neck Dissection	Neck Dissection	Neck and Dissection Radiotherapy	Hemilaryngectomy	Laser
Larynx	23/28	—	—	—	1/1	1/3[b]
Neck	—	—	1/1	2/2	—	—
Larynx and neck	—	0/2	—	—	—	—

[a]Entries indicate number of patients whose first recurrence was controlled over the number of patients treated.
[b]Although disease recurred in two patients treated by laser therapy, both recurrences were controlled by subsequent laser ablations.
From Howell-Burke D, Peters LK, Goepfert H, et al. T2 glottic cancer. Recurrence, salvage, and survival after definitive radiotherapy. *Arch Otolaryngol Head Neck Surg* 1990;116:830–835, with permission.

TABLE 10.12

CAUSES OF DEATH AFTER TREATMENT OF T2 GLOTTIC CARCINOMA IN 230 PATIENTS TREATED AT THE M.D. ANDERSON CANCER CENTER

Causes	No. of Patients
Index cancer	
Recurrence above clavicles	15[a]
Distant metastases	15
Surgical complications	3
Second cancers	32
Other intercurrent disease (or unknown)	55
Total	119

[a]One patient died with both local recurrence and distant disease.
Adapted from Garden AS, Forster K, Wong PF, et al. Results of radiotherapy for T2 N0 glottic carcinoma: does the "2" stand for twice-daily treatment? *Int J Radiat Oncol Biol Phys* 2003;55:322–328.

TABLE 10.13

FAILURES ABOVE THE CLAVICLES BY PRIMARY AND NODAL STAGING IN PATIENTS WITH ADVANCED GLOTTIC CARCINOMAS[a] TREATED WITH SURGERY (WITH OR WITHOUT POSTOPERATIVE RADIOTHERAPY)

T Stage N Stage	T3 (n = 185)		T4 (n = 57)	
	Surgery Alone	Combined Treatment	Surgery Alone	Combined Treatment
N0	22/135 (16)	2/22 (9)	10/32 (31)	1/16 (6)
N1	4/17 (24)	1/4 (25)	0/1 (0)	—
N2a	—	0/1 (0)	1/1 (100)	—
N2b	1/2 (50)	0/2 (0)	1/1 (100)	0/2 (0)
N3a	—	—	—	0/2 (0)
N3b	1/1 (100)	0/1 (0)	0/2 (0)	—
Total	28/155 (18)	3/30 (10)	12/37 (32.4)	1/20 (5)

Data from the M.D. Anderson Cancer Center.
[a]Values in parentheses are percentages.
From Yuen A, Medina. JE, Goepfert H, et al. Management of stage T3 and T4 glottic carcinomas. *Am J Surg* 1984;148:467–472, with permission.

TABLE 10.14

CONTROL OF T3 GLOTTIC CARCINOMA TREATED WITH DEFINITIVE RADIOTHERAPY (REVIEW)

Series	No. of Patients	Local Control (%)
Lundgren et al. (1988)	141	44
Harwood et al. (1979)	112	51
Mendenhall et al. (1997)	75	63
Wang (1997)	65	57
Bryant et al. (1995)	55	55

TABLE 10.15

RECURRENCE RATES FOLLOWING RADICAL RADIATION

Stage	No. Pts	Local Recurrence (%)		Regional Recurrence 5 yr (%)
		2 yr	5 yr	
T2 N0 M0	154	30	34	8
T3 N0 M0	68	52	55	3
T4 N0 M0	39	44	44	12

Data from the Princess Margaret Hospital.
From Harwood AR, Hawkins NV, Beale FA, et al. Management of advanced glottic cancer. *Int J Radiat Oncol Biol Phys* 1979;5:899–904, with permission.

SUGGESTED READINGS

Andrew JW, Eapen L, Kulkarni NS. Homogeneous irradiation of the "short-necked" laryngeal cancer patient. *Int J Radiat Oncol Biol Phys* 1984;10:549.

Ang KK, Peters LJ. Vocal cord cancer: 2b worse than not 2b? *Radiother Oncol* 1990;18:365.

Barton MB, Keane TJ, Gadalla T, et al. The effect of treatment time and treatment interruption on tumour control following radical radiotherapy of laryngeal cancer. *Radiother Oncol* 1992;23:137.

Bron LP, Soldati D, Zouhair A, et al. Treatment of early stage squamous-cell carcinoma of the glottic larynx: endoscopic surgery or cricohyoidoepiglottopexy versus radiotherapy. *Head Neck* 2001;23:823.

Bryant GP, Poulsen MG, Tripcony L, et al. Treatment decision in T3N0M0 glottic carcinoma. *Int J Radiat Oncol Biol Phys* 1995;31:285.

DeSanto LW. Cancer of the supraglottic larynx: a review of 260 patients. *Otolaryngol Head Neck Surg* 1985;93:705.

Fields JN, Marks JE. A technique for treatment of advanced carcinomas of the larynx and hypopharynx using low-megavoltage X-rays. *Radiother Oncol* 1986;7:281.

Fletcher GH. History of irradiation in squamous cell carcinomas of the larynx and hypopharynx. *Int J Radiat Oncol Biol Phys* 1986;12:2019.

Fletcher GH, Goepfert H. Larynx and pyriform sinus. In: Fletcher GH, ed. *Textbook of radiotherapy*, 3rd ed. Philadelphia, PA: Lea & Febiger, 1980.

Fletcher GH, Goepfert H. Irradiation in management of squamous cell carcinoma of the larynx. In: English GM, ed. *Otolaryngology*. Philadelphia, PA: Harper & Row, 1984.

Fletcher GH, Hamberger AD. Causes of failure in irradiation of squamous cell carcinoma of the supraglottic larynx. *Radiology* 1974;111:697.

Fletcher GH, Jesse RH, Lindberg RD, et al. The place of radiotherapy in the management of the squamous cell carcinoma of the supraglottic larynx. *Am J Roentgenol Radium Ther Nucl Med* 1970;108:19.

Fletcher GH, Lindberg RD, Hamberger A, et al. Reasons for irradiation failure in squamous cell carcinoma of the larynx. *Laryngoscope* 1975;85:987.

Forastiere AA, Goepfert H, Maor M, et al. Concurrent chemotherapy and radiotherapy for organ preservation in advanced laryngeal cancer. *N Engl J Med* 2003;349:2091.

Garden AS, Forster K, Wong PF, et al. Results of radiotherapy for T2 N0 glottic carcinoma: does the "2" stand for twice-daily treatment? *Int J Radiat Oncol Biol Phys* 2003;55:322.

Goepfert H, Jesse RH, Fletcher GH, et al. Optimal treatment for the technically resectable squamous cell carcinoma of the supraglottic larynx. *Laryngoscope* 1975;85:145.

Hahn SS, Spaulding CA, Kim JA, et al. The prognostic significance of lymph node involvement in pyriform sinus and supraglottic cancers. *Int J Radiat Oncol Biol Phys* 1987;13:1143.

Harwood AR, Beale FA, Cummings BJ, et al. Supraglottic laryngeal carcinoma: an analysis of dose-time-volume factors in 410 patients. *Int J Radiat Oncol Biol Phys* 1983;9:311.

Harwood AR, Hawkins NV, Beale FA, et al. Management of advanced glottic cancer. *Int J Radiat Oncol Biol Phys* 1979;5:899.

Harwood AR, Hawkins NV, Rider WD, et al. Radiotherapy of early glottic cancer—I. *Int J Radiat Oncol Biol Phys* 1979;5:473.

Hendrickson FR. Radiation therapy treatment of larynx cancers. *Cancer* 1985;55(Suppl. 9):2058.

Hinerman RW, Mendenhall WM, Amdur RJ, et al. Carcinoma of the supraglottic larynx: treatment results with radiotherapy alone or with planned neck dissection. *Head Neck* 2002;24:456.

Horiot JC, Fletcher GH, Ballantyne AJ, et al. Analysis of failures in early vocal-cord cancer. *Radiology* 1972;103:663.

Johansen LV, Grau C, Overgaard J. Supraglottic carcinoma: patterns of failure and salvage treatment after curatively intended radiotherapy in 410 consecutive patients. *Int J Radiat Oncol Biol Phys* 2002;53:948.

Johansen LV, Grau C, Overgaard J. Laryngeal carcinoma—multivariate analysis of prognostic factors in 1252 consecutive patients treated with primary radiotherapy. *Acta Oncol* 2003;42:771.

Johansen LV, Overgaard J, Hjelm-Hansen M, et al. Primary radiotherapy of T1 squamous cell carcinoma of the larynx: analysis of 478 patients treated from 1963 to 1985. *Int J Radiat Oncol Biol Phys* 1990;18:1307.

Karim AB, Kralendonk JH, Yap LY, et al. Heterogeneity of stage II glottic carcinoma and its therapeutic implications. *Int J Radiat Oncol Biol Phys* 1987;13:313.

Kazem I, van den Broek P, Huygen PL. Planned preoperative radiation therapy for advanced laryngeal carcinoma. *Int J Radiat Oncol Biol Phys* 1982;8:1533.

Keane T, Cummings BJ, O'Sullivan B, et al. A randomized trial of radiation therapy compared to split course radiation therapy combined with mitomycin C and 5 fluorouracil as initial treatment for advanced laryngeal and hypopharyngeal squamous carcinoma. *Int J Radiat Oncol Biol Phys* 1993;25:613.

Le QX, Fu KK, Kroll S, et al. Influence of fraction size, total dose, and overall time on local control of T1-T2 glottic carcinoma. *Int J Radiat Oncol Biol Phys* 1997;39:115.

Lee NK, Goepfert H, Wendt CD, et al. Supraglottic laryngectomy for intermediate-stage cancer: U.T. M.D. Anderson Cancer Center experience with combined therapy. *Laryngoscope* 1990;100:831.

Levendag PC, Hoekstra CJ, Eijkenboom WM, et al. Supraglottic larynx cancer, T1-4 N0, treated by radical radiation therapy. Problem of neck relapse. *Acta Oncol* 1988;27:253.

Levendag P, Vikram B. The problem of neck relapse in early stage supraglottic cancer—results of different treatment modalities for the clinically negative neck. *Int J Radiat Oncol Biol Phys* 1987;13:1621.

Lundgren JA, Gilbert RW, van Nostrand AW, et al. T3N0M0 glottic carcinoma—a failure analysis. *Clin Otolaryngol Allied Sci* 1988;13:455.

Lustig RA, MacLean CJ, Hanks GE, et al. The patterns of care outcome studies: results of the national practice in carcinoma of the larynx. *Int J Radiat Oncol Biol Phys* 1984;10:2357.

Marks JE, Breaux S, Smith PG, et al. The need for elective irradiation of occult lymphatic metastases from cancers of the larynx and pyriform sinus. *Head Neck Surg* 1985;8:3.

Mendenhall WM, Parsons JT, Brant TA, et al. Is elective neck treatment indicated for T2N0 squamous cell carcinoma of the glottic larynx? *Radiother Oncol* 1989;14:199.

Mendenhall WM, Parsons JT, Mancuso AA, et al. Definitive radiotherapy for T3 squamous cell carcinoma of the glottic larynx. *J Clin Oncol* 1997;15:2394.

Mendenhall WM, Werning JW, Hinerman RW, et al. Management of T1-T2 glottic carcinoma. *Cancer* 2004;100:1786.

Nguyen-Tan PF, Le QT, Quivey JM, et al. Treatment results and prognostic factors of advanced T3-T4 laryngeal carcinoma: the University of California, San Francisco (UCSF) and Stanford University Hospital experience. *Int J Radiat Oncol Biol Phys* 2001;50:1172.

Parsons JT, Mendenhall WM, Mancuso AA, et al. Twice-a-day radiotherapy for T3 squamous cell carcinoma of the glottic larynx. *Head Neck* 1989;11:123.

Parsons JT, Mendenhall WM, Stringer SP, et al. T4 laryngeal carcinoma: radiotherapy alone with surgery reserved for salvage. *Int J Radiat Oncol Biol Phys* 1998;40:54.

Peters LJ, Thames HD Jr. Dose-response relationship for supraglottic laryngeal carcinoma. *Int J Radiat Oncol Biol Phys* 1983;9:421.

Richard J, Sancho-Garnier H, Pessey JJ, et al. Randomized trial of induction chemotherapy in larynx carcinoma. *Oral Oncol* 1998;34:224.

Robbins KT, Davidson W, Peters LJ, et al. Conservation surgery for T2 and T3 carcinomas of the supraglottic larynx. *Arch Otolaryngol Head Neck Surg* 1988;114:421.

Sailer SL, Sherouse GW, Chaney EL, et al. A comparison of postoperative techniques for carcinomas of the larynx and hypopharynx using 3-D dose distributions. *Int J Radiat Oncol Biol Phys* 1991;21:767.

Stalpers LJ, Verbeek AL, van Daal WA. Radiotherapy or surgery for T2N0M0 glottic carcinoma? A decision-analytic approach. *Radiother Oncol* 1989;14:209.

Terhaard CH, Karim AB, Hoogenraad WJ, et al. Local control in T3 laryngeal cancer treated with radical radiotherapy, time dose relationship: the concept of nominal standard dose and linear quadratic model. *Int J Radiat Oncol Biol Phys* 1991;20:1207.

The Department of Veterans Affairs Laryngeal Cancer Study Group. Induction chemotherapy plus radiation compared with surgery plus radiation in patients with advanced laryngeal cancer. *N Engl J Med* 1991;324:1685.

Van den Bogaert W, Ostyn F, van der Schueren E. The different clinical presentation, behaviour and prognosis of carcinomas originating in the epilarynx and the lower supraglottis. *Radiother Oncol* 1983;1:117.

Wall TJ, Peters LJ, Brown BW, et al. Relationship between lymph nodal status and primary tumor control probability in tumors of the supraglottic larynx. *Int J Radiat Oncol Biol Phys* 1985;11:1895.

Wang CC. Carcinoma of the larynx. *Radiation therapy for head and neck neoplasms.* New York: Wiley-Liss, 1997.

Wang CC, McIntyre JT. Re-irradiation of laryngeal carcinoma—techniques and results. *Int J Radiat Oncol Biol Phys* 1993;26:783.

Wang CC, Nakfoor BM, Spiro IJ, et al. Role of accelerated fractionated irradiation for supraglottic carcinoma: assessment of results. *Cancer J Sci Am* 1997;3:88.

Warde P, Harwood A, Keane T. Carcinoma of the subglottis. Results of initial radical radiation. *Arch Otolaryngol Head Neck Surg* 1987;113:1228.

Weber RS, Berkey BA, Forastiere A, et al. Outcome of salvage total laryngectomy following organ preservation therapy: the Radiation Oncology Group trial 91-11. *Arch Otolaryngol Head Neck Surg* 2003;129:44.

Wendt CD, Peters LJ, Ang KK, et al. Hyperfractionated radiotherapy in the treatment of squamous cell carcinomas of the supraglottic larynx. *Int J Radiat Oncol Biol Phys* 1989;17:1057.

Yuen A, Medina JE, Goepfert H, et al. Management of stage T3 and T4 glottic carcinomas. *Am J Surg* 1984;148:467.

Hypopharynx

11

PYRIFORM SINUS

Treatment Strategy

Primary radiotherapy is preferred for T1 and T2, any N-stage tumor. Neck dissection is indicated in patients who have residual neck mass 6 weeks after completion of radiotherapy.

Extrapolating from trials on laryngeal cancer, concurrent radiation and chemotherapy is the preferred larynx-preserving treatment for T3 tumors.

The standard treatment for T4 tumors is pharyngolaryngectomy, usually with postoperative radiotherapy. Select patients may be enrolled into ongoing trials; for example, testing combination of antiepidermal growth factor receptor antibody, cetuximab, with concurrent radiation therapy–chemotherapy or induction chemotherapy followed by concurrent radiation therapy–chemotherapy.

Indications for postoperative radiotherapy and irradiation of the tracheal stoma are similar to those for carcinoma of the larynx.

Primary Radiotherapy

Target Volume

The initial target volume encompasses primary tumor with good margins and bilateral neck nodes, including the retropharyngeal nodes, and levels II, III, IV, and V nodes. The target volume also includes ipsilateral level IB in the presence of level II node (see Figs. 11.1 to 11.3).

The boost volume encompasses primary tumor and involved nodes with 1- to 2-cm margins.

Setup and Field Arrangement

Marking of shoulders and palpable nodes facilitates portal design. The patient is immobilized in a supine position, with the shoulders pulled down to the maximal extent. Lateral parallel–opposed photon fields are used to treat the primary tumor and upper and mid neck nodes.

- *Superior border:* at the level of the skull base to include the upper jugular and parapharyngeal lymphatics.
- *Anterior border:* 1-cm fall-off.
- *Posterior border:* behind the spinous processes or more posteriorly in the presence of large nodal mass.
- *Inferior border:* encompasses primary lesion with margin (as low as possible while avoiding the shoulders).

A matching anterior portal is used to treat the lower neck nodes. It may be necessary to use anterior and inferior tilts for patients with a short neck or for patients with inferior extent of the primary tumor or nodal mass. In this case, the supraclavicular fossae are included in the primary portal (see Fig. 10.8).

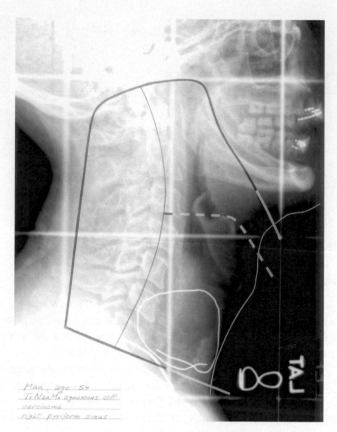

Man, age: 54
Ti N2a Mo squamous cell
carcinoma
right pyriform sinus

Figure 11.1 A 54-year-old man saw his physician for a routine checkup and was found to have a right jugular mass. He was referred for workup and treatment. Mirror examination showed discrete redness and mucosal irregularity in the medial and lateral walls of the right pyriform sinus without changes at the apex. There was a 5-cm firm node fixed to the sternocleidomastoid muscle, palpated in the right lower jugular area. A biopsy from the right pyriform sinus showed moderately to well-differentiated squamous cell carcinoma. Stage: T1 N2 aM0. The primary tumor, jugular, and retropharyngeal nodes were treated with lateral parallel–opposed photon fields. The inferior border was placed just above the shoulders to encompass the involved lower jugular node (wired). Because the disease was located on the right side, the fields were weighted 3:2 in favor of the right side. A total dose of 66.6 Gy was delivered to the isocenter, which resulted in a dose of 68 Gy to the primary and 72 Gy to the node in 7 weeks. Off-cord reduction was made at 45 Gy. The posterior cervical nodes were supplemented with electrons to 54 Gy. The supraclavicular nodes were treated with an anterior appositional photon field to 54 Gy. Tissues directly posterior and inferior to the palpable node received additional irradiation to a cumulative dose of 63 Gy. Physical examination 6 weeks after completion of radiotherapy revealed a complete response at the primary site. In the neck, however, a 3-cm residual node was noted. Therefore, patient subsequently underwent a right neck dissection. He was alive and healthy 2.5 years after therapy.

For boost volume, reduced lateral fields are used as follows:

- *Superior and inferior borders:* depends on the extent of the disease; at least include aryepiglottic folds superiorly and cricoid cartilage inferiorly.
- *Anterior border:* 1-cm fall-off, except when the primary lesion is confined to the posterior structures, where a small strip of anterior skin may be spared.
- *Posterior border:* mid vertebral bodies, or posterior one third of vertebral bodies when the primary involves posterior pharyngeal wall.

Involved upper and mid jugular nodes receive boost dose through lateral fields along with the primary tumor and lower neck nodes through a reduced anterior portal.

Nodes overlying the spinal cord can receive boost dose with electron beam(s) or, alternatively, the primary tumor and ipsilateral node can receive boost dose with oblique photon fields, depending on the location of the node(s).

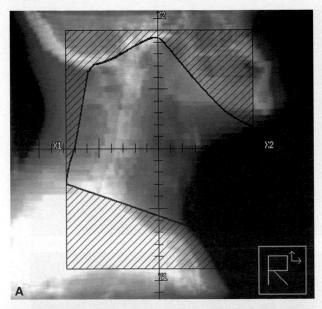

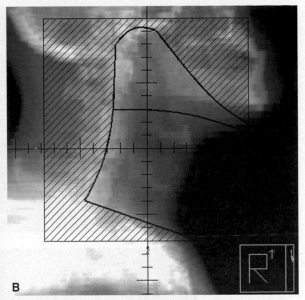

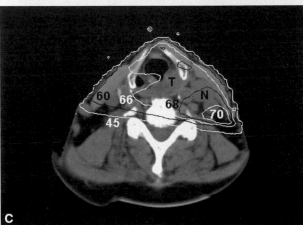

Figure 11.2 A 76-year-old man presented with a 10-month history of left-sided sore throat and otalgia. A 1.5-cm tumor was seen on the medial wall of the left pyriform sinus without extension to the apex. The larynx mobility was normal. A biopsy revealed moderately differentiated squamous cell carcinoma. A 1-cm lymph node was detected in level III in the left neck. Stage: T1 N1 M0. He was treated with 6-MV photons, with the primary tumor and upper and mid neck lymphatics, as well as the retropharyngeal nodes encompassed in parallel–opposed fields **(A)**. These portals received a dose of 42 Gy. An anterior supraclavicular and low neck field was matched on the skin and treated to a dose of 50 Gy. The upper fields were reduced off the spinal cord and continued to a dose of 54 Gy. An additional 12 Gy was delivered to coned-down portals to a final dose of 66 Gy. The off–spinal cord and boost fields were treated with parallel right anterior and left posterior oblique fields **(B)** to encompass the gross disease in the photon fields. The boost was preferentially weighted to the left. An isodose distribution through the central axis and primary tumor (*T*) and gross lymph node (*N*) is shown in **(C)**. Both posterior cervical strips received 12 Gy supplement in six fractions with 9-MeV electrons, then the left posterior strip received an additional boost of 12 Gy. The patient is without evidence of disease 24 months since diagnosis.

Dose

T1 tumors: 50 Gy in 25 fractions to the initial target volume, then 16 Gy in eight fractions to the primary tumor; neck nodes, when present, can receive higher doses appropriate for the size.

T2 tumors: concomitant boost or hyperfractionated regimen. Concomitant boost delivers 1.8-Gy fractions to 54 Gy in 30 fractions to the initial target volume and 1.5-Gy fractions to 15 to 18 Gy given as second daily fractions during the last 2 to 2.5 weeks; the spinal cord dose is limited to 45 Gy or less. Hyperfractionation delivers 55.2 Gy in 46 fractions to the initial target volume followed by 21.6 to 24 Gy in 18 to 20 fractions (1.2-Gy fractions, twice daily, 6-hour interval); the spinal cord dose is limited to 44.4 to 45.6 Gy or less, and uninvolved posterior cervical nodes are supplemented with 2 Gy daily to approximately 55 Gy.

Positive nodes receive doses appropriate for the size and the fractionation schedule used; for example, 66 to 70 Gy in 2-Gy fractions, 69 to 72 Gy with concomitant boost, or 74.4 to 79.2 Gy with hyperfractionation.

T3 tumors: in combination with three cycles of concurrent cisplatin, radiation is given in the conventional 2-Gy fractions to a dose of 50 Gy to the initial target volume and 70 Gy to the boost volume. The spinal cord dose is limited to 45 Gy or less.

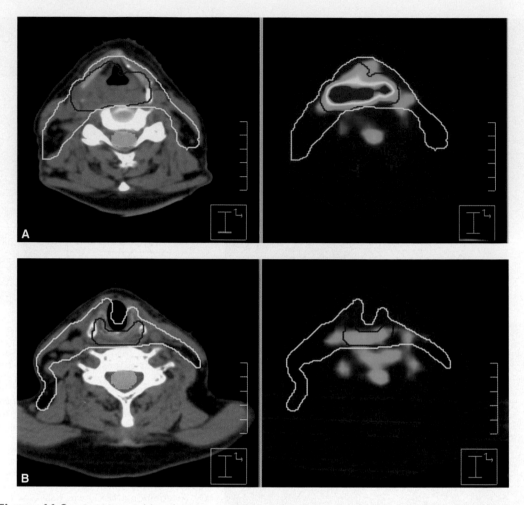

Figure 11.3 A 61-year-old male presented with sore throat, mild odynophagia, and weight loss. Examination revealed an extensive tumor of the oropharyngeal walls extending into the right pyriform sinus and postcricoid region, the biopsy of which showed squamous cell carcinoma. There was no clinical evidence of lymphadenopathy. He received concurrent radiation therapy and chemotherapy. Although bulky disease was seen filling the right pyriform sinus, the disease had significant superficial spread. A positron emission tomography–computed tomography (PET-CT) simulation was performed to assist in defining the targets, particularly the inferior extent of disease that could not be visualized clinically. An axial CT scan slice with adjacent fused PET image is shown **(A)**. The high-dose clinical target volume (*red*) and subclinical target volume (*yellow*) are shown on the CT scan. A more inferior slice through the postcricoid region **(B)** did not demonstrate increase in 2-[Fluorine 18]-fluoro-2-deoxy-D-glucose (FDG) uptake. A high-dose clinical volume was outlined for boost volume definition because this slice was approximately 1 cm below the identified gross target volume.

Dose Specification: See "General Principles"

Differential loading may be used for lateralized lesions with ipsilateral nodal disease only. In this situation, the dose is specified at an isodose line with a maximal allowable dose heterogeneity of ±2.5%.

Postoperative Radiotherapy

The indications and technique are similar to those for supraglottic carcinoma (see Fig. 11.4). The primary tumor bed, surgical bed, and bilateral retropharyngeal nodes; levels II, III, IV, and V nodes; and level IB in the presence of level II node are irradiated, which means that the superior border of the lateral fields are placed at the level of the base of skull.

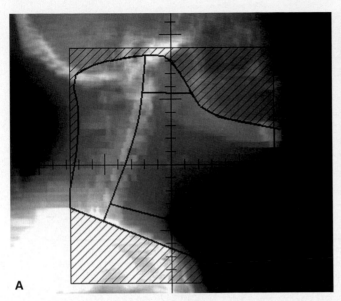

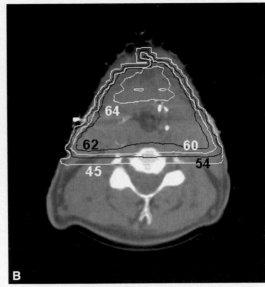

Figure 11.4 A 61-year-old man presented with several months of left otalgia and weight loss. A large mass was seen filling the left pyriform sinus and invading medially into the larynx. A biopsy revealed grade-2 squamous cell carcinoma. Because of the weight loss and near obstruction of the larynx, a gastrostomy tube was placed and tracheostomy was performed. He subsequently underwent total laryngectomy and partial pharyngectomy. The defect was repaired with a radial forearm graft. Additionally, bilateral neck dissections were performed. Histologic examination revealed a carcinoma of the left pyriform sinus invading the left aryepiglottic fold and thyroid cartilage. There was perineural and lymph–vascular space invasion. Seven of the 25 nodes recovered from the left neck dissection contained metastatic disease with extracapsular extension. Stage: T4 N2 bM0. He received postoperative radiation. Treatment began with parallel–opposed fields using ^{60}Co to a dose of 42 Gy. Fields were reduced off spinal cord and were continued to a dose of 56 Gy with 6-MV photons, with a final reduction bringing the areas deemed at high risk to a dose of 60 Gy **(A)**. An isodose distribution through the central axis is shown in **(B)**. The posterior cervical strips were supplemented with 12-MeV electrons to a dose of 56 Gy. An anterior field was used to treat the low neck and stoma to a dose of 50 Gy.

Background Data

TABLE 11.1

PYRIFORM SINUS: FAILURES ABOVE THE CLAVICLES, NED RATE AT 2 YEAR, AND CAUSES OF DEATH BETWEEN 2 AND 5 YEARS, 1949–DECEMBER 1976 (ANALYSIS, JANUARY 1981)

Treatment Modality	No. of Patients	Patients with Failure Above Clavicle No. (%)	Patients Alive NED 2 yr No. (%)	Cause of Death After 2 yr (No./Cause)
Surgery	203	80 (39%)[a]	81 (40%)[b]	8 DM 23 Other
Curative irradiation 250 Kv	9	4 (44%)	4 (44%)	1 Primary 1 DM
^{60}Co	48	10 (21%)	23 (48%)	1 Primary 4 DM 3 Other
Planned postoperative irradiation	125	14 (11%)[a]	63 (50%)[b]	1 Neck 6 DM 7 Other
Preoperative irradiation	17	5 (29%)	8 (47%)	2 DM 2 Other
Palliative irradiation	16	12 (75%)	0	0

Other, intercurrent disease or second primary; DM, distant metastases.
[a]$P < 0.0001$.
[b]$P = 0.04$.
From El Badawi SA, Goepfert H, Fletcher GH, et al. Squamous cell carcinoma of the pyriform sinus. *Laryngoscope* 1982;92:357, with permission.

TABLE 11.2

LOCAL CONTROL OF RADIATION ALONE FOR EARLY (T1–T2) SQUA-MOUS CELL CARCINOMA OF THE PYRIFORM SINUS (LITERATURE REVIEW)

Institution	Stage (No. of Patients)	5-year Actuarial Control (%)
University of Florida	T1 (19)	89
	T2 (67)	82
University of Texas M.D.	T1 (19)	89
Anderson Cancer Center[a]	T2 (63)	70
Massachusetts General	T1 (24)	74
Hospital	T2 (51)	76

[a]Includes all hypopharyngeal sites (69% of patients with pyriform sinus tumors).
Modified from Amdur RJ, Mendenhall WM, Stringer SP, et al. Organ preservation with radiotherapy for T1-T2 carcinoma of the pyriform sinus. *Head Neck* 2001;23:353; Garden AS, Morrison WH, Clayman GL, et al. Early squamous cell carcinoma of the hypopharynx: outcomes of treatment with radiation alone to the primary disease. *Head Neck* 1996;18:317; and Wang CC. Carcinoma of the hypopharynx. *Radiotherapy of head and neck neoplasms.* New York: Wiley-Liss, 1997;212, with permission.

TABLE 11.3

DISTRIBUTION OF INITIAL FAILURES IN PATIENTS WITH EARLY STAGE (T1–T2) CARCINOMA OF THE HYPOPHARYNX TREATED WITH RADIATION THERAPY

Type of Recurrence	T1 (n = 19)	T2 (n = 63)	Total (n = 82)
Primary relapse (P)	2	13	15
Nodal recurrence (N)	0	5	5
P + N	0	2	2
P + D	1	0	1
N + D	0	5	5
P + N + D	0	1	1
D	2	6	8
Failure above clavicles without D	2 (11%)	20 (32%)	22 (27%)
Total failures	5 (26%)	32 (51%)	37 (45%)

P, primary relapse; N, nodal recurrence; D, distant metastasis.
Modified from Garden AS, Morrison WH, Clayman GL, et al. Early squamous cell carcinoma of the hypopharynx: outcomes of treatment with radiation alone to the primary disease. *Head Neck* 1996;18:317, with permission.

TABLE 11.4

CANCER OF THE PYRIFORM SINUS TREATED BY RADICAL RADIOTHERAPY: SURVIVAL AND LOCAL CONTROL AT 2 YEARS ACCORDING TO THE SITE OF EXTENSION OF THE PRIMARY LESION IN PATIENTS WITH N0 TO N1B NODAL DISEASE

Site Involved	No. of Patients	Absolute Survival Free of Disease at 2nd yr: No. (%)	Determinate Group[a]: No. of Patients	Local Control: No. (%)
Larynx or epilarynx	120	63 (53%)	93	59/93 (63%)
Retrocricoid and/or hypopharyngeal wall	40	16 (40%)	29	15/29 (52%)
Oropharynx	58	21 (36%)	42	19/42 (45%)
Soft tissue and cartilage	23	6 (26%)	14	5/14 (36%)
Cervical esophagus	8	3 (38%)	6	3/6 (50%)
Total	249	109 (47%)	184	101/184 (55%)

[a]Excluded are patients who died of intercurrent disease, second cancer, or distant metastases, or lost to follow-up within 2 years of treatment.
Modified from Bataini P, Brugere J, Bernier J, et al. Results of radical radiotherapy treatment of carcinoma of the pyriform sinus: experience of the Institute Curie. *Int J Radiat Oncol Biol Phys* 1982;9:1277–1286, with permission.

TABLE 11.5

CANCER OF THE PYRIFORM SINUS TREATED BY RADICAL RADIOTHERAPY: LOCO-REGIONAL FAILURES ACCORDING TO STAGE OF PRIMARY AND NODAL DISEASE

Stage	No. of Patients	Recurrences			
		P: No. (%)	P + N: No. (%)	N: No. (%)	Total: No. (%)
T1–T2					
N0	33	10	—	—	10/33 (33%)
N1b	21	6	1	2	9/21 (43%)
N3	36	7	5	9	21/36 (58%)
Total	90	23 (26%)	6 (7%)	11 (12%)	40/90 (44%)
T3					
N0	90	27	6	3	36/90 (40%)
N1b	105	30	15	11	56/105 (53%)
N2b	9	5	—	6/9	—
N3	140	34	42	15	91/140 (65%)
Total	344	96 (28%)	64 (19%)	29 (8%)	189/344 (55%)
Overall total	434	119 (27%)	70 (16%)	40 (9%)	229/434 (53%)

Note: Minimal follow-up 2 years.
P, primary; N, node; P + N, primary + node.
Modified from Bataini P, Brugere J, Bernier J, et al. Results of radical radiotherapy treatment of carcinoma of the pyriform sinus: experience of the Institute Curie. *Int J Radiat Oncol Biol Phys* 1982;9:1277–1286, with permission.

TABLE 11.6

TABLE 11.6

CANCER OF THE PYRIFORM SINUS TREATED BY RADICAL RADIOTHERAPY: RADIOTHERAPY COMPLICATIONS IN 434 PATIENTS

Type of Complications	No. of Patients
Fatal	
Hemorrhage	7
Cachexia	2
Asphyxia due to laryngeal edema	1
Aspiration pneumonia	1
Total	11/434 (2.5%)
Major nonfatal (in 114 patients alive at 3 yr):	
Tracheostomy	6
Gastrostomy	1
Tracheostomy + gastrostomy	1
Soft tissue necrosis (treated conservatively)	4
Total	12/114 (11%)

From Bataini P, Brugere J, Bernier J, et al. Results of radical radiotherapy treatment of carcinoma of the pyriform sinus: experience of the Institute Curie. *Int J Radiat Oncol Biol Phys* 1982;9:1277–1286, with permission.

POSTERIOR HYPOPHARYNGEAL WALL

Treatment Strategy

Primary radiotherapy is preferred for T1 to T2 tumors. Combination of radiation with chemotherapy is the treatment of choice for T3 or N2 to N3 tumors. Outside the protocol study setting, the combination of conventional radiation fractionation (70 Gy in 35 fractions over 7 weeks) with cisplatin (100 mg per m^2 given on days 1, 22, and 43 of radiotherapy) is recommended. Neck dissection is indicated in patients who have residual neck mass 6 weeks after completion of therapy.

Occasionally, advanced tumors (T4) are treated with surgery and postoperative radiotherapy.

Primary Radiotherapy

Target Volume

The initial target volume encompasses the primary tumor with at least 2- to 3-cm margins (of note is that submucosal spread can be extensive) and bilateral retropharyngeal nodes; levels II, III, IV, and V nodes; and level IB in the presence of level II node (see Fig. 11.5).

The boost volume encompasses primary tumor and involved nodes with 1- to 2-cm margins.

Setup and Field Arrangement

Marking of palpable nodes and shoulders facilitates portal design. The patient is immobilized in a supine position with a thermoplastic mask with the shoulders pulled down as far as possible. Lateral parallel–opposed photon fields are used for treatment of the primary tumor and upper neck nodes.

- *Superior border:* at the base of skull to cover parapharyngeal lymphatics and upper jugular nodes.
- *Anterior border:* at least 2 cm anterior to the known extent of the tumor, but when feasible, short of fall-off anteriorly.
- *Posterior border:* just behind the spinous processes or more posteriorly in the presence of large nodal masses. After off-cord reduction, the posterior portal margin is at the posterior one third

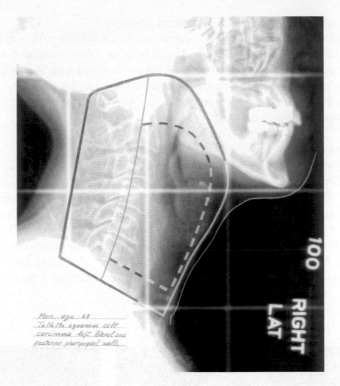

Figure 11.5 A 68-year-old man had a 1-year history of dysphagia. Mirror examination revealed a mass in the left lateral and posterior hypopharyngeal walls. The medial wall and apex of the pyriform sinus were free. There were no palpable neck nodes. A computed tomography (CT) scan confirmed the physical findings and in addition showed some thickening of the left aryepiglottic fold. Biopsy showed moderately differentiated squamous cell carcinoma. Stage: T2 N0 M0. This patient received radiotherapy with a hyperfractionation schedule. Lateral fields were designed to encompass the primary tumor and the majority of neck nodes while sparing a strip of anterior skin. The posterior border of the off-cord and boost portals at the level of the primary tumor was close to the posterior edge of the vertebral bodies to cover the lesion adequately. Supraclavicular nodes were treated with an anterior appositional photon field. The primary tumor received 76.6 Gy in 7 weeks (55.2 Gy in 46 fractions for 4.6 weeks + 21.6 Gy in 18 fractions for 2 weeks); uninvolved upper and mid jugular nodes received 55.2 Gy in 4.6 weeks and uninvolved posterior cervical nodes 54 Gy in 5 weeks. Supraclavicular nodes received 50 Gy in five fractions for 5 weeks. Physical examination 6 months after radiotherapy revealed fullness of the left pyriform sinus. Biopsy of this area showed squamous cell carcinoma. He underwent total laryngopharyngectomy with left modified neck dissection and pharyngeal reconstruction with jejunal free flap. Second local recurrence occurred 5 months after surgery and he died of uncontrolled local disease.

of vertebral bodies to include the retropharyngeal nodes and provide margin for the posterior pharyngeal wall.

- *Inferior border:* encompasses primary lesion with 3-cm or greater margin when possible.

A matching anterior appositional portal is used for treating lower neck nodes. However, it may be necessary to use anterior and inferior tilts for patients with short necks or because of the inferior extent of the primary tumor or nodal mass, in which case the supraclavicular fossa are included in the primary portal.

For boost volume, the lateral fields are reduced:

- *Superior and inferior borders:* depends on extent of the primary tumor.
- *Anterior border:* short of fall off.
- *Posterior border:* posterior one third of vertebral bodies.

Involved upper and mid jugular nodes are encompassed in lateral fields and lower neck nodes in a reduced anterior portal.

Nodes overlying the spinal cord can be boosted with electron beam(s) or, alternatively, the primary tumor and ipsilateral node can be boosted with oblique photon fields.

Intensity-Modulated Radiation Therapy

Conformal radiotherapy is best suited for treating tumors extending to the paravertebral region without overdosing the spinal cord because this technique can produce a horseshoe-shape isodose distribution. The patient is immobilized in a supine position with an extended thermoplastic mask. Thin-cut computed tomography scans are obtained in treatment position. The gross target volume, clinical target volume, and planning target volume are outlined for dosimetric planning (see Fig. 11.6).

Dose

T1 tumors: 50 Gy in 25 fractions to the initial target volume, then 16 Gy in eight fractions to the primary tumor.

T2 tumors: concomitant boost or hyperfractionated regimen. Concomitant boost delivers a dose of 1.8-Gy fractions to 54 Gy in 30 fractions to the initial target volume and a dose of 1.5-Gy fractions to 15 to 18 Gy given as second daily fractions during the last 2 to 2.5 weeks; the spinal cord dose is limited to 45 Gy or less. Hyperfractionation delivers a dose of 55.2 Gy in 46 fractions to the initial target volume, then 21.6 to 24 Gy in 18 to 20 fractions (1.2-Gy fractions, twice daily, at 6-hour interval); the spinal cord dose is limited to 44.4 to 45.6 Gy or less

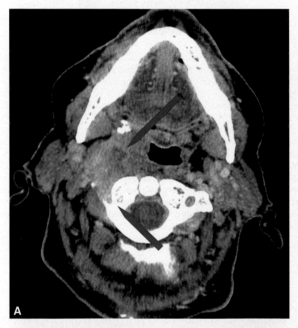

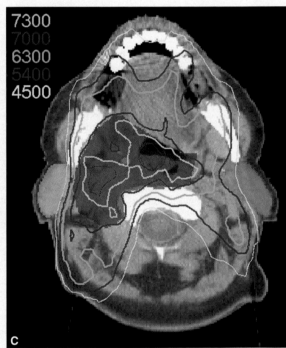

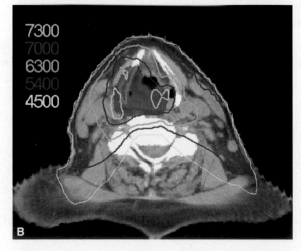

Figure 11.6 A 79-year-old man presented with odynophagia. Examination revealed an extensive pan-pharyngeal wall mass involving the right pyriform sinus and lateral oropharyngeal wall. In addition, there was a large necrotic right retropharyngeal lymph node **(A)** with extension into the paravertebral tissues. He received concurrent radiation therapy and chemotherapy. Intensity-modulated radiation therapy (IMRT) was chosen to improve target coverage, particularly of the paravertebral region. Representative axial isodose distributions are shown at the level of the pyriform sinus **(B)** and retropharyngeal nodal region at C1 **(C)**.

and uninvolved posterior cervical nodes are supplemented with a dose of 2 Gy daily to approximately 55 Gy.

Positive nodes, frequently present, receive doses appropriate for the size and the fractionation schedule used; for example, 66 to 70 Gy in 2-Gy fractions, 69 to 72 Gy with concomitant boost, or 74.4 to 79.2 Gy with hyperfractionation.

T3 tumors: in combination with three cycles of concurrent cisplatin, radiation is given in the conventional 2-Gy fractions to a dose of 50 Gy to the initial target volume and 70 Gy to the boost volume. The spinal cord dose is limited to 45 Gy or less.

Conformal radiotherapy consists of a dose of 66 to 70.4 Gy to the primary tumor and involved node(s) and a dose of 54 to 57.6 Gy to regions at risk for harboring subclinical disease given in 30 to 32 fractions. Therefore, the fraction size varies from 1.8 Gy to the subclinical region to 2.2 Gy to the gross disease.

Dose Specification: See "General Principles"

Postoperative Radiotherapy

Indications and technique for postoperative radiotherapy are similar to those for supraglottic cancer, with the exception that the posterior border of the off-cord and boost fields are brought closer to the posterior edge of the vertebral bodies to ensure good coverage of the prevertebral and paravertebral tissues.

Background Data

TABLE 11.7
LOCAL CONTROL OF RADIATION ALONE FOR SQUAMOUS CELL CARCINOMA OF THE HYPOPHARYNGEAL WALL

Institution	Stage (No. of Patients)	Actuarial Local Control (%)
University of Florida[a]	T1 (5)	100
	T2 (24)	76
	T3 (36)	51
	T4 (10)	25
Massachusetts General Hospital[b]	T1 (18)	88
	T2 (46)	55
	T3–4 (41)	49

[a]2-year actuarial control.
[b]5-year actuarial control.
Modified from Fein DA et al. *Int J Radiat Oncol Biol Phys* 1996; 26:751–757; and Wang CC. Carcinoma of the hypopharynx. *Radiotherapy of head and neck neoplasms.* New York: Wiley-Liss, 1997; 216, with permission.

POSTCRICOID AREA

Treatment Strategy

Surgery with or without postoperative radiotherapy is preferred for these rare tumors because they arise at a site that is difficult to visualize and technically challenging to irradiate.

Postoperative Radiotherapy

When confined to the postcricoid area, the technique of radiotherapy is similar to that of tumors of posterior pharyngeal wall. In patients in whom disease extends into the cervical esophagus, the postoperative "thyroid" technique is more suitable.

Background Data

TABLE 11.8
POSTCRICOID CARCINOMA: PATIENTS TREATED WITH RADIOTHERAPY, REVIEW

Authors	3-year Survival	5-yr Survival
Lederman (1958)	7/65 (11%)	5/57 (9%)
Lord et al. (1973)	1/18 (6%)	1/15 (7%)
Pearson (1966)	5/17 (29%)	5/17 (29%)
Macbeth (1969)	—	0/8 (0%)
Inoue et al. (1973)	1/5 (20%)	1/5 (20%)
Total	14/105 (13%)	12/102 (12%)

Modified from Stell PM, Ramadan MF, Dalby JE, et al. Management of post-cricoid carcinoma. *Clin Otolaryngol Allied Sci* 1982;7:145.

SUGGESTED READINGS

Amdur RJ, Mendenhall WM, Stringer SP, et al. Organ preservation with radiotherapy for T1-T2 carcinoma of the pyriform sinus. *Head Neck* 2001;23:353.

Bataini P, Brugere J, Bernier J, et al. Results of radical radiotherapy treatment of carcinoma of the pyriform sinus: experience of the Institute Curie. *Int J Radiat Oncol Biol Phys* 1982;9:1277.

Dubois JB, Guerrier B, Di Ruggiero JM, et al. Cancer of the piriform sinus: treatment by radiation therapy alone and with surgery. *Radiology* 1986;160:831.

El Badawi SA, Goepfert H, Fletcher GH, et al. Squamous cell carcinoma of the pyriform sinus. *Laryngoscope* 1982;92:357.

Fein DA, Mendenhall WM, Parsons JT, et al. Pharyngeal wall carcinoma treated with radiotherapy: impact of treatment technique and fractionation. *Int J Radiat Oncol Biol Phys* 1993;26:751.

Fletcher GH, Goepfert H. Larynx and pyriform sinus. In: Fletcher GH, ed. *Textbook of radiotherapy*, 3rd ed. Philadelphia, PA: Lea & Febiger, 1980.

Frank JL, Garb JL, Kay S, et al. Postoperative radiotherapy improves survival in squamous cell carcinoma of the hypopharynx. *Am J Surg* 1994;168:476.

Garden AS, Morrison WH, Clayman GL, et al. Early squamous cell carcinoma of the hypopharynx: outcomes of treatment with radiation alone to the primary disease. *Head Neck* 1996;18:317.

Garrett MJ. Megavoltage technique for treatment of carcinoma of the post cricoid region. *Clin Radiol* 1971;22:136.

Hinerman RW, Amdur RJ, Mendenhall WM, et al. Hypopharyngeal carcinoma. *Curr Treat Options Oncol* 2002;3:41.

Johansen LV, Grau C, Overgaard J. Hypopharyngeal squamous cell carcinoma—treatment results in 138 consecutively admitted patients. *Acta Oncol* 2000;39:529.

Keane TJ, Hawkins NV, Beale FA, et al. Carcinoma of the hypopharynx. Results of primary radical radiation therapy. *Int J Radiat Oncol Biol Phys* 1983;9:659.

Lefebvre JL, Castelain B, De la Torre JC, et al. Lymph node invasion in hypopharynx and lateral epilarynx carcinoma: a prognostic factor. *Head Neck Surg* 1987;10:14.

Lefebvre JL, Chevalier D, Luboinski B et al. EORTC Head and Neck Cancer Cooperative Group. Larynx preservation in pyriform sinus cancer: preliminary results of a European Organization for Research and Treatment of Cancer phase III trial. *J Natl Cancer Inst* 1996;88:890.

Marks JE, Freeman RB, Lee F, et al. Pharyngeal wall cancer: an analysis of treatment results complications and patterns of failure. *Int J Radiat Oncol Biol Phys* 1978;4:587.

Mendenhall WM, Parsons JT, Devine JW, et al. Squamous cell carcinoma of the pyriform sinus treated with surgery and/or radiotherapy. *Head Neck Surg* 1987;10:88.

Meoz-Mendez RT, Fletcher GH, Guillamondegui OM, et al. Analysis of the results of irradiation in the treatment of squamous cell carcinomas of the pharyngeal walls. *Int J Radiat Oncol Biol Phys* 1978;4:579.

Million RR, Cassisi NJ. Hypopharynx: pharyngeal walls, pyriform sinus, and postcricoid pharynx. In: Million RR, Cassisi NJ, eds. *Management of head and neck cancer: a multidisciplinary approach*. Philadelphia, PA: JB Lippincott Co, 1985.

Ogura JH, Marks JE, Freeman RB. Results of conservation surgery for cancers of the supraglottis and pyriform sinus. *Laryngoscope* 1980;90:591.

Pene F, Avedian V, Eschwege F, et al. A retrospective study of 131 cases of carcinoma of the posterior pharyngeal wall. *Cancer* 1978;42:2490.

Pingree TF, Davis RK, Reichman O, et al. Treatment of hypopharyngeal carcinoma: a 10-year review of 1,362 cases. *Laryngoscope* 1987;97:901.

Prades JM, Schmitt TM, Timoshenko AP, et al. Concomitant chemoradiotherapy in pyriform sinus carcinoma. *Arch Otolaryngol Head Neck Surg* 2002;128:384.

Pradhan SA. Post-cricoid cancer: an overview. *Semin Surg Oncol* 1989;5:331.

Samant S, Kumar P, Wan J, et al. Concomitant radiation therapy and targeted cisplatin chemotherapy for the treatment of advanced pyriform sinus carcinoma: disease control and preservation of organ function. *Head Neck* 1999;21:595.

Spaulding CA, Hahn SS, Constable WC. The effectiveness of treatment of lymph nodes in cancers of the pyriform sinus and supra-glottis. *Int J Radiat Oncol Biol Phys* 1987;13:963.

Stell PM, Ramadan MF, Dalby JE, et al. Management of post-cricoid carcinoma. *Clin Otolaryngol Allied Sci* 1982;7:145.

Vandenbrouck C, Eschwege F, De la Rochefordiere A, et al. Squamous cell carcinoma of the pyriform sinus: retrospective study of 351 cases treated at the Institut Gustave-Roussy. *Head Neck Surg* 1987;10:4.

Wang CC. Carcinoma of the hypopharynx. *Radiotherapy of head and neck neoplasms*. New York: Wiley-Liss, 1997.

Nasal Cavity

12

NASAL VESTIBULE

Treatment Strategy

Primary radiotherapy is preferred for smaller tumors for better cosmetic outcome. Combination of surgery and radiotherapy may be necessary for large, locally destructive tumors.

Primary Radiotherapy

Target Volume
Initial Target Volume
The initial target volume for well-differentiated tumors with diameters of 1.5 cm or less without extension into adjacent structures is primary tumor with approximately 2-cm margins. Radiation can be administered by brachytherapy, external beam, or a combination of both, depending on the location.

For poorly differentiated tumors or well-differentiated tumors greater than 1.5 cm in diameter without palpable nodes (N0), volume encompasses primary tumor with approximately 2-cm margins and bilateral facial lymphatics ("Manchu moustache area") and level IB (submandibular) and level II (subdigastric) nodes (see Fig. 12.1). Patients with involved node(s) also receive irradiation to the level III and IV nodes.

The boost volume encompasses primary tumor and, when present, involved nodes with 1- to 2-cm margins.

Setup and Field Arrangement
An intraoral stent containing cerrobend is used to displace the tongue posteriorly and to partially shield the upper alveolar ridge (see Fig. 3.8). The patient is immobilized in a supine position.

With external beam irradiation, an anterior appositional field (combination of electrons and photons usually in a ratio of 4:1) is used to treat the nasal vestibule (see Fig.12.2).

- *Superior border:* bridge of the nose or higher in large tumors.
- *Lateral borders:* approximately 1 cm lateral to the alae nasi.
- *Inferior border:* depends on the extent of upper lip invasion (e.g., from mid upper lip to the vermilion border).
- *Boost irradiation:* the anterior portal encompasses the primary tumor with 1- to 2-cm margins.

Technical details to improve the dose distribution are as follows:

- Nasal cavities are filled with bolus to reduce dose heterogeneity.
- Skin collimation is used and wax bolus is applied to smooth the contour for electron beam irradiations.
- If the overlying skin is involved, bolus is placed over the infiltrated area to eliminate the skin-sparing effect of photon irradiation.

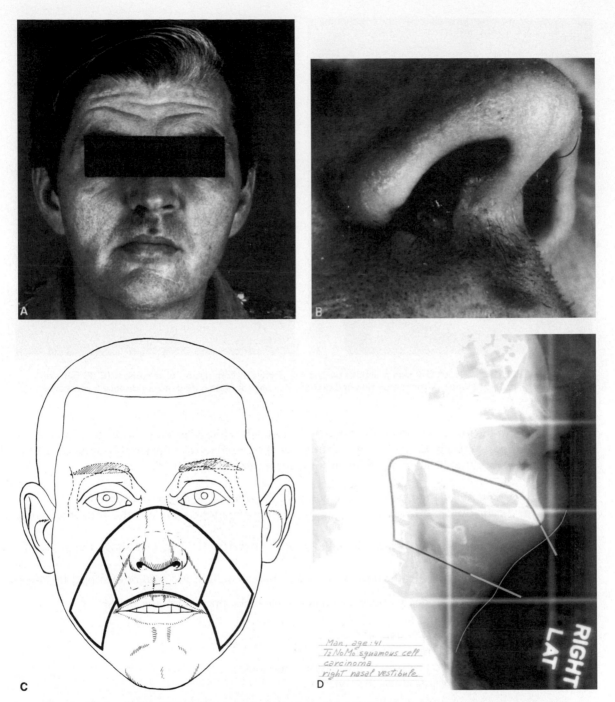

Figure 12.1   A 41-year-old man presented with a "pimple" at the junction of right nasal vestibule and upper lip. A generous biopsy was taken, which showed squamous cell carcinoma with perineural and lymphatic invasion. The patient was referred for treatment. Physical examination revealed a 2.5 × 1.5 cm ulcerative area in the nasal vestibule, extending halfway down the upper lip **(A, B)**. There was no palpable adenopathy. The diagram **(C)** illustrates the primary and moustache fields. The lower half of the nose and upper lip were treated with an anterior appositional field using 20-MeV electrons and 6-MV photons weighted in the ratio 4:1. The facial lymphatics were treated with anterior appositional (15-degree gantry rotation) 6-MeV electron fields. The upper neck nodes received irradiations with parallel–opposed lateral photon fields **(D)**. The primary tumor received 60 Gy (at 90%) in 30 fractions and facial lymphatics and upper neck nodes 50 Gy in 25 fractions.

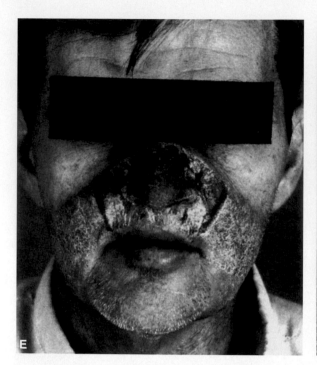
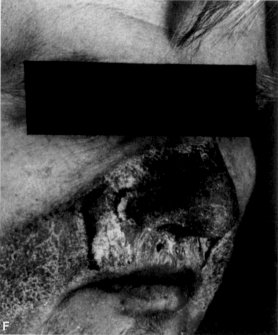

Figure 12.1 *(continued)* Dry skin reactions outline the portals at completion of treatment **(E, F)** but skin reactions subsided 3 weeks after completion of radiation. This patient had no evidence of disease 5 years after therapy.

For the moustache field, anterior right and left appositional electron fields (usually set up with an approximately 15- to 20-degree gantry angle) are used to treat the facial lymphatics. This field is set up clinically after approving the primary tumor and upper neck portals.

- *Medial border:* matches the lateral border of the anterior field (primary tumor).
- *Anterior border:* extends down from oral commissure to the middle of the horizontal ramus of the mandible.
- *Posterior border:* from the upper edge of the anterior field to just above the angle of the mandible.
- *Inferior border:* splits the horizontal ramus of the mandible and adjoins the upper neck field.

The upper neck nodes are treated with lateral parallel–opposed photon fields:

- *Anterior border:* 1 cm fall off.
- *Superior border:* matches moustache fields.
- *Posterior border:* just behind the mastoid processes.
- *Inferior border:* just above the arytenoids.

Patients with involved nodes receive irradiation to mid and lower neck nodes through an anterior portal. Involved nodes receive a boost dose with appositional electrons or glancing photon fields. Brachytherapy alone or a combination of external irradiation and brachytherapy is used to treat small lesions of the septum.

Dose
Small lesions (1.5 cm or less): 50 Gy in 25 fractions followed by 10 to 16 Gy in five to eight fractions boost by external irradiation (usually prescribed at 90% isodose line) or 60 to 65 Gy over 5 to 7 days by implants.

Larger lesions: 50 Gy in 25 fractions followed by 16 to 20 Gy in eight to ten fractions boost. Elective treatment of facial (moustache area) and upper neck nodes: 50 Gy in 25 fractions. Palpable nodes receive a total dose of 66 to 70 Gy depending on the size.

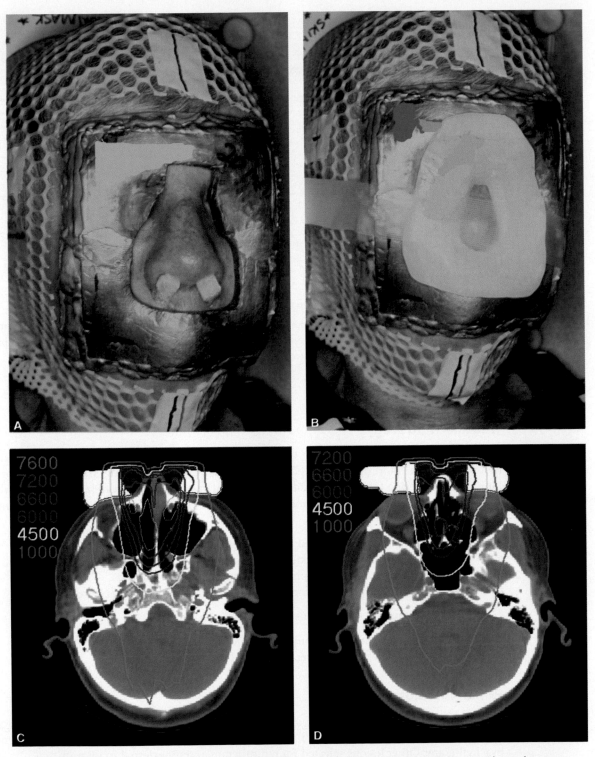

Figure 12.2 A 57-year-old woman presented with nasal fullness and epistaxis. Examination showed a tumor of the nasal septum, the biopsy of which revealed squamous cell carcinoma. Although the tumor was primarily at the anterior septum, the posterior and superior extent made it unfavorable for brachytherapy. Therefore, she was treated with external beam radiation. Lead skin collimation (see Fig. 3.15) with additional thickness over the eyes **(A)** and customized beeswax bolus **(B)** were made. Axial isodose distribution with simulated skin collimation (because the lead cannot be scanned) and the beeswax bolus are shown at the levels of the mid nose through the tumor **(C)** and through the inferior orbits **(D)**. A total dose of 66 Gy was delivered to a 90% isodose line (actual doses shown). Beams were a mix of 20-MeV electrons and 6-MV photons, in approximately 4.5:1 ratio. Small reductions were made inferiorly and superiorly to minimize hot spots in the palate and ethmoids. The patient remains without disease 3.5 years from treatment. However, she developed epiphora 2 years following therapy, which was resolved using dacryocystorhinostomy and silicone tube placement.

TABLE 12.1

TABLE 12.1

LOCOREGIONAL FAILURES OF RADIOTHERAPY OF NASAL VESTIBULE, 1983 TO 1984 (ANALYSIS, FEBRUARY 1986)

Treatment Category	No. of Patients	P	P + N	N	M ± N
Primary only Interstitial	11	—	—	—	—
External beam	7	—	1	1	1
Primary + moustache[a]	2	—	—	1	—
Primary + neck	2	—	—	—	—
Primary + moustache + neck	10	—	—	—	—

P, primary; N, neck; M, metastasis.
[a]Intervening tissues between the nasal vestibule and the neck.
From Chobe R, McNeese M, Weber R, et al. Radiation therapy for carcinoma of the nasal vestibule. *Otolaryngol Head Neck Surg* 1988;98:67–71, with permission.

Dose Specification: See "General Principles"
The electron beam to the nose should be of a sufficiently high energy (15 to 20 MeV) to provide an adequate deep margin. The dose is specified at an isodose line (usually 90%). Moustache fields are irradiated with 6-MeV electrons prescribed at D_{max}.

NASAL FOSSA PROPER

Treatment Strategy

There was no official American Joint Committee on Cancer (AJCC) staging for nasal carcinomas before the publication of the sixth edition of the AJCC Cancer Staging Manual. Therefore, the University of Florida (UF) staging system (stage I–III) was used. The correlation between the UF system and the T-classification criteria of the sixth edition of the AJCC Staging Systems are approximately as follows:

- Stage I represents tumors confined to nasal fossa; that is, T1 and T2.
- Stage II represents tumors with extension to adjacent sites (i.e., paranasal sinuses, skin, orbit, pterygomaxillary fossa, and nasopharynx); that is, T3 and small T4a.
- Stage III represents tumors extending beyond adjacent structures; that is, remaining T4.

   Our current treatment strategy is as follows:

- T1–T2 N0–N1: radiotherapy or surgery depending on the location and size.
- T3–T4 N2–N3: surgery + postoperative radiotherapy.

Primary Radiotherapy

The target volume encompasses primary tumor with 2- to 3-cm margins. Lesions of 1.5 cm or less in diameter that are located in the inferior nasal septum are generally treated with interstitial brachytherapy. Other lesions selected for radiotherapy receive external irradiation.

Setup and Field Arrangement for External Irradiation
Marking of lateral canthi, oral commissures, and limbus (particularly medial and inferior borders) facilitates portal design. An intraoral stent is used to open the mouth and to depress the tongue out of the radiation fields. The patient is immobilized in a supine position with the head positioned in such a way that the hard palate is perpendicular to the treatment couch.
   The location and size of the tumor determine the appropriate portal borders and arrangement (see Chapter 13). Tumors in the anterior nasal cavity not suited for brachytherapy (see subsequent text) may be treated with an appositional mixed beam arrangement (Fig. 12.2). This

requires careful CT scan-based treatment planning because it is very easy to underestimate the appropriate depth. Additionally, the isodose distribution can be heterogeneous in this location with irregular contours and significant bone and air interfaces, especially when using electron beam.

Three-field technique (see Chapter 13) is required for irradiation of primaries of the upper or posterior nasal cavity. This setup allows coverage of ethmoids without delivering high doses to the optic apparatus. CT scan-based treatment planning is necessary to determine the appropriate beam weighting and wedge sizes.

Intensity-Modulated Radiation Therapy

The complexity of the anatomy makes tumors located in these areas well-suited for intensity-modulated radiation therapy (IMRT), which has become our preferred technique. The patient is immobilized in a supine position, with an extended head and shoulder thermoplastic mask. Thin-cut CT scans are obtained in treatment position. The target volumes are outlined for dosimetric planning. Figures 12.3 and 12.4 show example cases.

Interstitial Brachytherapy

Because interstitial brachytherapy is applied for small lesions of the inferior nasal septum, it can be accomplished by a single-plane implant (see Figs. 12.5 and 12.6).

Dose

- *External irradiation:* dose of 50 Gy in 25 fractions to the initial target volume plus 16 to 20 Gy in eight to ten fractions to the boost volume depending on the size.
- *Brachytherapy:* approximately 60 to 65 Gy in 5 to 7 days specified at the margins of the lesion.

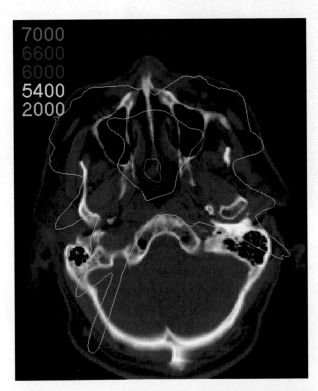

Figure 12.3 A 55-year-old male initially presented with T2 N0 squamous cell carcinoma of the oropharynx. He was treated with concomitant boost fractionation. Approximately 1 year later, a routine follow-up endoscopy discovered a mass in the posterior right nasal septum, biopsy positive for squamous cell carcinoma. The tumor was too deep for either brachytherapy or electron therapy. Given the previous radiotherapy, which encompassed the entire posterior pharynx, he was treated with intensity-modulated radiation therapy (IMRT). A total dose of 66 Gy was delivered in 30 fractions, and a representative axial isodose through the tumor is shown. He was without evidence of disease for both primary tumors.

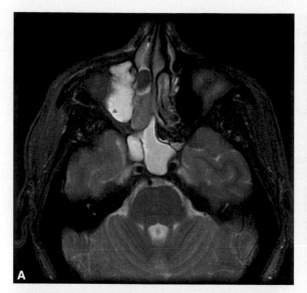

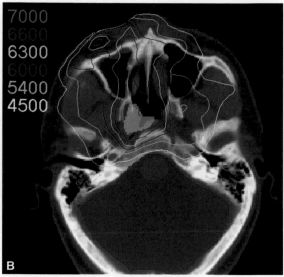

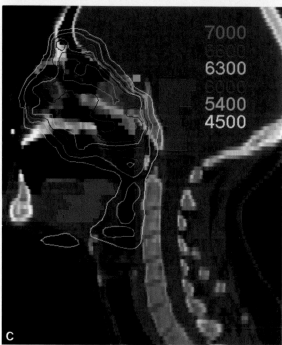

Figure 12.4   A 30-year-old man presented with nasal obstruction. Examination showed a right nasal mass, the biopsy of which revealed sinonasal undifferentiated carcinoma. A T2-weighted axial magnetic resonance imaging (MRI) reveals the lesion in the nasal cavity with secretions in the adjacent maxillary and sphenoid sinuses **(A)**. He was treated with neoadjuvant VP-16 and cisplatin for three cycles with a good response, with only questionable residual disease in the posterior nasal cavity. He subsequently received intensity-modulated radiation therapy (IMRT) with two additional cycles of single agent cisplatin. An axial dose distribution through the nasal cavity **(B)** and midsagittal view **(C)** are shown. The areas of residual abnormality (*yellow*) received 66 Gy, the pretreatment tumor volume (*teal*) received 63 Gy, and areas of potential microscopic spread including right level I and II nodes (not shown) received 54 Gy, all given in 30 fractions. Brain stem (*magenta*), optic chiasm (*blue*), and an oral avoidance volume (*orange*) are shown. He was free of recurrence at last follow-up, more than 3 years after completion of therapy.

Postoperative Radiotherapy

Target Volume

The initial target volume encompasses the entire surgical bed. The boost volume encompasses areas of known disease with 1- to 2-cm margins.

Setup and Field Arrangement

This setup is similar to that for the maxillary sinus; the field borders are adjusted to the location and extent of the tumor.

Dose

In general, 50 Gy in 25 fractions is delivered to the initial target volume and 10 Gy in five fractions (negative margins) to 16 Gy in eight fractions (positive margins) is delivered to the boost volume.

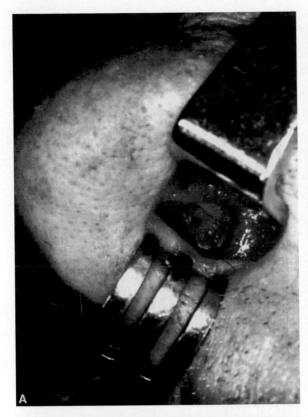

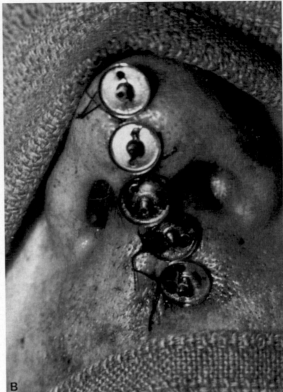

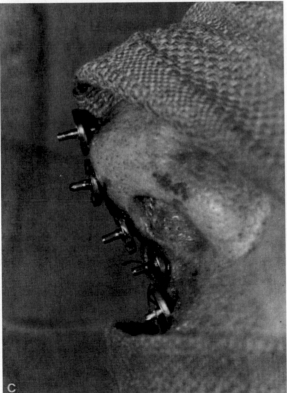

Figure 12.5 A 71-year-old man underwent a single-plane iridium implant of the nasal septum for a 1.5-cm squamous cell carcinoma in November 1976. Five 5-cm stainless-steel needles were loaded with 5-cm active-length iridium 192 wires (0.65 mg Ra equivalent per cm) to deliver a dose of 70 Gy at 5 mm in 127 hours. Note the primary lesion at the nasal septum **(A)** and the geometry of the iridium implant—(**B:** anterior view and **C:** lateral view). On follow-up, the patient had occasional nasal bleeding caused by changes in weather. Cancer of the prostate developed in June 1988 with bone metastasis and was treated with orchiectomy. The patient died in September 1989 from pneumonia and cardiac failure following surgery for an aneurysm of the aorta. He had no evidence of disease at the nasal septum. (From Delclos L. A second look at interstitial irradiation. In: Deeley TJ, ed. *Topical Reviews in Radiotherapy and Oncology*. Vol. II. Bristol: John Wright & Sons Ltd, 1982:190–191, with permission.)

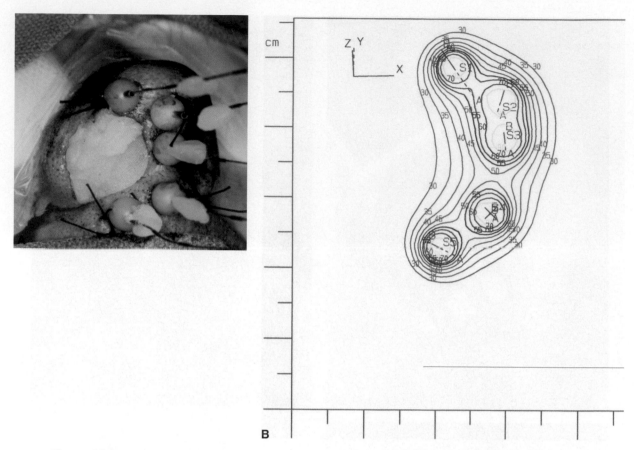

Figure 12.6 A 67-year-old man presented with T1 N0 squamous cell carcinoma of the right anterior nasal septum and received treatment with brachytherapy. Five needles were used with approximately 1-cm spacing **(A)**. The cavity was packed with Vaseline gauze and the needles were afterloaded with iridium 192. The active lengths varied between 3 and 3.5 cm, providing approximately 1-cm margin beyond the tumor. An isodose distribution through the midplane is shown. The total dose was 60 Gy specified to the 40 cGy per hour line. The patient was alive without disease 6 years later.

Dose Specification: See "General Principles"

Background Data

TABLE 12.2

LOCAL CONTROL AND REGIONAL RELAPSE FOR CARCINOMA OF THE NASAL VESTIBULE TREATED WITH RADIATION THERAPY (LITERATURE REVIEW)

Authors	Year of Publication	No. of Patients	Local Control	Neck Failure[a] (%)
Wong and Cummings	1986	56	80% (C)	4
Chobe et al.	1988	32	97% (C)	17
Mazeron et al.	1988	64	75% (C)	13
Levendag and Pomp	1990	63	86% (C)	6
Mendenhall et al.	1999	44	82% (C)	12
Wang	2000	54	81%—T1 79%—T2 53%—T3 (5 yr)	NS
Kummer et al.	2002	47	85% (C)	14
Langendijk et al.	2004	56	80% (2 yr)	12

C, crude; NS, not stated.
[a]Neck failure in patients who did not receive elective nodal irradiation.

TABLE 12.3
PATTERN OF FAILURE

Primary Site	Total No. of Patients	LR	RR	LR + DM	DM
After initial treatment					
Septum	14	2	2	0	0
Lateral wall and floor	31	9	0	1	2
After salvage treatment					
Septum	14	0	0	0	0
Lateral wall and floor	31	5	0	2	2

LR, local recurrence; RR, regional relapse; DM, distant metastases.
From Ang KK, Jiang GL, Frankenthaler RA, et al. Carcinomas of the nasal cavity. *Radiother Oncol* 1992;24:163, with permission.

TABLE 12.4
SURVIVAL RATES BY SITE OF PRIMARY DISEASE

Actuarial Rates	5 yr (%)	10 yr (%)	*P* value
Overall survival			
Septum	92	83	
Lateral wall and floor	67	49	0.03
Relapse-free survival			
Septum	69	69	
Lateral wall and floor	69	52	0.7
Disease-specific survival			
Septum	100	100	
Lateral wall and floor	76	71	0.04

From Ang KK, Jiang GL, Frankenthaler RA, et al. Carcinomas of the nasal cavity. *Radiother Oncol* 1992;24:163, with permission.

SUGGESTED READINGS

Ang KK, Jiang GL, Frankenthaler RA, et al. Carcinomas of the nasal cavity. *Radiother Oncol* 1992;24:163.

Bhattacharyya N. Cancer of the nasal cavity: survival and factors influencing prognosis. *Arch Otolaryngol Head Neck Surg* 2002;128:1079.

Chassagne D, Wilson JF. Brachytherapy of carcinomas of the nasal vestibule. *Int J Radiat Oncol Biol Phys* 1984;10:761.

Chobe R, McNeese M, Weber R, et al. Radiation therapy for carcinoma of the nasal vestibule. *Otolaryngol Head Neck Surg* 1988;98:67.

Fletcher GH, Goepfert H, Jesse RH. Nasal and paranasal sinus carcinoma. In: Fletcher GH, ed. *Textbook of radiotherapy*, 3rd ed. Philadelphia: Lea & Febiger, 1980.

Hawkins RB, Wynstra JH, Pilepich MV, et al. Carcinoma of the nasal cavity—results of primary and adjuvant radiotherapy. *Int J Radiat Oncol Biol Phys* 1988;15:1129.

Kummer E, Rasch CR, Keus RB, et al. T stage as prognostic factor in irradiated localized squamous cell carcinoma of the nasal vestibule. *Head Neck* 2002;24:268.

Langendijk JA, Poorter R, Leemans CR, et al. Radiotherapy of squamous cell carcinoma of the nasal vestibule. *Int J Radiat Oncol Biol Phys* 2004;59:1319.

LeLiever WC, Bailey BJ, Griffiths C. Carcinoma of the nasal septum. *Arch Otolaryngol* 1984;110:748.

Levendag PC, Pomp J. Radiation therapy of squamous cell carcinoma of the nasal vestibule. *Int J Radiat Oncol Biol Phys* 1990;19:1363.

Mazeron JJ, Chassagne D, Crook J, et al. Radiation therapy of carcinomas of the skin of nose and nasal vestibule: a report of 1676 cases by the Groupe Europeen de Curietherapie. *Radiother Oncol* 1988;13:165.

Mendenhall WM, Stringer SP, Cassisi NJ, et al. Squamous cell carcinoma of the nasal vestibule. *Head Neck* 1999;21:385.

Parsons JT, Mendenhall WM, Mancuso AA, et al. Malignant tumors of the nasal cavity and ethmoid and sphenoid sinuses. *Int J Radiat Oncol Biol Phys* 1988;14:11.

Schalekamp W, Hordijk GJ. Carcinoma of the nasal vestibule: prognostic factors in relation to lymph node metastasis. *Clin Otolaryngol* 1985;10:201.

Wong CS, Cummings BJ. The place of radiation therapy in the treatment of squamous cell carcinoma of the nasal vestibule. A review. *Acta Oncol* 1988;27:203.

Paranasal Sinuses

13

MAXILLARY SINUS

Treatment Strategy

Surgery alone is the preferred treatment of T1 tumors (uncommon). Postoperative radiotherapy is only indicated when the margin is close or positive. Surgery plus postoperative radiotherapy is the standard therapy for T2 to T4 tumors.

Patients with larger T3 and T4 tumors are occasionally selected for treatment with systemic therapy in an attempt to reduce the need for orbital exenteration. The response to chemotherapy determines the type of local-regional treatment. For complete or near-complete response, the treatment is radiotherapy with concurrent chemotherapy (uncommon), and for less than near-complete response, the treatment is surgery plus postoperative radiotherapy, with concurrent chemotherapy in case of the presence of positive margins or nodal disease with extracapsular extension.

Postoperative Radiotherapy

Target Volume

The initial target volume encompasses the entire surgical bed (see Figs. 13.1 and 13.2), ipsilateral levels IB and II (submandibular and subdigastric) nodes for patients with squamous cell or undifferentiated carcinoma with no clinical evidence of nodal involvement at diagnosis, or whole ipsilateral or bilateral neck for patients with N+ at diagnosis.

The boost volume encompasses areas of known disease with 1- to 2-cm margins.

Setup and Field Arrangement

An intraoral stent is used to open the mouth and depress the tongue. When surgical resection includes removal of the hard palate, the stent can be designed to hold a water-filled balloon to occlude the surgical defect (see Fig. 3.9). Orbital exenteration defect, if present, is filled directly with water-containing balloon (see Fig. 13.3) or other type of bolus material.

The patient is immobilized in a supine position with a slight hyperextension of the head to bring the floor of the orbit parallel to the axis of the anterior beam. This position allows delivery of the desired dose to the orbital floor without irradiating through a large volume of the ipsilateral eye.

Marking of lateral canthi, oral commissures, and external scar facilitates portal design. When there is no external scar (e.g., after craniofacial resection), a wire is placed on the premaxillary skin to indicate the slope of this structure. In addition, it is helpful to mark the position of the medial and inferior limbus with the eyes gazing forward for the purpose of corneal shielding. The location and size of the tumor determines the appropriate portal borders and arrangement.

For tumors of the **infrastructure with no extension into the orbit or ethmoids** (uncommon), anterior and ipsilateral wedge-pair (usually 45-degree wedges) photon fields are used (Fig. 13.1). The use of the "half-beam" technique (i.e., placing the isocenter at the level of the orbital floor and shielding of the upper half of the fields) prevents exposure of the contralateral eye by beam divergence.

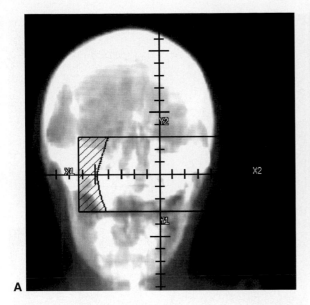

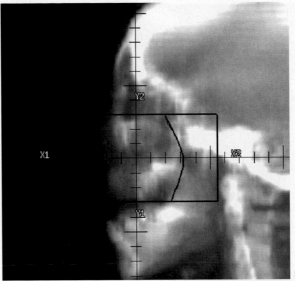

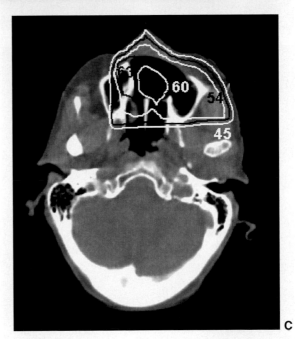

Figure 13.1 A 77-year-old woman presented with tingling of the left anterior maxillary gingiva. A mass in the gingiva was noted extending to the hard palate. Imaging studies revealed that the epicenter of the mass was in the inferior maxillary sinus, with extension to both the posterior wall and premaxillary soft tissue. She underwent an infrastructure maxillectomy. Histologic examination revealed grade-2 mucoepidermoid carcinoma. Postoperative radiation was delivered using anterior **(A)** and left lateral **(B)**, wedged-pair, portals with 45-degree wedges. The total dose was 60 Gy, with a serial reduction made at 54 Gy. An isodose distribution through the resected sinus is shown **(C)**.

Anterior portal borders:

- *Superior:* just above the floor of the orbit but below the cornea.
- *Lateral:* 1 cm beyond the lateral wall of the maxillary sinus (or falling off when there is tumor extension into the facial soft tissues).
- *Medial:* 1 to 2 cm across midline.
- *Inferior:* 1 cm below the floor of the maxillary sinus or below the surgical bed.

Lateral portal borders:

- *Superior and inferior:* same as the anterior portal.
- *Anterior:* in front of the anterior wall.
- *Posterior:* behind the pterygoid plates or more posteriorly depending on the extent of the contiguous tumor spread.

For tumors of the **infrastructure spreading across midline** through the hard palate, lateral-opposed photon fields are preferred. The use of the "half-beam" technique (i.e., placing the isocenter at the level of the orbital floor and shielding of the upper half of the fields) prevents exposure of the contralateral eye by beam divergence. The portal borders are similar to the lateral field described previously.

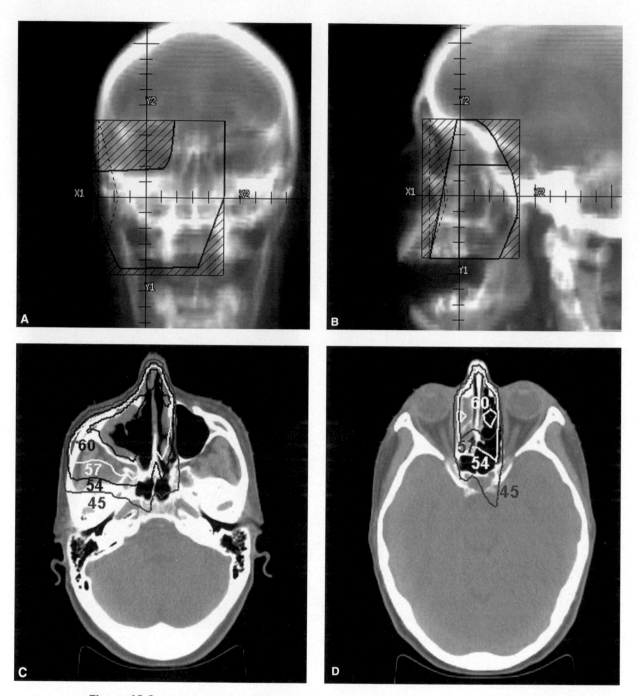

Figure 13.2   A 46-year-old woman was found to have a right nasal polyp, biopsy of which revealed neuroblastoma. Radiographic workup revealed the bulk of tumor in the medial wall of the right maxillary sinus. She underwent a medial maxillectomy and postoperative radiation. The radiation treatment was delivered through an anterior **(A)** and two lateral–opposed portals **(B)** with 6 MV photons. Sixty-degree wedges were used on the lateral fields with the heels oriented anterior. The loading of anterior to lateral-lateral was 1:0.07:0.07. The lateral fields were reduced after 40 Gy, and the total dose was 56 Gy specified at the 95% line. Representative isodose distributions through the maxillary sinus and between the orbits are shown **(C, D)**.

For tumors involving the **suprastructure or ethmoids**, a three-field technique is used (Figs. 13.2 and 13.3). An anterior portal is combined with right and left lateral fields. Loading varies from 1:0.15:0.15 to 1:0.07:0.07 depending on the tumor location and photon energy. The lateral fields have 60-degree wedges and can have a slight posterior tilt.

Anterior portal borders:

- *Superior:* above the crista galli to cover the ethmoids and, in the absence of orbital invasion, at the lower edge of the cornea to cover the orbital floor. When the orbit is involved, an attempt is

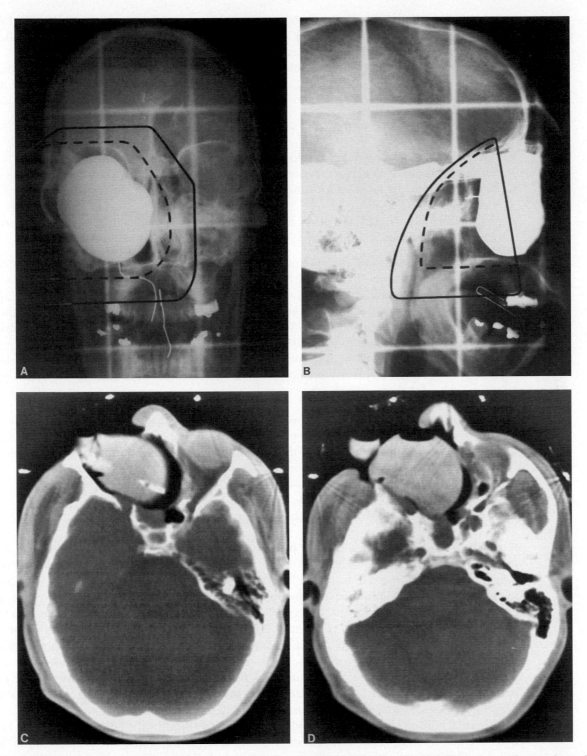

Figure 13.3 A 67-year-old man underwent a polypectomy from the right nasal cavity. Pathologic examination showed an inverted papilloma. Three years later he underwent a second polypectomy for recurrence. Pathologic examination revealed a small focus of carcinoma within inverted papilloma. Eight months after the second surgery this patient was referred to the M.D. Anderson Cancer Center for treatment of a large recurrence located in the right maxillary sinus, orbit, and infratemporal fossa. He underwent resection of this tumor with orbital exenteration. Pathologic examination revealed inverted papilloma with multiple foci of squamous cell carcinoma. The margins of resection contained papilloma but were free of invasive carcinoma. He received postoperative radiotherapy. The surgical bed was treated with an anterior **(A)** and right **(B)** and left lateral fields using 60Co beam loaded 1:0.15:0.15, respectively. A cork and tongue blade was used to depress the tongue. A water-filled balloon was placed in the surgical defect. The surgical scar, lateral orbital canthi, and oral commissures are indicated. The initial target volume received a dose of 50 Gy in 25 fractions, specified at the isocenter. Subsequently, the fields were reduced to administer a boost dose of 10 Gy in five fractions to the tumor bed. Computed tomography (CT) scan was obtained for treatment planning, which showed good filling of the surgical defect with the water-filled balloon **(C, D)**. This patient did well until 22 months later when a pedunculated lesion was noted in the right ethmoid remnant along with a firm area in the floor of the maxillary defect. Biopsy of both lesions revealed diffusely infiltrating inverting papilloma with focal squamous cell carcinomas.

made to shield the lacrimal gland whenever possible to avoid occurrence of dry, painful eye. Tumor extension into the frontal sinus or cranial fossa calls for more generous superior coverage.

■ *Inferior:* 1 cm below the floor of the maxillary sinus or below the surgical bed.
■ *Medial:* 1 to 2 cm, or farther, across midline to cover the contralateral ethmoidal extension.
■ *Lateral:* depends on the tumor extent (1 cm beyond lateral orbital wall when this structure is intact or falling off when there is tumor extension into facial soft tissues or infratemporal fossa).

Lateral portal borders:

■ *Superior:* follows the contour of the floor of the anterior cranial fossa.
■ *Inferior:* corresponds to that of anterior portal.
■ *Anterior:* behind the lateral bony canthus parallel to the slope of the face as marked by the wire.
■ *Posterior:* behind the pterygoid plates or more posteriorly, depending on the extent of the contiguous tumor spread and the surgery.

For boost volume, the portal size is reduced to encompass tumor bed and to exclude as much optic pathway as possible. The contralateral optic nerve and chiasm are excluded from the field after a dose of 54 Gy in 27 fractions. Sometimes, this requires two field reductions (i.e., after 50 Gy and 54 Gy, respectively). When the lesion abuts these structures, the benefits and risks of delivering a maximum dose of 60 Gy in 30 fractions, which carries a 5% to 10% risk of blindness resulting from nerve injury, are discussed with the patient.

For treatment of the **neck nodes,** ipsilateral upper neck irradiation is given to patients with squamous cell or undifferentiated carcinomas, stage T2 to T4 N0. This is accomplished through a lateral appositional electron field.

■ *Superior border:* sloping up from the horizontal ramus of the mandible anteriorly to match the inferior border of the primary portal posteriorly. This portal matching creates a small triangle over the cheek, which is irradiated with an abutting triangular, appositional electron field (6 MeV) when there is tumor extension into facial soft tissues.
■ *Anterior border:* just behind the oral commissures.
■ *Posterior border:* at the mastoid process.
■ *Inferior border:* at the thyroid notch (above the arytenoids).

Bilateral neck treatment is indicated in patients presenting with palpable node(s). Proper field matching technique should be selected in this setting to minimize dose heterogeneity, particularly to prevent overdosing in the depth by beam divergence. This can be accomplished by treating both the primary tumor bed and the upper neck with half-beam technique (shielding the caudal half of maxillary fields and the cephalad half of neck fields) to eliminate divergence and thereby prevent beam overlap. The central axis of the primary tumor portals and that of the opposed–lateral upper neck fields are placed at the axial plane of the inferior portal border of the maxillary fields (i.e., usually 1 cm below the floor of the maxillary sinus). It is prudent to move the junction line between the primary and neck fields during the course of treatment. The mid and lower neck is irradiated with an anterior appositional photon field matched to the inferior border of opposed–lateral upper neck fields (see "General Principles").

The portal borders of the maxillary fields are as defined previously. The borders of the upper neck fields are determined by the extent of the nodal disease. If the initial lateral fields are on the spinal cord, portal reduction is made after approximately 45 Gy. The posterior cervical areas are then irradiated to the desired dose with abutting electron fields.

Intensity-Modulated Radiation Therapy Planning

The complex anatomy of the paranasal sinuses makes it appealing to use high-precision conformal radiotherapy for the treatment of sinonasal tumors to reduce normal tissue toxicity without compromising the dose to the tumor bed. Intensity-modulated radiation generally yields better dose distribution for these tumors (see Figs. 13.4 and 13.5).

The patient is immobilized in a supine position with an extended head and shoulder thermoplastic mask. Thin-cut computed tomography (CT) scans are obtained in treatment position. The clinical target volume (CTV) and planning target volume are outlined for dosimetric planning.

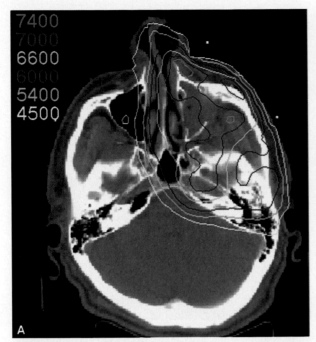

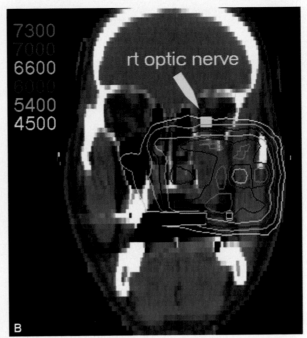

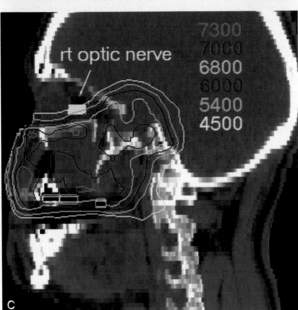

Figure 13.4 A 46-year-old man presented with maxillary tooth pain and numbness of the left palate and cheek. A left maxillary sinus mass was found, and a Caldwell-Luc procedure was performed. The tissue obtained was positive for sarcomatoid carcinoma. Magnetic resonance imaging revealed the maxillary sinus mass with perineural invasion through foramen rotundum extending to the cavernous sinus. He was treated with concurrent cisplatin (100 mg per m² given every 3 weeks) and radiation. Given the tumor shape, radiation was given with intensity-modulated radiation therapy (IMRT). A dose of 70 Gy in 35 fractions was prescribed to a clinical target volume (CTV) consisting of the gross disease and margin. The 66 Gy isodose line encompassed the entire volume at risk. Axial, coronal, and sagittal isodose distributions through the sinus are shown **(A, B, C)**. The left upper neck received 50 Gy in 25 fractions through a matching 12-MeV electron field. Postradiation imaging revealed residual abnormality in the maxillary sinus. A maxillectomy was performed revealing squamous cell carcinoma with extensive degenerative changes. The nerve specimens did not contain tumor. Three months after surgery, osteoradionecrosis of the anterior maxilla and palate developed. He was treated with hyperbaric oxygen and sequestrectomy. The patient remains without evidence of disease 2 years after treatment.

The high-risk target volume (CTV1) represents the original extent of disease with at least 1-cm margins. CTV1 includes at least the entire sinus, the nasal septum, and 1 cm of palate beyond the surgical defect. It also includes the pterygomaxillary space for posterior tumors. Although individualized, the lateral border often includes the masticator space beyond the sinus. The anterior border is just underneath the skin surface and bolus may be used when there is skin involvement. For squamous cell and undifferentiated carcinomas, subclinical target (CTV2) often includes ipsilateral or bilateral lymphatic pathways at the buccal tissues, facial nodes, and levels IB and II nodes.

Dose

Primary tumor bed: 50 Gy in 25 fractions to the initial target volume plus 10 Gy in five fractions (negative margins) to 16 Gy per eight fractions (positive margins) to the boost volume.

Elective nodal irradiation: 50 Gy in 25 fractions.

Involved nodal regions (particularly in the presence of extracapsular nodal disease): 60 to 66 Gy in 30 to 33 fractions.

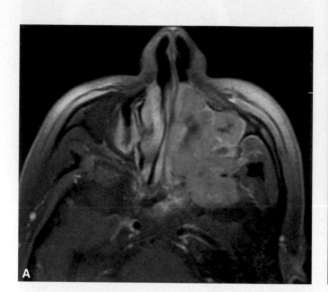
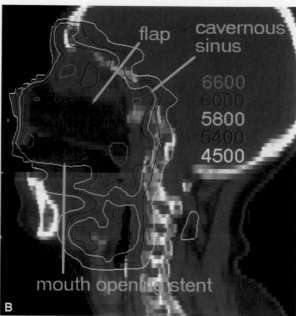

Figure 13.5   A 55-year-old woman who presented with loose maxillary teeth, decreased sensation of the left cheek, and visual changes was found to have a large left maxillary sinus mass as seen on an axial MRI image **(A)**. A biopsy revealed high-grade mucoepidermoid carcinoma. Tumor invaded the anterior and middle cranial fossa. She underwent left maxillectomy, orbital exenteration, and craniofacial resection, removing disease extension to the base of the anterior and middle skull. The resection margin was positive at the cavernous sinus. The operative bed was repaired with a rectus abdominus flap. She received postoperative intensity-modulated radiation therapy (IMRT). A sagittal dose distribution **(B)** is shown through the orbit filled with the flap. A dose of 60 Gy was delivered in 30 fractions. The ipsilateral levels IB and II nodes received 54 Gy in 30 fractions. A stereotactic boost (6 Gy in three fractions) was delivered to the left cavernous sinus. She remained without local disease, but developed bone metastases 1 year after therapy.

IMRT: 60 Gy to the primary tumor bed and 54 to 57 Gy to surgical bed in 30 fractions. In case of close or positive margins, a small volume that is delineated within CTV1 receives 66 Gy in 30 fractions (2.2 Gy per fraction). Therefore, the fraction size varies from 2.0 to 2.2 Gy to the tumor bed to 1.8 to 1.9 Gy to the surgical bed.

Instructing the patients to open the eye during irradiation to take advantage of photon dose buildup characteristics can minimize the dose to the cornea. The dose to the macula, optic nerve, and chiasm is limited to 54 Gy or less whenever possible to minimize the risk of blindness.

Dose Specification

For the primary tumor bed, specification is at an isodose line with dose heterogeneity of no more than ±5%. A planning CT scan is obtained and loading, wedges, and field margins are adjusted when necessary or for conformal radiation planning.

For the neck, see "General Principles."

Primary Radiotherapy

The radiation techniques are the same as those in the postoperative radiotherapy setting. Portal borders are determined by radiologically demonstrable tumor extent. The dose is 50 Gy in 25 fractions to the initial target volume plus 16 to 20 Gy in eight to ten fractions to the boost volume.

Intensity-Modulated Radiation Therapy Planning

A high dose CTV1 includes the gross tumor volume (GTV) with 1-cm margin and the entire sinus. The CTV2 adds additional margin and covers potential routes of extension dependent on the tumor location. For locally advanced disease, this often includes the ethmoids, nasal cavity, pterygomaxillary and masticator spaces, and sufficient margin on the hard palate. For tumor involving the suprastructure, it may be necessary to encompass the floor and/or medial wall of the orbit including portions of the globe. IMRT generally provides better dose distribution to the target volumes while sparing the optic structures.

A dose of 70 Gy is prescribed to CTV1 and 57 to 63 Gy to CTV2. The nodal volumes are the same as in the postoperative setting. The fraction number ranges from 33 to 35 and is usually determined by the volume of central nervous system (CNS) adjacent to the target encompassed in the high dose regions. It is desirable to keep the fraction size to the CNS below 2 Gy.

ETHMOID SINUSES

Treatment Strategy

Till recently, most patients have been treated with surgery and postoperative radiotherapy. Combination of chemotherapy and radiation has been used in select cases for organ preservation (see Fig. 13.6).

Postoperative Radiotherapy

The radiation techniques are the same as those for carcinoma of the suprastructure of the maxillary sinus (see Fig. 13.7). In the event of a craniofacial resection, no attempt is made to cover the incision site along the scalp.

The total dose usually does not exceed 54 Gy without detailed consent from the patient because it is extremely difficult to exclude optic nerves from the target volume because of the proximity. IMRT may occasionally provide better dose distribution in this setting. The dose to the chiasm may exceed 54 Gy if necessary for target coverage, again, provided a detailed consent is obtained from the patient. The fundamentals for target definition are similar to those applied for tumors of suprastructure.

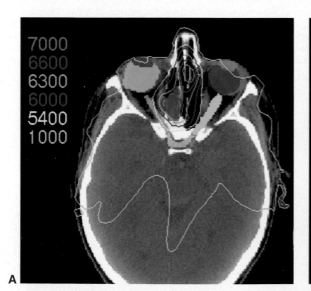
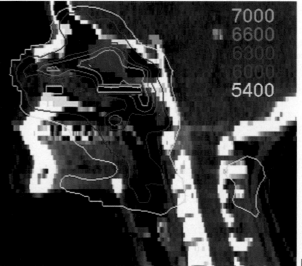

Figure 13.6 A 43-year-old woman presented with right periorbital pain and nasal obstruction. She underwent bilateral endoscopic surgery, and a mass removed from the right nasal cavity and ethmoids was positive for sinonasal-undifferentiated carcinoma. Magnetic resonance imaging revealed residual disease in the right nasoethmoidal region with extension to the nasopharynx. She was treated with three cycles of cisplatin and etoposide, with a partial response. This was followed by intensity-modulated radiation therapy (IMRT) using nine fields and dynamic multileaf collimation. The gross residual tumor received 70 Gy, the prechemotherapy volume received 60 Gy, and bilateral upper neck nodes received 56 Gy. Axial and sagittal isodose distributions are seen in **(A, B)**. The residual tumor and prechemotherapy tumor (*bright red* and *pale red*) and optic pathways (*yellow* for chiasm) are shown. Concurrent cisplatin was administered every 3 weeks. Posttreatment imaging revealed a residual mass. Therefore, a resection was performed. Histologic examination revealed fibrotic tissue only. She developed a solitary larynx metastasis 2 years later and received radiation and chemotherapy to the larynx only. She is without disease, 4 years from her initial diagnosis.

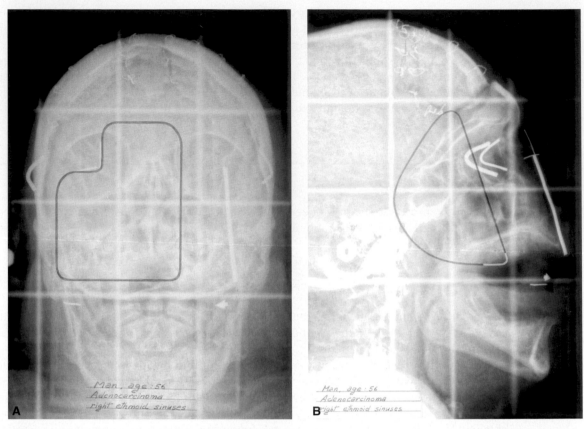

Figure 13.7 A 56-year-old man sought medical attention because of nasal stuffiness and pressure discomfort below the right eye. A polypoid mass was removed from the right nasal cavity, which was diagnosed as adenocarcinoma. CT scan revealed a tumor in the right ethmoid sinuses and upper part of the right nasal cavity. The floor of the right orbit was involved. The tumor was resected through a craniofacial approach. The right antrum and sphenoid sinus were inspected and found free of gross disease, but the mucosal lining was removed. Pathologic examination revealed an adenocarcinoma at the ethmoid sinuses spreading to the mucosa of the nasal septum. The patient received postoperative radiotherapy. The surgical bed was treated with an anterior field **(A)** and right **(B)** and left lateral fields using 6 MV photons. The lateral orbital canthi, external auditory canals, oral commissures, and position of the cornea of the right eye were marked at simulation. The thick, straight wire indicated the slope of the face. A dose of 56 Gy was delivered to the isocenter in 28 fractions.

Background Data

TABLE 13.1

INFLUENCE OF DISEASE AND THERAPY VARIABLES ON THE TREATMENT OUTCOME

Variables	No. of Patients	Local 5-yr Control (%)	Regional 5-yr Control (%)
Pathologic T stage[a]			
T1 + T2	12	91	71
T3	28	77	80
T4	29	65	93
N stage			
N0	67[b]	74	84
N1–N2	6	67	82
Histologic findings			
Squamous cell carcinoma	36	62	86

(continued)

TABLE 13.1
(continued)

Undifferentiated	9	89	67
Adenocarcinoma	6	80	67
Adenoid cystic carcinoma	20	82	94
Mucoepidermoid	2	(2/2)	(2/2)
Nerve invasion[a]			
No	29	90[c]	86
Yes	42	64	80
Margin of resection[a]			
Negative	54	74	86
Positive	17	77	76
Elective nodal treatment	50	77	80

[a]Excluding patients whose pathologic reports were not complete.
[b]Including 11 patients, who did not receive elective neck treatment, and developed nodal recurrence.
[c]Significant at 0.05 level.
From Jiang GL, Ang KK, Peters LJ, et al. Maxillary sinus carcinomas: natural history and results of postoperative radiotherapy. *Radiother Oncol* 1991;21:193, with permission.

TABLE 13.2
INFLUENCE OF DISEASE AND THERAPY VARIABLES ON THE TREATMENT OUTCOME

Variables	Incidence of DM at 5 yr (%)	5-yr RFS (%)	5-yr DSS (%)
Pathologic T stage[a]			
T1 + 2	17	64	75
T3	25	57	69
T4	37	44	59
N stage			
N0	27[b]	53	66[b]
N1–2	48[c]	33	33
Histologic findings			
Squamous cell carcinoma	17[b]	49	53
Undifferentiated	50	53	42
Adenocarcinoma	39	42	60
Adenoid cystic carcinoma	31	60	84
Mucoepidermoid	(0/2)	(2/2)	(2/2)
Nerve invasion[a]			
No	20	74[b]	78
Yes	36	37	57
Margin of resection[a]			
Negative	17	58	66
Positive	32	38	66
Elective nodal treatment	—	51	58

DM, distant metastasis; RFS, relapse-free survival; DSS, disease-specific survival.
[a]Excluding patients whose pathologic reports were not complete.
[b]Significant at 0.05 level.
[c]Including 11 patients, who did not receive elective neck treatment, and in whom nodal recurrence developed.
From Jiang GL, Ang KK, Peters LJ, et al. Maxillary sinus carcinomas: natural history and results of postoperative radiotherapy. *Radiother Oncol* 1991;21:193, with permission.

CANCER OF THE PARANASAL SINUSES AND NASAL CAVITIES TREATED BY RADIOTHERAPY AND SURGERY OR BY RADIOTHERAPY ALONE: 5-YEAR DETERMINATE SURVIVAL RATE ACCORDING TO HISTOLOGIC AND SITE FINDINGS

Site	Antrum	Ethmoid Frontal Sphenoid	Antroethmoid	Total Sinuses	Nasal Cavities
Squamous carcinoma					
Number	103	27	18	148	50
Survival	22%	22%	28%	24%	58%
Undifferentiated carcinoma					
Number	36	28	15	79	13
Survival	14%	36%	20%	23%	23%
Adenocarcinoma					
Number	8	18	7	33	7
Survival	12%	28%	43%	27%	29%
Adenoid cystic carcinoma					
Number	13	6	6	25	5
Survival	31%	1/6	4/6	36%	3/5
Transitional cell carcinoma					
Number	14	17	18	49	12
Survival	39%	77%	39%	51%	75%
Malignant melanoma					
Number	3	6	4	13	26
Survival	0%	18%	25%	15%	35%

Modified from McNicoll W, Hopkin N, Dalley VM, et al. Cancer of the paranasal sinuses and nasal cavities. Part II. Results of treatment. *J Laryngol Otol* 1984;98:707, with permission.

INFLUENCE OF DISEASE AND THERAPY VARIABLES ON THE TREATMENT OUTCOME OF 34 PATIENTS IRRADIATED FOR CARCINOMA OF THE ETHMOID SINUSES

Variables	No. of Patients	5-yr Actuarial Local Control (%)	5-yr Actuarial Disease-Specific Survival (%)
T stage			
T1	6	100	100
T2	13	79	62
T3	15	53	51
Dura invasion[a]			
No	13	100	83
Yes	5	30	40
Histologic findings[b]			
Undifferentiated carcinoma	12	82	72
Squamous cell carcinoma	8	53	70
Adenoid cystic and adenocarcinoma	13	73	50
Local treatment			
Surgery + radiation	21	74	68
Radiation alone	13	64	56
Chemotherapy			
No	25	80	62
Yes	9	50	67

[a]Patients treated with postoperative irradiation only.
[b]Excludes one patient with transitional cell carcinoma.
Modified from Jiang GL, Morrison WH, Garden AS, et al. Ethmoid sinus carcinomas: natural history and treatment results. *Radiother Oncol* 1998;49:21–27, with permission.

TABLE 13.5

PATTERNS OF FAILURE IN PATIENTS WITH SINONASAL CARCINOMAS WITH NEUROENDOCRINE DIFFERENTIATION

Histology	Patient No.	Local Failure[a] (%)	Regional Failure[a] (%)	Distant Failure[a] (%)
Esthesioneuroblastoma	31	4	9	0
Neuroendocrine carcinoma	18	27	13	12
Sinonasal-undifferentiated carcinoma	16	21	16	25
Small cell carcinoma	7	33	44	75

[a]5-yr actuarial rates
Data from the M.D. Anderson Cancer Center.
Modified from Rosenthal DI, Barker JL Jr, El-Naggar AK, et al. Sinonasal malignancies with neuroendocrine differentiation: patterns of failure according to histologic phenotype. *Cancer* 2004;101:2567, with permission.

SUGGESTED READINGS

Beale FA, Garrett PG. Cancer of the paranasal sinuses with particular reference to maxillary sinus cancer. *J Otolaryngol* 1983;12:377.

Claus F, De Gersem W, De Wagter C, et al. An implementation strategy for IMRT of ethmoid sinus cancer with bilateral sparing of the optic pathways. *Int J Radiat Oncol Biol Phys* 2001;51:318.

Fletcher GH, Goepfert H, Jesse RH. Nasal and paranasal sinus carcinoma. In: Fletcher GH, ed. *Textbook of radiotherapy*, 3rd ed. Philadelphia: Lea & Febiger, 1980.

Jesse RH, Goepfert H, Lindberg RD. Carcinoma of the sinuses: a review of treatment. In: Chambers RG, Janssen de Limpens AM, Jaques DA et al., eds. *Cancer of the head and neck*. Amsterdam: Excerpta Medica, 1975.

Jiang GL, Ang KK, Peters LJ, et al. Maxillary sinus carcinomas: natural history and results of postoperative radiotherapy. *Radiother Oncol* 1991;21:193.

Jiang GL, Morrison WH, Garden AS, et al. Ethmoid sinus carcinomas: natural history and treatment results. *Radiother Oncol* 1998;49:21.

Klintenberg C, Olofsson J, Hellquist H, et al. Adenocarcinoma of the ethmoid sinuses. A review of 28 cases with special reference to wood dust exposure. *Cancer* 1984;54:482.

Knegt PP, de Jong PC, van Ander JG, et al. Carcinoma of the paranasal sinuses. Results of a prospective pilot study. *Cancer* 1985;56:57.

Le QT, Fu KK, Kaplan M, et al. Treatment of maxillary sinus carcinoma: a comparison of the 1997 and 1977 American Joint Committee on cancer staging systems. *Cancer* 1999;86:1700.

Le QT, Fu KK, Kaplan MJ, et al. Lymph node metastasis in maxillary sinus carcinoma. *Int J Radiat Oncol Biol Phys* 2000;46:541.

Logue JP, Slevin NJ. Carcinoma of the nasal cavity and paranasal sinuses: an analysis of radical radiotherapy. *Clin Oncol* 1991;3:84.

McNicoll W, Hopkin N, Dalley VM, et al. Cancer of the paranasal sinuses and nasal cavities. Part II. Results of treatment. *J Laryngol Otol* 1984;98:707.

Mock U, Georg D, Bogner J, et al. Treatment planning comparison of conventional, 3D conformal and intensity-modulated photon (IMRT) and proton therapy for paranasal sinus carcinoma. *Int J Radiat Oncol Biol Phys* 2004;58:147.

Papadimitrakopoulou VA, Ginsberg LE, Garden AS, et al. Intrarterial cisplatin with intravenous paclitaxel and ifosfamide as an organ-preservation approach in patients with paranasal sinus carcinoma. *Cancer* 2003;98:2214.

Parsons JT, Stringer SP, Mancuso AA, et al. Nasal vestibule, nasal cavity and paranasal sinuses. In: Million RR, Cassisi NJ, eds. *Management of head and neck cancer: a multidisciplinary approach*, 2nd ed. Philadelphia: JB Lippincott Co, 1994.

Paulino AC, Fisher SG, Marks JE. Is prophylactic neck irradiation indicated in patients with squamous cell carcinoma of the maxillary sinus? *Int J Radiat Oncol Biol Phys* 1997;39:283.

Paulino AC, Marks JE, Bricker P, et al. Results of treatment of patients with maxillary sinus carcinoma. *Cancer* 1998;83:457.

Pommier P, Ginestet C, Sunyach M, et al. Conformal radiotherapy for paranasal sinus and nasal cavity tumors: three-dimensional treatment planning and preliminary results in 40 patients. *Int J Radiat Oncol Biol Phys* 2000;48:485.

Roa WHY, Hazuka MB, Sandler HM, et al. Results of primary and adjuvant CT-based 3-dimensional radiotherapy for malignant tumors of the maxillary sinus. *Int J Radiat Oncol Biol Phys* 1994;28:857.

Robin PE, Powell DJ. Treatment of carcinoma of the nasal cavity and paranasal sinuses. *Clin Otolaryngol* 1981;6:401.

Rosenthal DI, Barker JL Jr, El-Naggar AK, et al. Sinonasal malignancies with neuroendocrine differentiation: patterns of failure according to histologic phenotype. *Cancer* 2004;101:2567.

Sakai S, Hohki A, Fuchihata H, et al. Multidisciplinary treatment of maxillary sinus carcinoma. *Cancer* 1983;52:1360.

Sato Y, Morita M, Takahashi H, et al. Combined surgery, radiotherapy, and regional chemotherapy in carcinoma of the paranasal sinuses. *Cancer* 1970;25:571.

Shibuya H, Horiuchi J, Suzuki S, et al. Maxillary sinus carcinoma: result of radiation therapy. *Int J Radiat Oncol Biol Phys* 1984;10:1021.

Tsien C, Eisbruch A, McShan D, et al. Intensity-modulated radiation therapy (IMRT) for locally advanced paranasal sinus tumors: incorporating clinical decisions in the optimization process. *Int J Radiat Oncol Biol Phys* 2003;55:776.

Waldron JN, O'Sullivan B, Gullane P, et al. Carcinoma of the maxillary antrum: a retrospective analysis of 110 cases. *Radiother Oncol* 2000;57:167.

Waldron JN, O'Sullivan B, Warde P, et al. Ethmoid sinus cancer: twenty-nine cases managed with primary radiation therapy. *Int J Radiat Oncol Biol Phys* 1998;41:361.

Salivary Glands

14

PAROTID

Treatment Strategy

Surgery is the preferred treatment for operable cases. Postoperative radiotherapy is indicated in the following clinical settings: high-grade tumors (mucoepidermoid carcinomas, malignant mixed tumors, adenocarcinomas, and squamous cell carcinomas); close or positive surgical margins (including incompletely resected recurrent pleomorphic adenoma); tumor adherence to or invasion of the facial nerve, or presence of histologic evidence of perineural spread; bone and/or connective tissue involvement; lymph node metastases (particularly with extracapsular extension); or after resection of recurrent disease even with negative margins.

Postoperative Radiotherapy

Target Volume
Initial Target Volume
The volume for benign tumors and low-grade tumors without lymph node involvement is the parotid bed only. For high-grade tumors and tumors with lymph node involvement, the volume encompasses the parotid bed and ipsilateral neck. For gross invasion of the facial nerve, more generous coverage of facial canal to geniculate ganglion is desired.

The boost volume encompasses the tumor bed and involved nodal bed.

Setup and Field Arrangement
Target volume 5 cm or less deep (superficial lobe and deep lobe in thin patients) (see Figs. 14.1 and 14.2).

An intraoral stent containing cerrobend is used to shield the posterior oral tongue (see Fig. 3.4).

Marking of the surgical scar and lateral canthus of the ipsilateral orbit facilitates portal design.

Patient is immobilized in an open neck position with a thermoplastic mask. Flattening of the ipsilateral ear against the mastoid process minimizes dose heterogeneity resulting from electron perturbation. For the same reason, the external auditory canal is filled with Domeboro fluid prior to each electron treatment.

Bolus is used to cover the superior aspect of the portal when it extends above the zygomatic arch to minimize the dose to the temporal lobe of the brain.

A lateral appositional field is used to cover the parotid bed and upper neck nodes. Radiation is delivered with a combination of electrons (16 to 20 MeV depending on the depth) and photons (6 MV) usually in the ratio of 4:1.

Portal borders are as follows:

- *Superior:* zygomatic arch or higher as indicated by tumor extent or surgical scar.
- *Anterior:* anterior edge of the masseter muscle.
- *Inferior:* thyroid notch.
- *Posterior:* just behind the mastoid process.

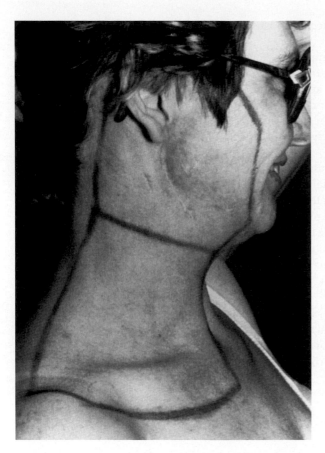

Figure 14.1 A 39-year-old woman presented with a 4-month history of a right parotid swelling. She underwent a surgical exploration, which revealed a large mass extending from the base of skull to the subdigastric muscle inferiorly. This lesion was dissected off the facial nerve and removed in two major pieces. Pathologic examination showed a pleomorphic adenoma. Five months later she presented with a recurrent nodule in the upper posterior cervical region. This was excised and was also found to contain pleomorphic adenoma. Four months after the second intervention, a small mass developed at the posterior auricular region. Fine needle aspiration showed carcinoma. She was then referred to M.D. Anderson Cancer Center. Review of the slides revealed carcinoma ex-pleomorphic adenoma in the specimens of the first and second surgical procedures. Physical examination upon referral revealed no palpable gross disease and an intact facial nerve. It was decided to deliver postoperative radiotherapy to the parotid bed and upper neck with a lateral appositional field using a combination of electrons and photons (20 MeV and 6 MV, respectively). An intraoral stent was used to protect the mucosa of the oral tongue and contralateral oral cavity. The mid and lower neck nodes on the ipsilateral side were treated with a separate electron field. The tumor bed received a dose of 60 Gy in 30 fractions prescribed to the 90% isodose line and the mid and lower neck prescribed a dose of 50 Gy in 25 fractions.

Off-cord reduction is made after reaching a dose of approximately 44 Gy and the posterior strip is supplemented with lower energy electrons (usually 9 MeV).

Field reduction takes place after 50 to 54 Gy in 25 to 27 fractions to deliver the boost dose when indicated. If the anterior edge of the portal is close to the eye, skin collimation is applied

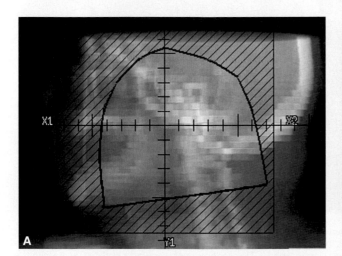

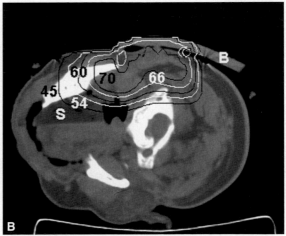

Figure 14.2 This 66-year-old man presented with a 2-cm left preauricular mass. Radiographic imaging revealed a mass in the superficial lobe of the left parotid gland. He underwent a superficial parotidectomy and upper neck dissection. Histologic examination revealed an adenoid cystic carcinoma with positive anterior and deep margins but none of five lymph-nodes harbored metastases. The patient was irradiated postoperatively in the open neck position. A tongue displacing stent (*S*) was used, and bolus material (*B*) applied to modulate the depth of the electron range. An initial 50 Gy was delivered to the parotid bed and upper neck **(A)** with a 4:1 mix of 16 MeV electrons and 6 MV photons. A boost of 16 Gy to the high-risk area was delivered with 12 MeV electrons. A representative axial isodose distribution is shown in **(B)**.

and the beam may be angled 5 to 10 degrees posteriorly to minimize the dose to the orbital content.

A 1.5- to 2-cm bevelled bolus or a computer-generated custom bolus is placed at the superior part of the portal (above the line connecting the orbital floor and the mastoid process) to reduce the dose to the temporal lobe. A lateral appositional electron field is used to treat the mid and lower neck nodes when indicated (for borders of neck field, see "General Principles").

For more deep-seated tumors or when facial canal is part of the target volume, a wedge-pair technique (see Figs. 14.3 and 14.4) or intensity-modulated radiation therapy (IMRT) (see Fig. 14.5) with photon beams are often preferable.

With these techniques, the patient is immobilized in a supine position with the head hyperextended with thermoplastic mask. The axial plane of the fields is chosen so that the posterolateral portal does not exit through the contralateral eye. A relatively simple wedge-pair technique uses anterolateral and posterolateral oblique photon fields (the anterolateral oblique field is on the spinal cord and the posterolateral oblique field is off cord). The simulation focuses on marking of the surgical scar and both inferior orbital rims and selection of provisional isocenter. The provisional isocenter is generally placed at the center of the square defined by the zygomatic arch, anterior edge of the masseter, thyroid notch, and mastoid, and halfway between the skin and the oropharyngeal wall.

Thin-slice computed tomography (CT) scan is obtained in the treatment position for outlining the target volume and planning the portal sizes, hinge angle, and thickness of wedges using treatment planning system. No off–spinal cord reduction is required with a wedged-pair technique because the posterolateral field is off the cord from the beginning. Field reduction for boost dose, when indicated, occurs after 50 to 54 Gy.

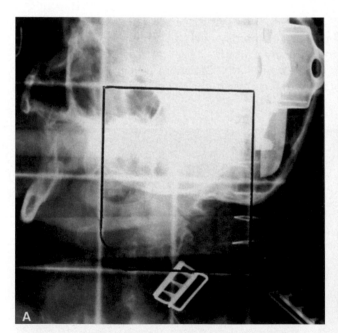
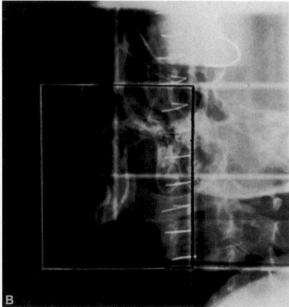

Figure 14.3 A 46-year-old woman presented with a 1-year history of intermittent left facial swelling and left parietal headache. Physical examination of the parotid region and other head and neck areas was unremarkable. The facial nerve was intact. A computed tomography (CT) scan, however, showed a soft-tissue mass in the deep lobe of the parotid. The patient underwent a total parotidectomy with sparing of the facial nerve. The tumor was removed from beneath the facial nerve with some difficulty. Pathologic studies revealed pleomorphic adenoma measuring 3.5 × 3 × 2.5 cm. The deep margin of resection was positive. Two intraparotid lymph nodes and 16 periparotid nodes, removed to gain access to the parotid, were all free of tumor. It was decided to treat this patient with postoperative radiotherapy because of difficult and incomplete resection. The target volume extended to 6 cm from the surface, which was too deep for the highest available electron energy (20 MeV). Therefore, it was elected to treat with wedge-pair fields. A total dose of 50 Gy was delivered to the 95%-isodose line in 25 fractions.

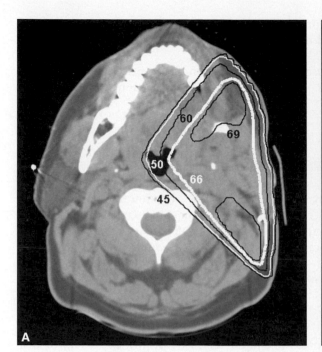
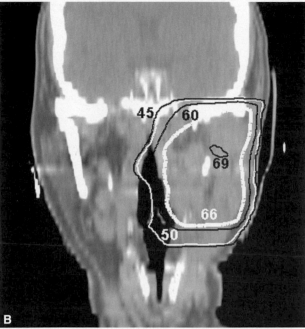

Figure 14.4   A 46-year-old man presented with a left parotid mass associated with facial pain and facial palsy. Magnetic resonance imaging (MRI) showed a mass occupying most of the superficial lobe and extending into the deep lobe, measuring 5 cm in greatest dimension. He underwent a resection of the mass consisting of left total parotidectomy, left parapharyngeal space dissection, left upper neck dissection, and left segmental mandibulectomy. Histopathologic evaluation of resected tumor showed adenoid cystic carcinoma, 5.5 × 4.0 × 3.0 cm, extending to the surgical margin, cribriform, grade 2. None of 11 lymph nodes contained metastatic deposits. The patient was irradiated postoperatively with a left anterior oblique and left posterior oblique pair of portals with 60-degree wedges. This was chosen because of the disease deep in the dissected parapharyngeal space. A field reduction was made at 50 Gy. The total dose was 66 Gy in 33 fractions. Axial and coronal isodose distributions are shown in **(A, B)**. The patient remains free of disease 30 months from diagnosis.

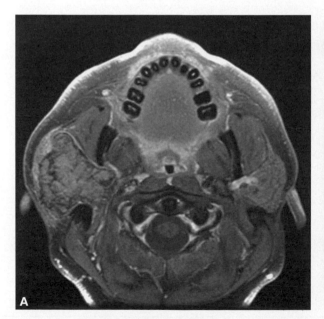
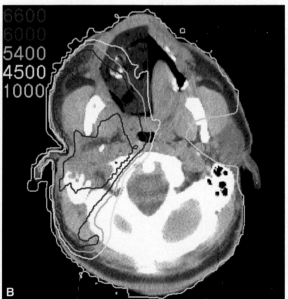

Figure 14.5   A 31-year-old man presented with a slow-growing right parotid mass. A magnetic resonance imaging (MRI) **(A)** revealed the right parotid mass, involving the deep lobe and abutting the mastoid. He underwent a total parotidectomy with facial nerve sparing, partial mastoidectomy, and lateral skull base dissection. Histologic examination revealed acinic cell carcinoma, with tumor at the margins. He received postoperative radiotherapy using intensity-modulated radiation therapy (IMRT) to conform better to the postoperative bed, including the resected temporal bone. An axial isodose distribution **(B)** is shown at approximately the same level as the preoperative MRI image **(A)**. Postoperative changes including the partial mastoidectomy are evident. A total dose of 60 Gy was delivered in 30 fractions. Note the oral cavity has a tongue-displacing stent, and the high-dose isodose lines encompass the stent rather than the tongue.

With IMRT, target volumes to receive different doses are delineated as outlined in previous chapters. Treatment is delivered in a fixed number of fractions and higher-risk regions receive a higher dose per fraction.

A matching anterior photon portal is used to treat the mid and lower neck nodes when indicated (for borders, see "General Principles"). In this case, a half-beam matching technique might be preferable.

Dose

For benign and low-grade tumors with negative section margins, a dose of 50 to 54 Gy in 25 to 27 fractions is prescribed.

For high-grade tumors and those with lymph node metastases, the commonly prescribed dose is 60 Gy in 30 fractions after complete resection or 64 to 66 Gy in 32 to 33 fractions in the presence of positive margin or extracapsular tumor extension (ECE). Off cord reduction, with ipsilateral electron–photon technique, takes place at approximately 44 Gy and field reduction after 50 to 54 Gy.

For elective neck irradiation, a dose of 50 Gy in 25 fractions is prescribed.

Dose Specification

For lateral appositional field, the dose is prescribed at the 90%-isodose line. The energy of electrons is chosen according to the depth of the tumor bed.

For wedge-pair technique or IMRT, the dose is prescribed at the isodose line encompassing the target volume.

Background Data

TABLE 14.1
HISTOLOGIC DISTRIBUTION OF SALIVARY NEOPLASMS BY SITE

Site	Benign	Mucoepi-dermoid	Adenoid Cystic	Adenocar-cinoma	MMT	Acinic	Epidermoid	Anaplastic
Parotid	1,342	272	54	62	107	75	45	8
Submandibular	106	37	45	9	24	2	8	—
Palate	60	37	67	41	18	1	—	4
Lip/cheek	13	23	12	20	2	3	—	—
Antrum	—	13	31	23	3	1	—	1
Tongue	2	14	30	12	2	—	—	3
Nasal cavity	4	12	17	23	—	1	—	3
Gingiva	—	13	10	6	3	1	—	1
Floor of mouth	1	6	7	8	—	—	—	—
Larynx	—	3	3	7	—	—	—	8[a]
Tonsil	—	4	3	3	1	—	—	2
Ethmoid	—	1	1	6	—	—	—	1
Nasopharynx	—	2	1	5	1	—	—	—
Pharyngeal wall	1	2	—	—	—	—	—	—

MMT, malignant mixed tumor.
[a]All neuroendocrine carcinomas.
From Spiro RH. Salivary neoplasms: overview of a 35-year experience with 2,807 patients. *Head Neck Surg* 1986;8:177–184, with permission.

TABLE 14.2

LOCAL FAILURE OF ADENOID CYSTIC CARCINOMAS TREATED WITH SURGERY AND POST-OPERATIVE IRRADIATION STRATIFIED BY POSITIVE MARGINS AND NAMED NERVE INVOLVEMENT

Site	No. of Failures/ No. of Patients (%)	No. of Failures/No. of Patients with Positive Margins (%)	No. of Failures/No. of Patients with Named Nerve Involvement (%)
Minor salivary gland	16/122 (13)	10/54 (19)	5/31 (16)
Submandibular /sublingual gland	1/41 (2)	1/11 (9)	1/14 (7)
Parotid gland	4/30 (13)	3/15 (20)	4/10 (40)
All patients	21/193 (11)	14/80 (18)	10/55 (18)

Data from the M.D. Anderson Cancer Center.
Modified from Garden AS, Weber RS, Morrison WH, et al. The influence of positive margins and nerve invasion in adenoid cystic carcinoma of the head and neck treated with surgery and radiation. *Int J Radiat Oncol Biol Phys* 1995;32:619, with permission.

TABLE 14.3

FIVE-YEAR ACTUARIAL LOCAL–REGIONAL CONTROL OF ADENOID CYSTIC CARCINOMAS TREATED WITH NEUTRON THERAPY

Site	No. of Patients	Local–Regional Control (%)
Paranasal sinus	32	43
Oral cavity	26	68
Oropharynx	19	75
Nasopharynx	15	21
Submandibular-sublingual gland	15	59
Parotid	27	67

Modified from Douglas JG, Laramore GE, Austin-Seymour M, et al. Treatment of locally advanced adenoid cystic carcinoma of the head and neck with neutron radiotherapy. *Int J Radiat Oncol Biol Phys* 2000;46:551, with permission.

TABLE 14.4

LOCAL–REGIONAL FAILURES AFTER POSTOPERATIVE RADIOTHERAPY FOR PAROTID GLAND NEOPLASMS BY EXTENT OF RESIDUAL DISEASE

Residual Disease	No. of Patients	Mean Tumor Dose (Rad)	Failures		
			Primary Site	Neck	Primary Site + Neck
Gross (any grade)	14	5,825	1 (5,250)[a]	1 (5,000)[a]	0
Microscopic (any grade)	26	5,543	2 (6,000; 5,535)	1 (5,000)	0
High grade (good margin)	16	5,569	1 (6,000)	2 (6,000; 5,500)	0
Unknown grade (good margin)	17	5,591	1 (6,000)	0	1 (5,500)[a]
Low grade (questionable margin)	4	5,632	0	0	0
Total	77	—	5	4	1

[a]Numbers in parentheses are the tumor doses in the patients who experienced a failure.
From McNaney D, McNeese MD, Guillamondegui OM, et al. Postoperative irradiation in malignant epithelial tumor of the parotid. *Int J Radiat Oncol Biol Phys* 1983;9:1289–1295, with permission.

TABLE 14.5

LOCAL FAILURES AFTER POSTOPERATIVE RADIOTHERAPY FOR PAROTID GLAND MALIGNANCIES BY PATIENT, SURGICAL, AND PATHOLOGIC FEATURES

Feature	No. of Patients	No. of Failures
Facial nerve sacrificed	42	9 (21%)
Positive margins	37	6 (16%)
Close or uncertain margins	66	5 (8%)
Low histologic grade	46	1 (2%)
Focal perineural invasion	36	4 (11%)
Named nerve involvement	20	5 (25%)
Extraglandular disease extension	78	11 (14%)
All patients	166	15 (9%)

Data from M.D. Anderson Cancer Center.
Modified from Garden AS, El-Naggar AK, Morrison WH, et al. Postoperative radiotherapy for malignant tumors of the parotid gland. *Int J Radiat Oncol Biol Phys* 1997;37:79–85.

SUBMANDIBULAR GLAND

Treatment Strategy

As in parotid gland tumor, surgery is the preferred treatment for submandibular gland neoplasms. Indications of postoperative radiotherapy are as listed in the "Parotid" section.

Postoperative Radiotherapy

Target Volume
The initial target volume for low-grade tumors without lymph node involvement encompasses the surgical bed (see Fig. 14.6); the volume for high-grade tumors or presence of lymph node involvement encompasses the surgical bed and ipsilateral neck nodes.

For perineural invasion (usually adenoid cystic carcinoma): when limited to focal involvement of small unnamed nerves, the volume encompasses the neural track more generously (additional 2- to 3-cm margins); invasion of lingual or hypoglossal nerve requires coverage of nerve pathway to the skull base.

The boost volume encompasses the tumor bed and involved nodal bed.

When skull base irradiation is required, IMRT may be preferable to minimize dose to the brain and contralateral parotid gland. The typical nerves involved with submandibular gland tumors are branches of V3 (particularly the lingual nerve) and the hypoglossal nerve. The mandibular nerve exits foramen ovale. The lingual nerve branches off medial to the lateral pterygoid muscle and lies anterior to the inferior alveolar nerve (also a branch of V3). While the inferior alveolar nerve enters its respective canal in the mandible, the lingual nerve continues between the pterygoid muscle and the ramus of the mandible. Eventually, prior to giving off its terminal branches in the tongue, it crosses the submandibular duct and is the point most vulnerable to invasion and perineural spread (see Fig. 14.7).

Setup and Field Arrangement
Ipsilateral irradiation is sufficient for most patients (exceptions: medial extent of primary tumor or coverage of the skull base beyond the range of electrons). The patient is immobilized in the open neck position with a thermoplastic mask. Marking of the scar and oral commissure facilitates portal design.

A lateral appositional field encompasses the tumor bed and upper neck nodes. Radiation is delivered with a combination of electrons (12 to 20 MeV depending on the depth) and photons (6 MV) in a ratio of 4:1. Portal borders are as follows:

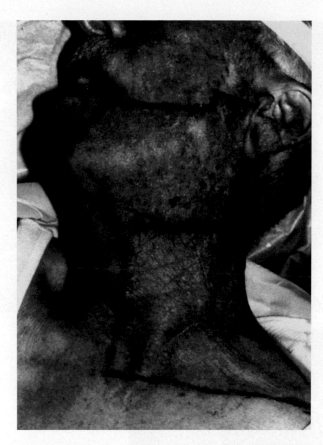

Figure 14.6 An 82-year-old man noted an asymptomatic mass in the left submandibular area and sought medical attention immediately. Examination revealed a 3-cm left submandibular mass. This tumor was resected along with a left modified neck dissection, and histologic examination revealed an adenoid cystic carcinoma in the submandibular gland measuring 2.5 × 2 × 2 cm with perineural invasion. One of the eight nodes (a subdigastric node) in the specimen contained metastatic disease. The lingual and hypoglossal nerves were free of gross tumor invasion. Postoperative radiotherapy was delivered through a left lateral appositional field encompassing the tumor bed, the proximal extension of the nerves at risk, and the upper neck. A combination of 20 MeV electrons and 6 MV photons was used weighted 4 to 1. A dose of 50 Gy in 25 fractions was delivered, after which the field was reduced to administer an additional 10 Gy in five fractions boost to the tumor bed. The mid and lower neck nodes were treated with a matching 9-MeV electron field to a dose of 50 Gy in 25 fractions.

- *Superior:* from the oral commissure sloping up to cover the ascending ramus of the mandible just short of the temporomandibular joint. The field is extended up to the base of the skull when there is perineural invasion of a major nerve.
- *Anterior:* determined by the extent of surgery; the oral commissure and skin of the chin are shielded when possible.
- *Inferior:* thyroid notch.
- *Posterior:* just behind the mastoid process.

Off-cord reduction is made at approximately 44 Gy and the posterior strip is supplemented with lower energy electrons. A lateral appositional electron field is used for irradiation of the mid and lower neck nodes when indicated (see "General Principles").

For IMRT, the patient is immobilized in a supine position with extended thermoplastic head and shoulder mask. Thin-slice CT scan is obtained in the treatment position for outlining the target volumes.

Dose

For high-grade tumors and those with lymph node metastases, the commonly prescribed dose is 60 Gy in 30 fractions after complete resection or 64 to 66 Gy in 32 to 33 fractions in the presence of positive margin or ECE. Field reduction is made after 50 to 54 Gy.

For elective neck irradiation, a dose of 50 Gy in 25 fractions is prescribed.

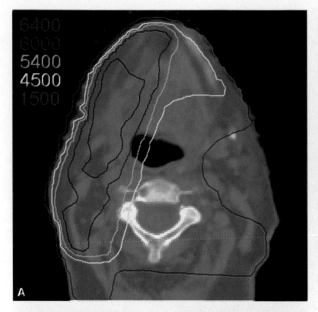

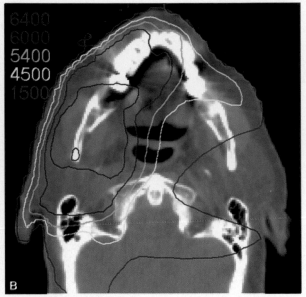

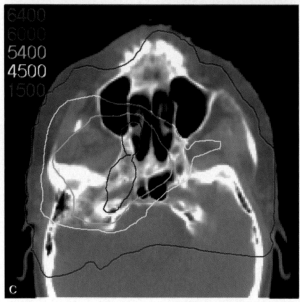

Figure 14.7 A 68-year-old woman presented with right lower facial numbness and a submandibular mass. She underwent resection of the mass, which was an adenoid cystic carcinoma. The lingual nerve was involved and encased by the tumor and five nodes (levels I and II) were involved. Because the neural pathways to foramen ovale needed radiation, she was treated with postoperative intensity-modulated radiation therapy (IMRT). Axial isodose distributions are shown at the level of the removed gland and upper neck **(A)**, superior oral cavity, including the lingual nerve pathway along the ascending ramus, and high jugular region **(B)** and the skull base **(C)**.

Background Data

TABLE 14.6	
HISTOLOGIC FINDINGS OF SUBMANDIBULAR GLAND TUMORS	
Type of Tumors	**No. of Patients**
Benign	
Pleomorphic adenoma	21
Other[a]	3
Malignant	
Adenoid cystic	37
Tubular	5
Cribriform	17
Solid	15

(continued)

TABLE 14.6
(continued)

Type of Tumors	No. of Patients
Mucoepidermoid	15
High grade	5
Intermediate grade	3
Low grade	6
Not specified	1
Adenocarcinoma	9
Carcinoma ex-mixed tumor	8
Squamous carcinoma	8
Undifferentiated	4
Other[b]	5
Total	110

[a]Oncocytoma (1), sebaceous adenoma (1), and benign lymphoepithelial lesion (1).
[b]Acinic cell (1), lymphoepithelioma (1), unclassified (2), and carcinoma ex monomorphic adenoma (1).
From Weber RS, Byers RM, Petit B, et al. Submandibular gland tumors. Adverse histologic factors and therapeutic implications. *Arch Otolaryngol Head Neck Surg* 1990;116:1055, with permission.

TABLE 14.7

EFFECT OF THERAPY ON FAILURE SITE FOR PATIENTS WITH MALIGNANT LESIONS EXTENDING INTO PERIGLANDULAR SOFT TISSUE

Treatment Modality	No. of Patients	No Evidence of Disease	Local–Regional Relapse	Distant Metastases
Surgery	23	9	12[a]	2
Surgery and radiotherapy	22	13	4[a]	5

[a]P <0.034. Includes four patients from group 2 with previous excisional biopsy and soft-tissue extension treated with radiotherapy after referral.
From Weber RS, Byers RM, Petit B, et al. Submandibular gland tumors. Adverse histologic factors and therapeutic implications. *Arch Otolaryngol Head Neck Surg* 1990;116:1055, with permission.

TABLE 14.8

SUBMANDIBULAR GLAND NEOPLASMS: 5-YEAR LOCAL–REGIONAL CONTROL RATES (STRATIFIED BY RISK VARIABLES) OF SURGERY AND POSTOPERATIVE IRRADIATION

Variable	No. of Patients	Control (%)
Adenocarcinoma	10	41
Adenoid cystic carcinoma	50	98
High grade	23	69
Positive resection margin	19	79
Perineural invasion	54	94
Named nerve involvement	17	88
Positive nodes	21	78
Extraglandular extension	58	85
All patients	83	88

Data from the M.D. Anderson Cancer Center.
Modified from Storey MR, Garden AS, Morrison WH, et al. Postoperative radiotherapy for malignant tumors of the submandibular gland. *Int J Radiat Oncol Biol Phys* 2001;51:952, with permission.

MINOR SALIVARY GLAND TUMORS

Treatment Strategy

Surgery is the preferred treatment for operable patients if the cosmetic and functional repercussions are not too severe. Occasional patients with small tumors may be treated with radiation. Indications for postoperative radiotherapy are listed in the "Parotid" section.

Postoperative Radiotherapy

Target Volume
Initial Target Volume
- Low-grade tumors without lymph node involvement: surgical bed.
- High-grade tumors or lymph node involvement: surgical bed and neck nodes. The extent of elective neck treatment varies with histology and the anatomical site of the primary lesion.
- Adenoid cystic carcinoma or presence of perineural invasion: more generous coverage of the neural track (see Figs. 14.8 and 14.9).

The boost volume encompasses the tumor bed and involved nodal bed.

Setup and Field Arrangement
Varies with the site of the primary lesion (see respective sites). If conformal therapy is chosen, intricate understanding of the nerves at risk and their specific proximal pathways to the respective foramina in the base of skull are essential.

Dose: See "Parotid" section

Dose Specification: See "General Principles"

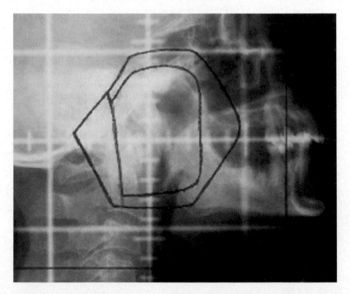

Figure 14.8 A 59-year-old man presented with obstructive right ear symptoms. A mass was found in the posterior wall of the right nasopharynx. A transoral piecemeal excision was performed and histologic examination revealed adenoid cystic carcinoma with perineural invasion and positive margins. Examination was suspicious for a residual mass, so a wide reexcision using a transpalatal approach was performed. The pathologic studies on the reexcision were negative, but because of the original findings and location of disease, postoperative radiation was recommended. Radiation was delivered through a pair of parallel–opposed beams. The initial fields encompassed the primary tumor and operative bed. The generous margin superiorly allowed for coverage of the perineural pathways. The fields were reduced off the spinal cord at 42 Gy, and reduced further at 50 Gy to boost the tumor bed to 60 Gy. The patient remains free of disease 10 years from his therapy.

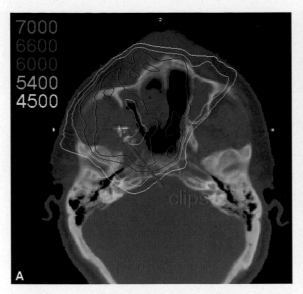
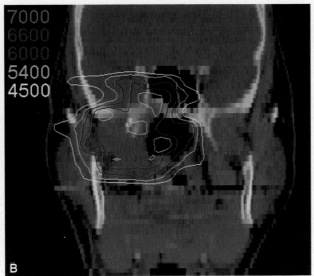

Figure 14.9 A 51-year-old man presented with an asymptomatic hard palate mass. Tumor biopsy revealed adenoid cystic carcinoma, cribiform, and tubular type. He underwent resection, which included an infrastructure maxillectomy and drill-out of the maxillary nerve. Tumor was present at the proximal section margin of the nerve, where clips were placed. He received postoperative intensity-modulated radiation therapy (IMRT). The region of positive margin and V2 through foramen rotundum received 66 Gy and a more generous margin including the operative bed received 60 Gy in 30 fractions. Isodose distributions through the clipped margin are shown on axial **(A)** and coronal **(B)** views.

Background Data

TABLE 14.9
MINOR SALIVARY GLAND TUMORS OF THE LIP AND BUCCAL MUCOSA: HISTOLOGIC DISTRIBUTION

Histologic Findings	Site		Total
	Lip	Buccal Mucosa	
Adenoid cystic carcinoma	9	12	21
Mucoepidermoid carcinoma			
High grade	—	1	1
Low grade	—	5	5
Not specified	3	1	4
Adenocarcinoma	1	5	6
Acinic cell carcinoma	—	4	4
Terminal duct carcinoma	1	2	3
Clear cell carcinoma	1	1	2
Carcinoma ex-pleomorphic adenoma	1	—	1
Pleomorphic adenoma	2	—	2
Papillary sialoadenoma	1	—	1
Total	19	31	50

Data from the M.D. Anderson Cancer Center.
From Weber RS, Palmer JM, El-Naggar AE, et al. Minor salivary gland tumors of the lip and buccal mucosa. *Laryngoscope* 1989;99:6, with permission.

TABLE 14.10

CERVICAL NODE METASTASES IN 434 PATIENTS WITH MALIGNANT TUMORS OF MINOR SALIVARY GLAND ORIGIN

Distribution by	No. of Patients	Metastases Previously Excised	Present on Admission	Appeared Later	Total with Metastases
By histologic findings					
Adenoidcystic	174	1	13	10	24 (14%)
Mucoepidermoid	76	—	12	11	23 (30%)
Solid duct					
Adenocarcinoma	106	—	19	11	30 (28%)
Variants of duct					
Adenocarcinoma	37	1	4	4	9 (24%)
Malignant mixed	13	1	3	1	5 (38%)
Acinic cell	2	—	—	—	—
Oat cell	14	—	5	2	7 (50%)
Colonic type	12	—	1	—	1 (8%)
Anatomic site					
Palate	140	—	10	12	22 (16%)
Sinuses or nasal	127	1	9	9	19 (15%)
Tongue	52	1	15	6	22 (42%)
Cheek or lips	40	—	4	2	6 (15%)
Gingivae	29	—	2	4	6 (21%)
Floor of the mouth	17	—	5	2	7 (41%)
Larynx	15	1	5	4	10 (67%)
Tonsil	11	—	7	—	7 (65%)
Pharynx	3	—	—	—	—
Total	434	3	57	39	99 (23%)

Modified from Spiro RH, Koss LG, Hajdu SI, et al. Tumors of minor salivary origin. A clinicopathologic study of 492 cases. *Cancer* 1973;31:117, with permission.

TABLE 14.11

LOCAL CONTROL OF MINOR SALIVARY GLAND CARCINOMAS TREATED WITH RADIATION STRATIFIED BY SITE OF DISEASE

Site	Local Control/Total Patients; Radiation Alone	Local Control/Total Patients; Surgery + Radiation
Oral cavity	7/11	18/19
Oropharynx	5/6	4/5
Larynx and hypopharynx	4/4	1/1
Nasopharynx, nasal cavity, and sinuses	4/18	12/15
All sites	20/39 (51%)	35/40 (88%)

Modified from Parsons JT, Mendenhall WM, Stringer SP, et al. Management of minor salivary gland carcinomas. *Int J Radiat Oncol Biol Phys* 1996;35:43, with permission.

SUGGESTED READINGS

Armstrong JG, Harrison LB, Thaler HT, et al. The indications for elective treatment of the neck in cancer of the major salivary glands. *Cancer* 1992;69:615.

Barton J, Slevin NJ, Gleave EN. Radiotherapy for pleomorphic adenoma of the parotid gland. *Int J Radiat Oncol Biol Phys* 1992;22:925.

Batsakis JG. Neoplasms of the minor and lesser major salivary glands. *Surg Gynecol Obstet* 1972;135:289.

Batsakis JG, Luna MA. Low-grade and high-grade adenocarcinomas of the salivary duct system. *Ann Otol Rhinol Laryngol* 1989;98:162.

Batsakis JG, Luna MA, El-Naggar AK. Histopathologic grading of salivary gland neoplasms: II. Acinic cell carcinomas. *Ann Otol Rhinol Laryngol* 1990;99:929.

Bissett RJ, Fitzpatrick PJ. Malignant submandibular gland tumors. A review of 91 patients. *Am J Clin Oncol* 1988;11:46.

Byers RM, Jesse RH, Guillamondegui OM, et al. Malignant tumors of the submaxillary gland. *Am J Surg* 1973;126:458.

Cohen J, Guillamondegui OM, Batsakis JG, et al. Cancer of the minor salivary glands of the larynx. *Am J Surg* 1985;150:513.

Douglas JG, Koh WJ, Austin-Seymour M, et al. Treatment of salivary gland neoplasms with fast neutron radiotherapy. *Arch Otolaryngol Head Neck Surg* 2003;129:944.

Douglas JG, Laramore GE, Austin-Seymour M, et al. Treatment of locally advanced adenoid cystic carcinoma of the head and neck with neutron radiotherapy. *Int J Radiat Oncol Biol Phys* 2000;46:551.

Eversole LR. Mucoepidermoid carcinoma: review of 815 reported cases. *J Oral Surg* 1970;28:490.

Eveson JW, Cawson RA. Tumours of the minor (oropharyngeal) salivary glands: a demographic study of 336 cases. *J Oral Pathol* 1985;14:500.

Fitzpatrick PJ, Theriault C. Malignant salivary gland tumors. *Int J Radiat Oncol Biol Phys* 1986;12:1743.

Fordice J, Kershaw C, El-Naggar A, et al. Adenoid cystic carcinoma of the head and neck: predictors of morbidity and mortality. *Arch Otolaryngol Head Neck Surg* 1999;125:149.

Frankenthaler RA, Luna MA, Lee SS, et al. Prognostic variables in parotid gland cancer. *Arch Otolaryngol Head Neck Surg* 1991;117:1251.

Fu KK, Leibel SA, Levine ML, et al. Carcinoma of the major and minor salivary glands: analysis of treatment results and sites and causes of failures. *Cancer* 1977;40:2882.

Garden AS, El-Naggar AK, Morrison WH, et al. Postoperative radiotherapy for malignant tumors of the parotid gland. *Int J Radiat Oncol Biol Phys* 1997;37:79.

Garden AS, Weber RS, Morrison WH, et al. The influence of positive margins and nerve invasion in adenoid cystic carcinoma of the head and neck treated with surgery and radiation. *Int J Radiat Oncol Biol Phys* 1995;32:619.

Goepfert H, Luna MA, Lindberg RD, et al. Malignant salivary gland tumors of the paranasal sinuses and nasal cavity. *Arch Otolaryngol* 1983;109:662.

Griffin TW. Optimal treatment for salivary gland tumors. *Int J Radiat Oncol Biol Phys* 1991;21:857.

Guillamondegui OM, Byers RM, Luna MA, et al. Aggressive surgery in treatment for parotid cancer: the role of adjunctive postoperative radiotherapy. *AJR Am J Roentgenol* 1975;123:49.

Hicks MJ, El-Naggar AK, Flaitz CM, et al. Histocytologic grading of mucoepidermoid carcinoma of major salivary glands in prognosis and survival: a clinicopathologic and flow cytometric investigation. *Head Neck* 1995;17:89.

Huber PE, Debus J, Latz D, et al. Radiotherapy for advanced adenoid cystic carcinoma: neutrons, photons or mixed beam? *Radiother Oncol* 2001;59:161.

King JJ, Fletcher GH. Malignant tumors of the major salivary glands. *Radiology* 1971;100:381.

Laramore GE, Krall JM, Griffin TW, et al. Neutron versus photon irradiation for unresectable salivary gland tumors: final report of an RTOG-MRC randomized clinical trial. *Int J Radiat Oncol Biol Phys* 1993;27:235.

Liu F-F, Rotstein L, Davison AJ, et al. Benign parotid adenomas: a review of the Princess Margaret Hospital experience. *Head Neck* 1995;17:177.

Luna MA. Pathology of tumors of the salivary glands. In: Thawley SE, Panje WR, Batsakis JG et al., eds. *Comprehensive management of head and neck tumors*, 2nd ed. Philadelphia, PA: WB Saunders, 1999.

McNaney D, McNeese MD, Guillamondegui OM, et al. Postoperative irradiation in malignant epithelial tumor of the parotid. *Int J Radiat Oncol Biol Phys* 1983;9:1289.

Olsen KD, Devine KD, Weiland LH. Mucoepidermoid carcinoma of the oral cavity. *Otolaryngol Head Neck Surg* 1981;89:783.

Parsons JT, Mendenhall WM, Stringer SP, et al. Management of minor salivary gland carcinomas. *Int J Radiat Oncol Biol Phys* 1996;35:443.

Rentschler R, Burgess MA, Byers R. Chemotherapy of malignant major salivary gland neoplasms: a 25-year review of M.D. Anderson Hospital experience. *Cancer* 1977;40:619.

Roper PR, Wolf PF, Luna MA, et al. Malignant salivary gland tumors of the base of the tongue. *South Med J* 1987;80:605.

Spiro RH. Salivary neoplasms: overview of a 35-year experience with 2,807 patients. *Head Neck Surg* 1986;8:177.

Spiro RH, Armstrong J, Harrison L, et al. Carcinoma of major salivary glands. Recent trends. *Arch Otolaryngol Head Neck Surg* 1989;115:316.

Spiro RH, Dubner S. Salivary gland tumors. *Curr Opin Oncol* 1990;2:589.

Spiro RH, Hajdu SI, Strong EW. Tumors of the submaxillary gland. *Am J Surg* 1976;132:463.

Spiro RH, Koss LG, Hajdu SI, et al. Tumors of minor salivary origin. A clinicopathologic study of 492 cases. *Cancer* 1973;31:117.

Storey MR, Garden AS, Morrison WH, et al. Postoperative radiotherapy for malignant tumors of the submandibular gland. *Int J Radiat Oncol Biol Phys* 2001;51:952.

Terhaard CHJ, Lubsen H, VanderTweel I, et al. Salivary gland carcinoma: independent prognostic factors for locoregional control, distant metastases, and overall survival: results of the Dutch Head and Neck Oncology Cooperative Group. *Head Neck* 2004;26:681.

Tran L, Sidrys J, Sadeghi A, et al. Salivary gland tumors of the oral cavity. *Int J Radiat Oncol Biol Phys* 1990;18:413.

Waldron CA, El-Mofty SK, Gnepp DR. Tumors of the intraoral minor salivary glands: a demographic and histologic study of 426 cases. *Oral Surg Oral Med Oral Pathol* 1988;66:323.

Wang CC, Goodman M. Photon irradiation of unresectable carcinomas of salivary glands. *Int J Radiat Oncol Biol Phys* 1991;21:569.

Weber RS, Byers RM, Petit B, et al. Submandibular gland tumors. Adverse histologic factors and therapeutic implications. *Arch Otolaryngol Head Neck Surg* 1990;116:1055.

Weber RS, Palmer JM, El-Naggar AE, et al. Minor salivary gland tumors of the lip and buccal mucosa. *Laryngoscope* 1989;99:6.

Thyroid

15

TREATMENT STRATEGY

The primary treatment for thyroid cancers is surgery. Radioactive iodine (RAI) is a generally accepted adjuvant therapy to surgery for most functioning thyroid cancers.

Relative indications for postoperative external beam radiotherapy depend on tumor histology. For differentiated (follicular/papillary) cancers that do not take up RAI, the indications include incomplete resection, direct invasion of adjacent structures (trachea, nerve, muscle, etc.), extracapsular extension of nodal disease, extensive mediastinal nodal involvement, and resection of recurrent disease at primary site.

Medullary carcinoma has the same indications as that of differentiated cancer plus persistent elevation of calcitonin levels after surgery, without demonstrable distant metastatic disease.

For anaplastic carcinoma, all patients receive irradiation after maximal surgical debulking. Patients with locally advanced anaplastic carcinoma are generally enrolled into ongoing Phase II protocols testing combination of chemotherapy (varies with protocol) and local–regional treatment.

POSTOPERATIVE RADIOTHERAPY

Target Volume

The initial target volume encompasses the surgical bed, neck nodes at risk, upper mediastinum, and midmediastinal area when upper mediastinum is involved (see Fig. 15.1). The boost volume encompasses the area of known disease locations with 1- to 2-cm margins.

Intensity-modulated radiation therapy (IMRT) generally offers better coverage of the rather complex anatomy and geometry. An example of the former is the difference in tissue thickness between the neck and mediastinum, and the target is often a horse-shoe shaped tumor bed. The high-risk target volume (clinical target volume [CTV]1) encompasses the thyroid bed, central compartment (including tracheal wall and tracheoesophageal groove), and involved nodal regions. This volume is often estimated on the basis of surgical and pathologic findings because contrast computed tomography (CT) scans are rarely done for well-differentiated thyroid carcinoma to avoid interference with RAI therapy when indicated postoperatively. It is therefore crucial to be familiar with the anatomy and the routes of spread, particularly to the trachea, esophagus, larynx, and adjacent muscles. CTV2 consists of nodal levels at risk, which include clinically negative paratracheal nodes to the carina and levels III and IV nodes. When level III node is positive, CTV2 also includes ipsilateral level II node.

Setup and Field Arrangement

Marking of surgical scar facilitates portal design. The patient is immobilized with thermoplastic mask in a supine position, with the head hyperextended to minimize inclusion of oral cavity in the portal. If the patient is unable to hyperextend the neck, a cephalad gantry tilt can be used to

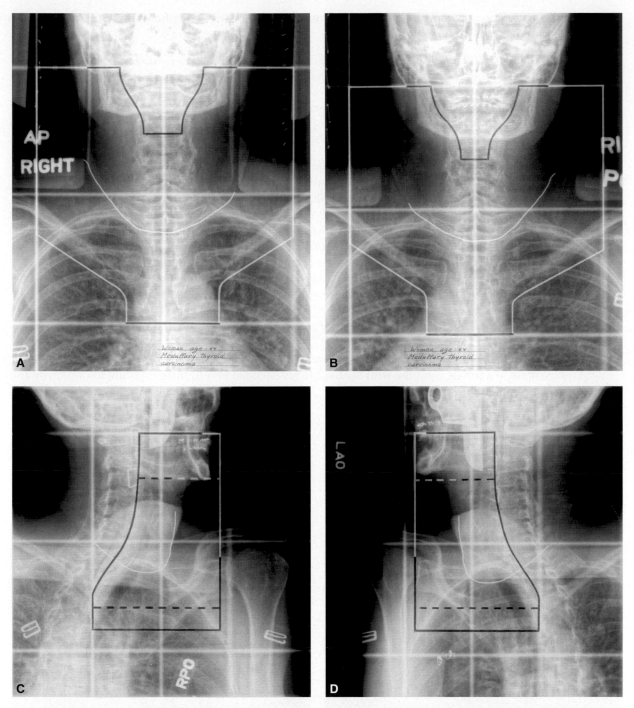

Figure 15.1 A 64-year-old woman was found to have a thyroid nodule on routine physical examination. She had no family history of thyroid cancer and had never received radiotherapy. Computed tomography (CT) scan showed a mass in the right lobe of the thyroid gland. There was no evidence of associated lymph adenopathy or disease in the mediastinum. Fine-needle aspiration showed medullary thyroid carcinoma. Serum calcitonin levels were elevated. Carcinoembryonic antigen level was normal. Metastatic workup results were negative. The patient underwent a thyroidectomy and right neck dissection. Histologic examination showed a 2-cm medullary carcinoma of the right lobe. Eight right paratracheal nodes and four jugular nodes were positive, the largest measuring 1.2 cm. Postoperatively, serum calcitonin levels remained elevated. Because of extensive nodal involvement and persistent elevated serum calcitonin level, it was decided to deliver postoperative radiotherapy. An opposed anterior and posterior (AP–PA) technique with a compensating filter for the anterior field was used to treat the initial target volume **(A, B)**. The wire indicates the surgical scar. A dose of 44 Gy was delivered in 22 fractions following which the left anterior and right posterior oblique fields **(C, D)** were used to boost the tumor bed and right neck. After reaching a tumor dose of 50 Gy, the length of the oblique fields was reduced to encompass the areas of known tumor involvement for an additional 10 Gy. Therefore, the primary tumor bed and involved nodal areas received a total dose of 60 Gy, the right neck received a dose of 50 Gy, and the contralateral neck and mediastinum received a dose of 44 Gy, all delivered in 2 Gy per fraction. This patient was alive without evidence of disease and without complications 6 years after completion of therapy.

achieve the same goal. Opposed anterior and posterior (AP–PA) photon fields are used for the initial target volume:

- *Superior border:* at the level of the mastoid processes. It can be lower on the side of the neck that has a low risk for microscopic nodal involvement to spare the ipsilateral submandibular gland.
- *Lateral borders:* covering the medial two thirds of the clavicles.
- *Inferior border:* just below the carina (when upper mediastinum is involved, it is 3 to 4 cm below the mediastinal component).

The use of missing tissue compensating filter or field-in-field technique (see Chapter 3) minimizes dose heterogeneity, and therefore potential overdose to a segment of the spinal cord, because of the large differences in the diameter of the patient at different anatomic levels.

The oral cavity and oropharynx can be shielded to the extent possible without compromising on the coverage of the tumor bed and neck.

The boost dose is usually delivered through opposed anterior-oblique and posterior-oblique off-cord photon fields encompassing the tumor bed and the side of the neck with nodal involvement. A planning CT scan is obtained to determine the angle and width of these fields. The superior and inferior borders are chosen according to the extent of the disease.

If the contralateral neck or thyroid bed is also at high risk, it can receive boost dose through an appositional electron field with a gantry angle corresponding to that of the anterior-oblique photon field to avoid overlap (see Fig. 15.2).

With IMRT, the patient is immobilized with an extended head and shoulder thermoplastic mask in a supine position, with the head hyperextended to minimize exposure to oral cavity and

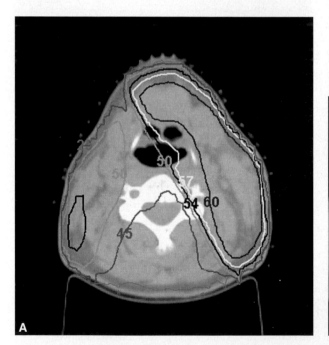
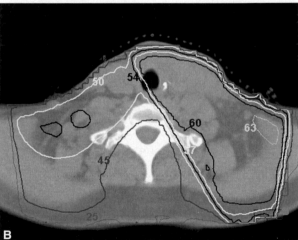

Figure 15.2 A 48-year-old woman underwent a total thyroidectomy for papillary carcinoma followed by postoperative iodine 131 ablation. A year later, she re-presented with a 2-cm left neck mass. Fine-needle aspiration confirmed recurrence, and she underwent a left neck and central compartment dissection. Histologic examination revealed recurrent thyroid carcinoma in the connective tissues of the neck. A postoperative iodine scan was negative. She received postoperative external beam radiation. The initial fields were parallel–opposed, with 6-MV photons from anterior and 18 MV from posterior. The portals covered the entire neck and upper mediastinum. After a dose of 42 Gy, the fields were reduced off spinal cord by using parallel–opposed right anterior and left posterior oblique fields. At 50 Gy, a reduction was made off the superior and inferior borders, and the areas felt to be at the highest risk were irradiated to 60 Gy. The right neck was supplemented with 12-MeV electron beam to bring the dose to the mid and lower right neck to 50 Gy. **A, B:** Representative axial isodose distribution through the mid and lower neck, respectively.

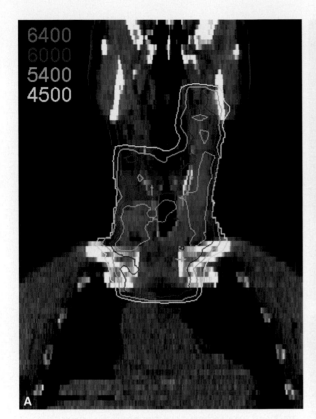

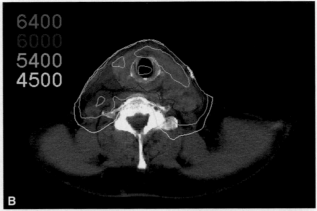

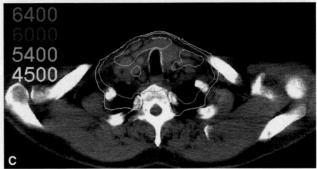

Figure 15.3 A 57-year-old man presented with left neck swelling. A fine-needle aspiration revealed papillary carcinoma of the thyroid gland. Preoperative imaging was limited to ultrasonography. He underwent a total thyroidectomy with selective dissection of the left levels II, III, IV, and Vb and a left superior mediastinum nodal dissection. The primary tumor was 3.5 cm in size, multifocal, and extending into the extrathyroidal tissues. All nodal levels dissected were positive, including seven out of seven paratracheal nodes. Because a postoperative iodine scan revealed residual activity in the thyroid bed, he received 150 mCi ^{131}I to ablate the residual thyroid tissue. This was followed by external beam intensity-modulated radiation therapy (IMRT), recommended because of the extent of the disease. Contours of CTV1 (60 Gy, *green*) and CTV2 (54 Gy, *blue*) and isodose curves are shown on a coronal image **(A)**, an axial image at the level of the cricoid **(B)**, and an axial image at the paratracheal level **(C)**. Note that the involved left neck was defined as CTV1, whereas posterior level III and level IV on the right were uninvolved and were defined as CTV2. Because the right neck was uninvolved, right level II was excluded. He remains without recurrence 2 years post-therapy.

oropharynx. Thin-slice CT scan is obtained for delineation of target volumes (see Figs. 15.3 and Fig. 15.4).

Dose

With conventional 3-D approach, the initial target volume dose is 44 Gy in 22 fractions. The boost volume dose is 16 Gy in eight fractions. An additional boost dose of 4 to 6 Gy in two to three fractions may be given to a relatively small high-risk region.

With IMRT, the doses prescribed to CTV1 and CTV2 are usually 60 Gy and 54 Gy, respectively, given in 30 fractions. A total dose of 63 to 66 Gy (given in 2.1 to 2.2 Gy per fraction) may be prescribed to a region having additional risk feature (e.g., positive margin). If this high-dose target involves the esophagus, therapy may be given in 33 fractions to limit the fraction size to no more than 2 Gy because esophageal stenosis is a risk factor in this population.

Dose Specification

With conventional or 3-D approaches, treatment is usually given with 6-MV photons for the anterior field and with 18-MV photons for the posterior field. A 3-mm bolus is placed over the thyroidectomy scar. Loading for AP–PA fields is usually 3:2. A CT treatment plan is obtained and adjustment can be made where necessary. The dose is prescribed at the isocenter or an isodose line.

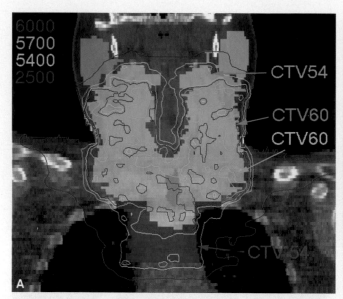

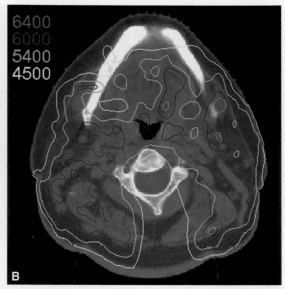

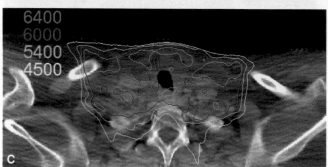

Figure 15.4 A 56-year-old man presented with cough and was found to have a thyroid mass. He underwent partial thyroidectomy, which revealed a 6.5 cm mass with positive margins and six of six positive nodes. Microscopic residual disease persisted even after a subsequent completion of thyroidectomy. On presentation to the M.D. Anderson Cancer Center, restaging with ultrasonography revealed bilateral adenopathy. He underwent bilateral neck and paratracheal dissections including exploration of level I. Histologic examination revealed multiple positive nodes with extracapsular extension and soft tissue involvement. He received ^{131}I followed by intensity-modulated radiation therapy (IMRT). Contours of CTV1 and CTV2 and isodose curves are shown on a coronal image (**A**), an axial image at level II in the neck (**B**), and an axial image at the paratracheal level (**C**). It is noted that because of the extent of the disease in level II and in the operative bed, the plan has generous anterior coverage including level Ib (**B**), and the tracheoesophageal groove, which is covered in CTV1 (**C**). He remains without recurrence of the disease 2 years since completing his radiation.

Background Data

TABLE 15.1

FIVE-YEAR SURVIVAL AFTER EXTERNAL RADIOTHERAPY IN PATIENTS WITH DIFFERENTIATED THYROID CARCINOMA: REVIEW OF THE LITERATURE

References	Complete Surgery	Incomplete Surgery	Inoperable Tumors
Portmann	24/31 (77%)	10/30 (33%)	—
Mabille	17/19 (90%)	9/20 (45%)	5/22 (23%)
Smedal et al.	24/24 (100%)	25/31 (81%)	—
Sheline et al.	—	11/17 (65%)	—
McWhirter	54/61 (89%)	20/63 (32%)	—
Jacobsson	28/29 (97%)	16/27 (59%)	—
Windeyer	5/6 (83%)	11/20 (55%)	—
Simpson	—	23/54 (43%)	—
Staunton and Martin	—	—	3/14 (21%)
Tubiana et al.	62/66 (94%)	76/97 (78%)	11/17 (65%)

From Tubiana M, Haddad E, Schlumberger M, et al. External radiotherapy in thyroid cancers. *Cancer* 1985;55: 2062–2071, with permission.

SUGGESTED READINGS

Benker G, Olbricht T, Reinwein D, et al. Survival rates in patients with differentiated thyroid carcinoma. Influence of postoperative external radiotherapy. *Cancer* 1990;65:1517.

Brierley J, Tsang R, Simpson WJ, et al. Medullary thyroid cancer: analyses of survival and prognostic factors and the role of radiation therapy in local control. *Thyroid* 1996;6:305.

Farahati J, Reiners C, Stuschke M, et al. Differentiated thyroid cancer. Impact of adjuvant external radiotherapy in patients with perithyroidal tumor infiltration (stage T4). *Cancer* 1996;77:172.

Hill CS Jr, Ibanez ML, Samaan NA, et al. Medullary (solid) carcinoma of the thyroid gland: an analysis of the M.D. Anderson Hospital experience with patients with the tumor, its special features, and its histogenesis. *Medicine* 1973;52:141.

Kim JH, Leeper RD. Treatment of locally advanced thyroid carcinoma with combination doxorubicin and radiation therapy. *Cancer* 1987;60:2372.

Leeper RD. Thyroid cancer. *Med Clin North Am* 1985;69:1079.

Levendag PC, De Porre PM, van Putten WL. Anaplastic carcinoma of the thyroid gland treated by radiation therapy. *Int J Radiat Oncol Biol Phys* 1993;26(1):125.

Nguyen TD, Chassard JL, Lagarde P, et al. Results of postoperative radiation therapy in medullary carcinoma of the thyroid: a retrospective study by the French Federation of Cancer Institutes—the Radiotherapy Cooperative Group. *Radiother Oncol* 1992;23:1.

Nutting CM, Convery DJ, Cosgrove VP, et al. Improvements in target coverage and reduced spinal cord irradiation using intensity-modulated radiotherapy (IMRT) in patients with carcinoma of the thyroid gland. *Radiother Oncol* 2001;60:173.

O'Connell ME, A'Hern RP, Harmer CL. Results of external beam radiotherapy in differentiated thyroid carcinoma: a retrospective study from the Royal Marsden Hospital. *Eur J Cancer* 1994;30A:733.

Rougier P, Pannentier C, Laplance A, et al. Medullary thyroid carcinoma: prognostic factors and treatment. *Int J Radiat Oncol Biol Phys* 1983;9:161.

Samaan NA, Maheshwari YK, Nader S, et al. Impact of therapy for differentiated carcinoma of the thyroid: an analysis of 706 cases. *J Clin Endocrinol Metab* 1983;56:1131.

Samaan NA, Schultz PN, Hickey RC. Medullary thyroid carcinoma: prognosis of familial versus nonfamilial disease and the role of radiotherapy. *Horm Metab Res Suppl* 1989;21:21.

Simpson WJ. Anaplastic thyroid carcinoma: a new approach. *Can J Surg* 1980;23:25.

Simpson WJ. Radioiodine and radiotherapy in the management of thyroid cancers. *Otolaryngol Clin North Am* 1990;23:509.

Simpson WJ, Palmer JA, Rosen IB, et al. Management of medullary carcinoma of the thyroid. *Am J Surg* 1982;144:420.

Strong EW. The treatment of thyroid cancer: a summary. In: Najarian JS, Delaney JP, eds. *Advances in cancer surgery*. New York: Stratton, 1976.

Tennvall J, Lundell G, Hallquist A et al, The Swedish Anaplastic Thyroid Cancer Group. Combined doxorubicin, hyperfractionated radiotherapy, and surgery in anaplastic thyroid carcinoma. Report on two protocols. *Cancer* 1994;74:1348.

Tsang RW, Brierley JD, Simpson WJ, et al. The effects of surgery, radioiodine, and external radiation therapy on the clinical outcome of patients with differentiated thyroid carcinoma. *Cancer* 1998;82:375.

Tubiana M, Haddad E, Schlumberger M, et al. External radiotherapy in thyroid cancers. *Cancer* 1985;55:2062.

Tubiana M, Lacour J, Monnier JP, et al. External radiotherapy and radioiodine in the treatment of 359 thyroid cancers. *Br J Radiol* 1975;48:894.

Wilson PC, Millar BM, Brierley JD. The management of advanced thyroid cancer. *Clin Oncol* 2004;16:561.

Wu XL, Hu YH, Li QH, et al. Value of postoperative radiotherapy for thyroid cancer. *Head Neck Surg* 1987;10:107.

Skin

16

SQUAMOUS CELL CARCINOMA AND BASAL CELL CARCINOMA

Treatment Strategy

Surgery and radiotherapy are equally effective in curing most skin cancers. The choice of treatment modality is determined by several factors, such as functional and cosmetic results, patient age and occupation, treatment time, and cost. Surgery is preferred for most patients, particularly for younger patients who have years of exposure to sunlight ahead of them.

Primary radiotherapy is most often indicated for lesions on and around the nose, lower eyelids, and ear, where it can usually attain better functional and cosmetic results than surgery. Extensive lesions of the cheek and oral commissures, which would require full thickness resection, may also show better results on irradiation.

Postoperative radiotherapy is indicated for positive surgical margins, perineural invasion, and invasion of bone, cartilage, and skeletal muscle.

Rarely, patients have adenopathy at diagnosis. The choice of treatment of the nodal disease is determined by the type of therapy selected for the primary lesion and by the size of the node. A combination of surgery and radiotherapy is indicated when nodal disease is >3 cm or when extracapsular extension (ECE) is present.

Primary Radiotherapy

Target Volume

The initial target volume encompasses primary tumor with 1- to 2-cm margins, depending on the size, location, and type of tumor (well-circumscribed versus ill-defined border). Elective nodal irradiation is not indicated except when the primary is a large, infiltrative squamous cell carcinoma (SCC) or adnexal tumor.

The boost volume encompasses primary tumor with 0.5- to 1-cm margins, depending on the size, location, and type of tumor.

Setup and Field Arrangement

The patient is immobilized in a position that gives the best access to irradiate the tumor (preferably the plane of the skin to be treated is parallel to the surface of the treatment couch to avoid the need for gantry rotation) (see Fig. 16.1).

An appositional field is used in most cases. The borders of the field are chosen to include a 1- to 2-cm margin of normal skin around the tumor (up to 1 cm for lesions <1-cm tumor and 1 to 2 cm for larger tumors). Margins may be smaller when treating areas close to the eye. More generous margins are appropriate for lesions with an ill-defined border.

Radiation treatment is given with orthovoltage x-rays (usually 75 to 125 kilovolt potential [kVp]) or electrons (usually 6 to 12 MeV). The energy of x-rays or electrons is chosen on the basis

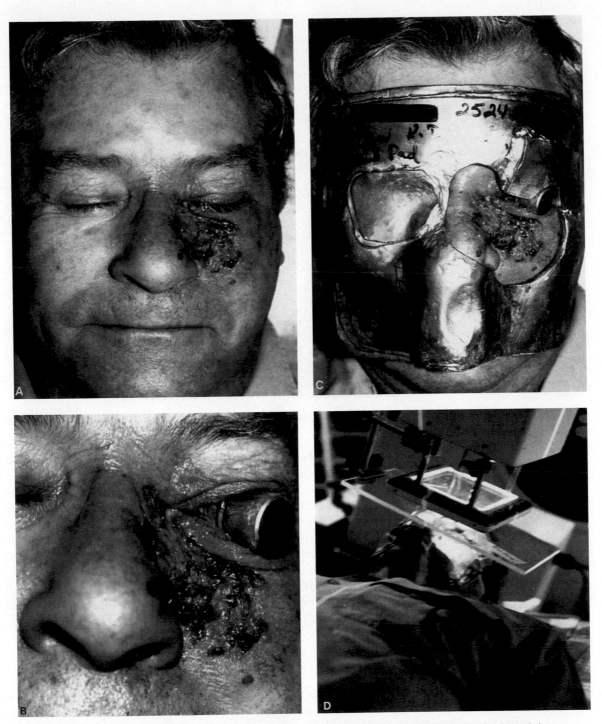

Figure 16.1   A 59-year-old man sought medical attention because of a small ulcer at the left lateral dorsum of the nose that gradually increased in size over a 4-year period. Physical examination showed a 5 × 3 cm ulcerating lesion with raised borders, involving the left lateral dorsum of the nose, the medial aspect of the cheek, and the medial canthus **(A)**. The thickest part of the tumor was close to the medial canthus. Biopsy revealed basal cell carcinoma. Computed tomography (CT) scans showed a small soft tissue mass in the medial canthus of the left orbit. The deepest point of this mass was 1.5 cm from the surface. Stage: T2 N0 M0. The lesion was treated with an appositional left anterior oblique field of 9-MeV electrons. A custom-made eye shield mounted on a contact lens was used to protect the cornea and lens **(B)**. A lead mask with extra layers over the contralateral eye was used for skin collimation **(C)**. A 1/4-inch scatter plate was placed in the beam to eliminate the skin-sparing effect **(D)**.

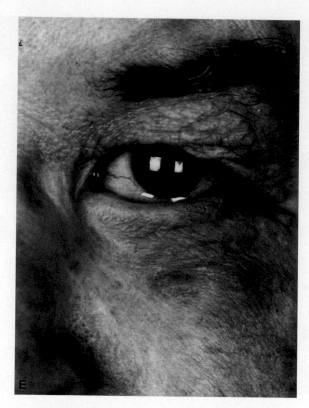

Figure 16.1 (*continued*) A dose of 60 Gy was delivered in 2-Gy fractions. Local control with good cosmetic and functional results was obtained **(E)**.

of the thickness of tumor. The energy of electron beams should be selected so that the distal 90% isodose line is a few millimeters deeper than the base of the tumor, including surface bolus.

The treatment distance for x-rays also depends on the thickness of the lesion. A 23-cm focus skin distance (FSD) cone is appropriate for superficial tumors, whereas a 50-cm FSD with open fields and skin collimation is preferable for thicker lesions to avoid a large dose gradient across the lesion. The FSD for electrons is usually 100 cm.

A custom-made lead cutout is used for skin collimation. The cutout should be large enough so that the portal size for an electron beam is at least 4 × 4 cm.

Skin bolus or a perspex scatter plate is used with electrons to ensure full surface dose.

An internal eye shield is inserted when treating an eyelid lesion with orthovoltage x-rays or with electrons of 8 MeV or less. (Note: Eye shields should be individually calibrated with respect to the electron attenuating properties.)

Dose

Effective regimens for treating most skin cancers include a dose of 50 to 55 Gy in 20 fractions, a dose of 45 Gy in 15 fractions, or a dose of 40 Gy in ten fractions. In general, protracted treatment provides better cosmetic results.

For large tumors close to crucial structures (e.g., eye), maximum tolerance is obtained with a dose of 60 to 70 Gy in 30 to 35 fractions (Fig. 16.1).

If the patient is in poor general condition, hypofractionation (e.g., four fractions of 8 Gy) may be used.

Dose Specification

X-rays are prescribed at D_{max}, with electrons at the 90% line. This difference in prescription accounts for the relative biologic effectiveness (RBE) difference between the two beam qualities.

Postoperative Radiotherapy

Most frequent indications are lymphatic spread to the parotid gland, upper neck nodes, or both, and perineural extension along the branches of the trigeminal nerves, facial nerves, or both.

Target Volume

The initial target volume encompasses the primary tumor bed and ipsilateral parotid and neck nodes, or trigeminal or facial nerve pathways, depending on the indication.

The boost volume encompasses areas of known disease with 1- to 2-cm margins.

Setup and Field Arrangement

For the treatment of parotid and neck nodes or branches of the facial nerve, the technique is similar to that for primary parotid tumors (see Chapter 14). The patient is immobilized in an open neck position. The anterior margin of the parotid portal can be slightly less generous because there is no need to encompass the parotid duct. Treatment is given with an electron beam of appropriate energy (e.g., 12 MeV for parotid and upper neck nodes and 9 MeV for lower neck nodes).

For the treatment of perineural extension through the supraorbital, infraorbital, or mandibular branches of the trigeminal nerve, the patient is immobilized in a supine position. The head is slightly hyperextended for irradiation of the infraorbital and mandibular nerves and is slightly flexed for the supraorbital nerve. A wedge-pair technique using 6-MV x-rays is usually suitable for these situations, which allows irradiation of the nerve track to the gasserian ganglion, with sparing of most of the eye. The portal margins depend on the tumor extent.

Intensity-modulated radiation therapy (IMRT) may provide better coverage for more convoluted target volumes.

Dose

The dose consists of 50 to 54 Gy in 25 to 27 fractions to the initial target volume followed by a dose of 6 to 12 Gy in three to six fractions to the boost volume.

Dose Specification: See "General Principles"

Background Data

TABLE 16.1
CONTROL OF MALIGNANT SKIN LESIONS WITH RADIATION THERAPY: HAHNEMANN UNIVERSITY EXPERIENCE, 1960 TO 1980

Diagnosis	No. Irradiated	No. of Treatment Failures	No. of Recurrences Controlled by Reirradiation	No Evidence of Disease 4-yr or Longer
Basal cell carcinoma	444	20	2	426/444 (95.9%)
Squamous cell carcinoma	156	12	—	144/156 (92.3%)
Keratoacanthoma	12	0	—	12/12 (100%)

From Solan MJ, Brady LW, Binnick SA, et al. Skin cancer. In: Perez CA, Brady LW, eds. *Principles and practice of radiation oncology.* 2nd ed. Philadelphia: JB Lippincott, 1992:479–495, with permission.

TABLE 16.2

CLINICAL EXPERIENCE WITH 1,166 EYELID TUMORS TREATED BY RADIOTHERAPY (1958 to 1978)[a]

Histologic Finding	Primary Tumors	Recurrent Tumors	Total	5-yr Control	%
Basal cell carcinoma	686	376	1,062	1,009	95.0
Squamous cell carcinoma	62	42	104	97	93.3
Total	748	418	1,166	1,106	94.8

[a]Most of the primary tumors were controlled and the few failures were salvaged by surgery. Of the 1,166 tumors, 745 (64 %) were <2 cm in diameter.
Adapted from Fitzpatrick PJ. Skin cancer of the head—treatment by radiotherapy. *Int J Radiat Oncol Biol Phys* 1984;10:450, with permission.

TABLE 16.3

CARCINOMA OF THE EYELIDS, PINNA, AND NOSE TREATED WITH RADIOTHERAPY: DISTRIBUTION OF PATIENTS AND TREATMENT FAILURE BY LESION SIZE

Size	No. of Patients	Failures	%
<2 cm	602	42	7
2–5 cm	32	12	37
>5 cm	12	6	50
Total	646	60	9

Modified from Petrovich Z, Kuisk H, Langholz B, et al. Treatment results and patterns of failure in 646 patients with carcinoma of the eyelids, pinna, and nose. *Am J Surg* 1987;154:447, with permission.

MELANOMA

Treatment Strategy

The primary treatment for cutaneous melanoma is complete local excision (which is essential for tissue diagnosis and microstaging) and, for palpable nodes, neck dissection. An exception is large facial lentigo maligna melanoma, which can be treated effectively with primary radiotherapy when wide surgical resection requires extensive reconstruction or is anticipated to yield poor cosmetic outcome.

Our indications for adjuvant postoperative radiotherapy following therapeutic nodal dissections are as follows:

- Lymph node >3 cm or multiple lymph nodes.
- Extracapsular extension.
- Nodal recurrence without distant metastases.
- Local excision of macroscopic disease only.

Sentinel lymph node biopsy (SLNB) with directed lymphadenectomy has replaced routine elective regional radiotherapy following wide local excision of primary lesions 1.5 mm thick or greater (American Joint Committee on Cancer [AJCC] stage II or III) or Clark's level IV or higher without clinical evidence of lymphadenopathy. Elective nodal irradiation is indicated if the procedure cannot detect the sentinel basin or if the patient's condition precludes a therapeutic dissection.

Postoperative Radiotherapy

Target Volume

For stage II and III, the target volume encompasses the primary tumor bed and ipsilateral draining lymph nodes down to the supraclavicular nodes.

For nodal recurrence, the entire ipsilateral neck is included. The primary tumor bed is also irradiated if excision was carried out <1 year before the nodal recurrence.

Setup and Field Arrangement

Setup and field arrangement varies with the site of the primary lesion. Most patients are treated with electrons of appropriate energies (see Fig. 16.2). Patients are usually immobilized in an open neck position. Cutaneous melanoma of frontal, temporal, and preauricular areas; auricle; and cheek are usually treated with two or three fields depending on the distance between the primary and parotid nodes. A field, similar to that of parotid gland tumors, is used to irradiate intraparotid and upper neck nodes with 12-MeV electrons. This field covers most of the tumor beds of lesions arising in these locations. An adjoining field is added to irradiate the tumor bed with 6- to 9-MeV electrons if the site of the primary tumor is outside the boundary of the parotid field. A matching portal is used to treat the lower neck nodes, as described in the subsequent text.

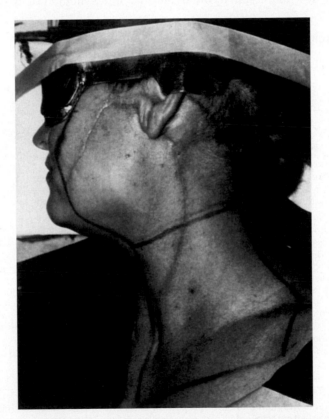

Figure 16.2 A 51-year-old woman underwent excision of a 2.3-cm skin lesion located in the left cheek. Histologic examination revealed a 6.5-mm thick malignant melanoma. She was referred for further treatment. Physical examination showed a 2-cm excision scar with surrounding erythema and a 1-cm left subdigastric node. Workup for distant metastasis was negative. She then underwent a wide re-excision of the skin of the left cheek along with a left superficial parotidectomy and supraomohyoid neck dissection. Examination of the specimens revealed presence of residual melanoma in the dermis of the cheek and metastatic deposit in three subdigastric and one midjugular node. She received adjunctive radiotherapy to the tumor bed and ipsilateral neck nodes through two abutting appositional fields to a given dose of 30 Gy in five fractions (6 Gy per fraction). The left cheek and upper neck nodal basin were irradiated with 12-MeV electrons and the lower neck with 9-MeV electrons. Skin collimation was used around the eye and a 0.5-cm bolus was placed on the cheek. The field junction was moved twice during treatment. She did well until a right parietal brain metastasis was diagnosed 3 years later. There was no evidence of local–regional disease.

Cutaneous melanoma of the nose and nasolabial fold is irradiated with the technique described for nasal vestibule, except that lower-energy electrons ($< 9\,$MeV) are used for the tumor bed. Field borders encompass nodal areas and the surgical bed with approximately 2-cm margins. Bolus is used to prevent underdosage to the primary tumor bed when 9-MeV electrons or lower-energy electrons are used.

An appositional electron or photon field may be used to treat the mid and lower neck nodes when indicated. The junctions between the fields are moved after the second and fourth radiation fractions to improve dose homogeneity.

Melanoma of some locations, such as lip or suboccipital region, may require irradiation with opposed–lateral photon portal (see Fig. 16.3). The use of missing tissue compensator or field-in-field technique is necessary in this setting to avoid hot spots, which can dramatically increase the risk of normal tissue injury by increasing both the fraction size and total dose ("double trouble").

Dose

The dose consists of 30 Gy in five fractions, two fractions per week, for elective irradiation. An additional fraction of 6 Gy may be added to a total dose of 36 Gy in six fractions for residual disease (see Fig. 16.4).

Dose Specification: at D_{max}

The dose to the spinal cord or brachial plexus should not exceed 24 Gy in four fractions.

Background Data

TABLE 16.4

PATTERN OF FAILURE AFTER ELECTIVE OR ADJUNCTIVE RADIOTHERAPY FOR CUTANEOUS MELANOMA

Status	D	N	D + N	DM	Median Follow-up	Total
Elective[a]	4	10	5	57	68 mo	157
Adjunctive[b]	5	5	3	81	78 mo	160
Total	9	15	8	138	—	317

D, dermal recurrence; N, nodal relapse; DM, distant metastasis.
[a]Stage I or II cutaneous melanoma treated with wide local excision of the primary followed by elective regional radiation.
[b]Patients with cervical nodal metastases treated with surgery and radiation.
Modified from Ballo MT, Bonnen MD, Garden AS, et al. Adjuvant irradiation for cervical lymph node metastases from melanoma. *Cancer* 2003;97:1789–1796; and Bonnen MD, Ballo MT, Myers JN, et al. Elective radiotherapy provides regional control for patients with cutaneous melanoma of the head and neck. *Cancer* 2004;100:383–389, with permission.

Figure 16.3 A 75-year-old man underwent repeated excisions of a lesion in the middle of the lower lip over a period of 1.5 years. Final diagnosis, after review of all slides, was melanoma, and the patient was referred to M.D. Anderson Cancer Center for further therapy. Review of the record of the latest surgery revealed that the excision margin was microscopically positive. It was thought that wide excision would involve removal of most of the lower lip, and therefore, the patient was offered radiotherapy. On physical examination, there was a scar in the center of the lower lip but no evidence of gross residual disease **(A).** There was no palpable adenopathy. An intraoral stent was used to separate the lips and to displace the tongue posteriorly and cranially **(B, C).** The lower lip and bilateral upper neck nodes (i.e., submental, submandibular, and subdigastric) were irradiated through left and right parallel–opposed cobalt 60 (^{60}Co) γ-rays fields. **D:** shows that with the aid of the stent the commissures (wired) and the oral tongue could be excluded from the portals. A maximum dose of 30 Gy was delivered in five fractions, twice a week, through the lateral fields. Following this, an additional fraction of 6 Gy was delivered to the tumor bed through an anterior appositional 8-MeV electron beam. A second intraoral stent was constructed; it served to flatten the lower lip and to open the mouth; in addition, lead alloy was inserted in the anterior part of the stent to shield the lower gum **(E, F).**

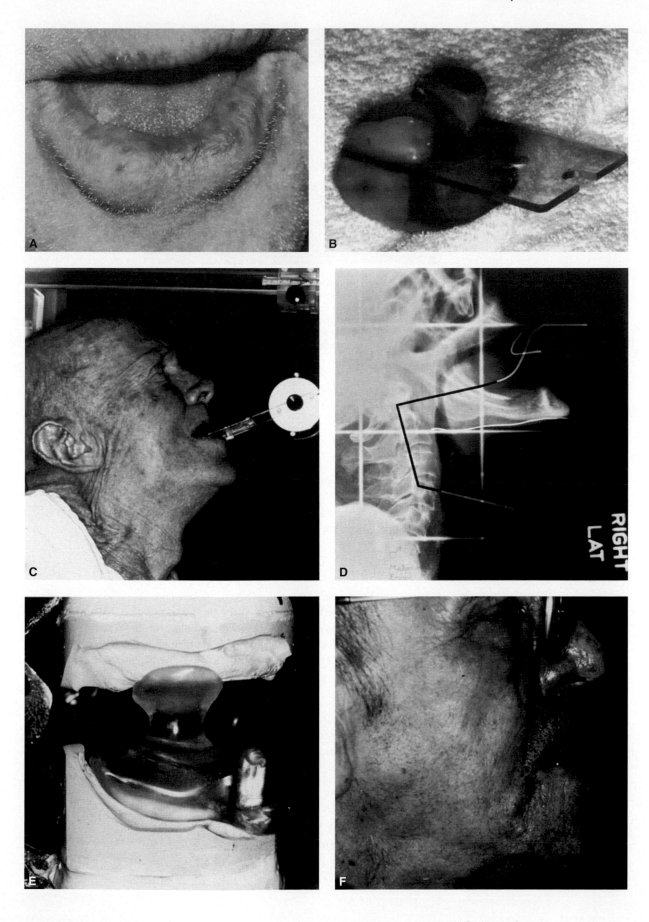

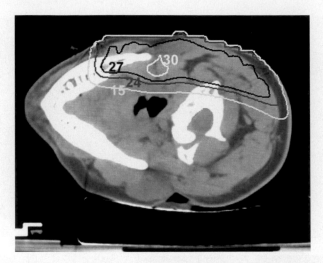

Figure 16.4 A 50-year-old man presented with a melanoma located 2 cm below the right earlobe. It was excised with negative margins. Histologic review showed spread of melanoma into the subcutaneous tissue. An additional lesion adjacent to the scar was found and excised as well. This second lesion was a satellite metastasis invading connective tissue. He had no palpable lymphadenopathy. He received adjuvant radiation to the right neck delivered with 12-MeV electrons to a dose of 30 Gy given in five fractions. The patient was treated in an open neck position. A representative axial isodose through the upper neck is shown.

MERKEL CELL CARCINOMA

Treatment Strategy

The primary therapy for Merkel cell carcinoma is surgery to establish tissue diagnosis and resect primary tumor and nodal masses.

Adjunctive postoperative radiotherapy is recommended in most patients because the rate of local–regional relapse after surgery is high.

Postoperative Radiotherapy

Target Volume

The initial target volume encompasses the surgical bed with 4- to 5-cm margins, except when the lesion is situated at or close to crucial structures (e.g., optic apparatus) and the draining lymphatics. For Merkel cell carcinoma of the head and neck region, the whole ipsilateral neck is irradiated.

The boost volume encompasses areas of known disease with 1- to 2-cm margins.

Setup and Field Arrangement

Setup and field arrangement varies with the site of the primary lesion. Most patients are treated with electron beams of appropriate energies, with patients immobilized in an open neck position, as described for cutaneous melanoma of the head and neck region.

Dose

The dose for the initial target volume is 46 Gy in 23 fractions.

The dose for the boost volume is 10 Gy in five fractions to the tumor bed, 14 Gy in seven fractions to positive section margins, or 20 Gy in ten fractions to bulky macroscopic disease.

Dose Specification: See "General Principles"

Background Data

TABLE 16.5

PATTERN OF FAILURE OF MERKEL CELL CARCINOMA BY TREATMENT METHODS

Method	No. of Patients	Local Recurrence	Regional Recurrence	Distant Recurrence	No. Recurrence
Surgery only	34	15 (44%)	29 (85%)	11 (32%)	1 (3%)
Surgery and radiation	26	3 (12%)	7 (27%)	11 (42%)	13 (50%)
Radiation only	6	1 (17%)	4 (44%)	2 (33%)	1 (17%)
P (radiation vs. no radiation)		0.01	<0.001	0.59	<0.001

Adapted from Gillenwater AM, Hessel AC, Morrison WH, et al. Merkel cell carcinoma of the head and neck: effect of surgical excision and radiation on recurrence and survival. *Arch Otolaryngol Head Neck Surg* 2001;127:149.

SUGGESTED READINGS

Abbatucci JS, Boulier N, Laforge T, et al. Radiation therapy of skin carcinomas: results of a hypofractionated irradiation schedule in 675 cases followed more than 2 years. *Radiother Oncol* 1989;14:113.

Ang KK, Peters LJ, Weber RS, et al. Postoperative radiotherapy for cutaneous melanoma of the head and neck region. *Int J Radiat Oncol Biol Phys* 1994;30:795.

Ashby MA, Pacella JA, De Groot R, et al. Use of a radon mould technique for skin cancer: results from the Peter MacCallum Cancer Institute (1975–1984). *Br J Radiol* 1989;62:608.

Ballo MT, Bonnen MD, Garden AS, et al. Adjuvant irradiation for cervical lymph node metastases from melanoma. *Cancer* 2003;97:1789.

Bentzen SM, Overgaard J, Thames HD, et al. Clinical radiobiology of malignant melanoma. *Radiother Oncol* 1989;16:169.

Bonnen MD, Ballo MT, Myers JN, et al. Elective radiotherapy provides regional control for patients with cutaneous melanoma of the head and neck. *Cancer* 2004;100:383.

Byers RM. The role of modified neck dissection in the treatment of cutaneous melanoma of the head and neck. *Arch Surg* 1986;121:1338.

Creagan ET, Cupps RE, Ivins JC, et al. Adjuvant radiation therapy for regional nodal metastases from malignant melanoma: a randomized, prospective study. *Cancer* 1978;42:2206.

de Wilt JH, Thompson JF, Uren RF, et al. Correlation between preoperative lymphscintigraphy and metastatic nodal disease sites in 362 patients with cutaneous melanomas of the head and neck. *Ann Surg* 2004;239:544.

Del Charco JO, Mendenhall WM, Parsons JT, et al. Carcinoma of the skin metastatic to the parotid area lymph nodes. *Head Neck* 1998;20:369.

Fitzpatrick PJ. Skin cancer of the head—treatment by radiotherapy. *J Otolaryngol* 1984;13:261.

Fitzpatrick PJ. Radiation therapy for tumors of the skin of the head and neck. In: Thawley SE, Panje WR, eds. *Comprehensive management of head and neck tumors*. Philadelphia: WB Saunders, 1987.

Fitzpatrick PJ, Thompson GA, Easterbrook WM, et al. Basal and squamous cell carcinoma of the eyelids and their treatment by radiotherapy. *Int J Radiat Oncol Biol Phys* 1984;10:449.

Gillenwater AM, Hessel AC, Morrison WH, et al. Merkel cell carcinoma of the head and neck: effect of surgical excision and radiation on recurrence and survival. *Arch Otolaryngol Head Neck Surg* 2001;127:149.

Harwood AR. Conventional fractionated radiotherapy for 51 patients with lentigo maligna and lentigo maligna melanoma. *Int J Radiat Oncol Biol Phys* 1983;9:1019.

Hietanen T, Nieminen S, Ekfors T, et al. Elective treatment of regional lymph nodes in malignant melanoma. *Strahlentherapie* 1985;161:1.

Hliniak A, Maciejewski B, Trott KR. The influence of the number of fractions, overall treatment time and field size on the local control of cancer of the skin. *Br J Radiol* 1983;56:596.

Kearsley JH, Harris TJ, Bourne RG. Radiotherapy for superficial skin cancer at the Queensland Radium Institute: famine in the land of plenty. *Int J Radiat Oncol Biol Phys* 1988;15:995.

Lejeune FJ. Surgery and radiotherapy for melanoma and skin neoplasms. *Curr Opin Oncol* 1990;2:407.

Lovett RD, Pérez CA, Shapiro SJ, et al. External irradiation of epithelial skin cancer. *Int J Radiat Oncol Biol Phys* 1990;19:235.

Mameghan H, Knittel T. Response of melanoma to heat and radiation therapy—a review of the literature and experience from The Prince of Wales Hospital, Sydney. *Med J Aust* 1988;149:474.

McCord MW, Mendenhall WM, Parsons JT, et al. Skin cancer of the head and neck with clinical perineural invasion. *Int J Radiat Oncol Biol Phys* 2000;47:89.

Medina JE, Ferlito A, Brandwein MS, et al. Current management of cutaneous malignant melanoma of the head and neck. *Acta Otolaryngol* 2002;122:900.

Mendenhall WM, Parsons JT, Mendenhall NP, et al. T2-T4 carcinoma of the skin of the head and neck treated with radical irradiation. *Int J Radiat Oncol Biol Phys* 1987;13:975.

Morrison WH, Garden AS, Ang KK. Radiation therapy for nonmelanoma skin carcinomas. *Clin Plast Surg* 1997;24:719.

Morrison WH, Peters LJ, Silva EG, et al. The essential role of radiation therapy in securing locoregional control of Merkel cell carcinoma. *Int J Radiat Oncol Biol Phys* 1990;19:583.

O'Brien CJ, Petersen-Schaefer K, Stevens G, et al. Adjuvant radiotherapy following neck dissection and parotidectomy for metastatic malignant melanoma. *Head Neck* 1997;19:589.

Overgaard J, Hansen PV, Von der Maase H. Some factors of importance in the radiation treatment of malignant melanoma. *Radiother Oncol* 1986;5:183.

Perez CA. Management of incompletely excised carcinoma of the skin. *Int J Radiat Oncol Biol Phys* 1991;20:903.

Petrovich Z, Kuisk H, Langholz B, et al. Treatment results and patterns of failure in 646 patients with carcinoma of the eyelids, pinna, and nose. *Am J Surg* 1987;154:447.

Petrovich Z, Parker R, Luxton G, et al. Carcinoma of the lip and selected sites of head and neck skin. A clinical study of 896 patients. *Radiother Oncol* 1987;8:11.

Sause WT, Cooper JS, Rush S, et al. Fraction size in external beam radiation therapy in the treatment of melanoma. *Int J Radiat Oncol Biol Phys* 1991;20:429.

Silva JJ, Tsang RW, Panzarella T, et al. Results of radiotherapy for epithelial skin cancer of the pinna: the Princess Margaret Hospital experience, 1982–1993. *Int J Radiat Oncol Biol Phys* 2000;47:451.

Solan MJ, Brady LW, Binnick SA, et al. Skin cancer. In: Perez CA, Brady LW, eds. *Principles and practice of radiation oncology*, 2nd ed. Philadelphia: JB Lippincott Co, 1992.

Stevens G, Thompson JF, Firth I, et al. Locally advanced melanoma: results of postoperative hypofractionated radiation therapy. *Cancer* 2000;88:88.

Tapley N. Radiation therapy with the electron beam. *Semin Oncol* 1981;8:49.

Tapley N, Fletcher GH. Applications of the electron beam in the treatment of cancer of the skin and lips. *Radiology* 1973;109:423.

Trott KR, Maciejewski B, Preuss-Bayer G, et al. Dose-response curve and split-dose recovery in human skin cancer. *Radiother Oncol* 1984;2:123.

Neck Node Metastasis from Unknown Primary

17

TREATMENT STRATEGY

The diagnosis is established by a nodal biopsy or aspiration, which is usually followed by a neck dissection and an examination under anesthesia, with biopsy of suspicious potential primary sites. Tonsillectomy is usually performed in the absence of suspicious lesions.

No further treatment is given when no occult primary is found and when there is only one small node (<3 cm) involved without extracapsular extension (ECE). Such patients are subjected to close follow-up to attempt early detection of a primary lesion that may manifest later on. The probability of primary tumor manifestation is estimated to be approximately 20%.

Irradiation to the ipsilateral neck alone is indicated if the probability of recurrence in the neck is high (e.g., presence of extracapsular nodal disease) but the histologic findings (e.g., adenocarcinoma) or nodal location (e.g., submental, submandibular, supraclavicular) indicate a low probability of a primary along the pharyngeal axis. It may also be considered when, because of advanced age or poor medical condition, the patient is not expected to tolerate large-volume irradiation to the pharyngeal axis.

Many centers currently recommend irradiation to the pharyngeal axis and the bilateral neck in all other cases. However, improvement in imaging techniques for detecting occult primary tumors, better characterization of the incidence of second primary tumors in patients with head and neck cancer, and the possibility to administer reirradiation using conformal radiotherapy technology bring into question the cost (including acute and long-term morbidity) *versus* benefit advantage of this strategy. Unfortunately, it is not feasible to conduct a randomized trial to address this issue, given the rarity of the disease.

Intensity-modulated radiation therapy (IMRT) may allow comprehensive bilateral therapy while providing parotid sparing.

COMPREHENSIVE RADIOTHERAPY

Target Volume

Initial Target Volume
The initial target volume is composed of nasopharynx, oropharynx, and bilateral neck nodes when the location of the involved nodes is indicative of a nasopharyngeal primary (upper posterior cervical chain) or when the clinical or histologic features suggest primary site origin from the oropharynx or nasopharynx, for example, a nonsmoker with a level II node, particularly with cystic squamous cell carcinoma, non-keratinizing "nasopharyngeal-like," or undifferentiated carcinoma.

In other cases, the initial target volume encompasses nasopharynx, oropharynx, hypopharynx, and bilateral neck nodes (see Figs. 17.1 and 17.2).

The boost volume encompasses the involved nodal bed.

Setup and Field Arrangement

The patient is immobilized in a supine position with a thermoplastic mask. Marking of surgical scar and shoulders facilitates portal design. The initial target volume is irradiated with lateral–opposed photon fields.

- *Superior border:* at mid sphenoid sinus or at the bottom of the pituitary fossa to encompass the roof of the nasopharynx.
- *Anterior border:* include posterior third of the nasal cavities and the anterior tonsillar pillars; 1-cm fall-off for the dissected neck.
- *Posterior border:* behind the spinous processes or more posteriorly to encompass the scar.
- *Inferior border:* just above the arytenoids or above the shoulders, depending on whether hypopharynx is part of the target volume.

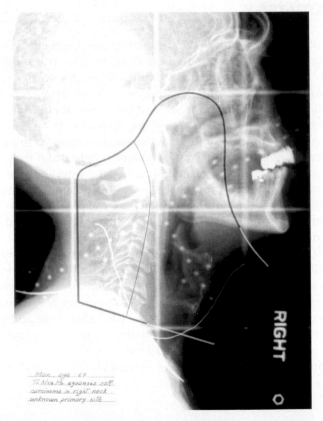

Figure 17.1 A 67-year-old man consulted his physician for mild hoarseness. He was found to have leuko-plakia on both true vocal cords. Examination of the neck revealed a 2-cm mobile lymph node in the right mid-jugular region. A fine-needle aspiration from this node showed poorly differentiated squamous cell carcinoma. A computed tomography (CT) scan confirmed the lymphadenopathy in the right jugular chain. An examination under anesthesia showed no abnormalities except for leukoplakia on both true vocal cords. Biopsy specimens were taken from the nasopharynx, tonsils, base of tongue, and both true vocal cords. All results were negative for malignancy. The biopsy specimens of the vocal cords showed only hyperkeratosis. The patient then under-went a right modified radical neck dissection. Histologic examination showed poorly differentiated squamous cell carcinoma in two of the 13 lymph nodes, one located in the midjugular area and the other one at the mid-posterior cervical chain. There was extracapsular extension (ECE) from the midjugular node. Stage: T0 N2b M0. Subsequently, this patient received postoperative radiotherapy. The entire pharyngeal axis and the upper and mid neck were treated bilaterally with opposed–lateral fields, as shown in the figure. The lower neck nodes were treated with an anterior appositional field. A total dose of 54 Gy was delivered, then the right neck received an additional irradiation dose of 63 Gy with an appositional electron field.

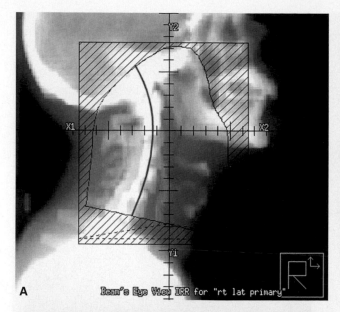

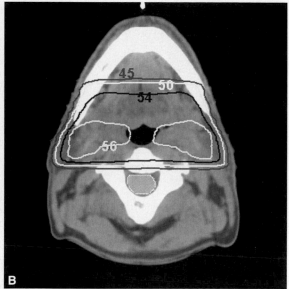

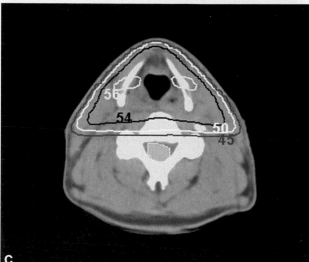

Figure 17.2 A 50-year-old man presented with bilateral jugular adenopathy, multiple left neck nodes, and a 1.5-cm right neck node. He underwent an examination under anesthesia, which did not reveal any primary tumor. Biopsy specimens of both tonsils, the nasopharynx, base of tongue, vallecula, and pyriform sinuses were negative for neoplasm. The patient then underwent bilateral neck dissections. The left neck dissection revealed four of 34 nodes positive for poorly differentiated carcinoma (levels 2 and 3), whereas the right neck dissection was negative for metastases. Stage: T0 pN2b M0. He received radiotherapy to both necks and the pharyngeal axis. A digitally reconstructed radiograph of the opposed–lateral field is shown **(A)**. Radiation was delivered with 6-MV photons in 1.8-Gy fractions to a dose of 54 Gy, with an off–spinal cord reduction to 41.4 Gy. A 3-mm tissue equivalent bolus material was placed over the scar. The posterior strips were supplemented with 9-MeV electron beams. Wedges were used to obtain a more homogenous distribution. Isodose distribution of the parallel photon beams at the level of the upper **(B)** and mid necks **(C)** are shown. The low neck was treated with a separate anterior field.

A matching anterior appositional photon field is used to treat the jugular nodes below the lateral portals and supraclavicular nodes.

The boost dose is usually delivered through one or two lateral appositional electron fields. The field borders are dictated by the extent of the nodal disease and surgery.

The upper neck nodal basin is treated with 12-MeV electron beams and the mid and lower neck nodes with 9-MeV electron beams or glancing photon fields.

Intensity-Modulated Radiation Therapy Planning

Most patients are now treated with IMRT to spare parotid function (see Fig. 17.3). In the event of gross nodal disease, the node(s) with 1-cm margin are outlined as clinical target volume 1 (CTV1). The neck compartments outside CTV1 with a 2-cm margin are delineated as CTV2. The remaining levels (IB, II, III, IV, and V) on the ipsilateral side, retropharyngeal nodes, and

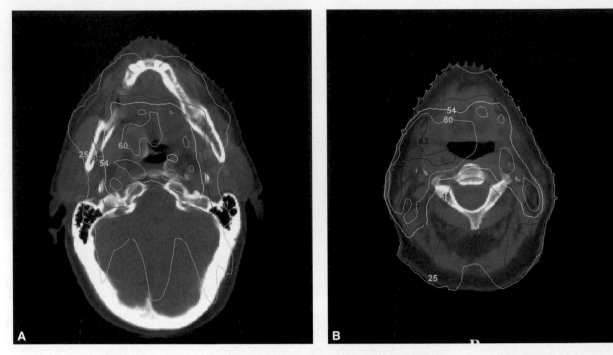

Figure 17.3 A 55-year-old woman presented with an asymptomatic right neck mass. Excision of this mass revealed moderately differentiated squamous cell carcinoma. An examination under anesthesia, with biopsies of the larynx, base of tongue, pharyngeal wall, and nasopharynx revealed several areas of dysplasia but no invasive carcinoma. Physical examination and CT scan showed changes related to the neck biopsy but no gross disease. Stage: T0 Nx M0. She was treated with intensity-modulated radiation therapy (IMRT) to a dose of 60 Gy to the involved nodal bed and a dose of 54 Gy to clinically uninvolved nodes and mucosa of the pharyngeal axis in 30 fractions. The spinal cord dose was limited to <45 Gy. Isodose distribution through the level of the parotid glands **(A)** and upper neck **(B)** are shown. The dose to a large volume of the parotid glands was <25 Gy.

contralateral levels II to V are contoured as CTV3. The pharyngeal axis (including the hypopharynx and larynx when indicated) is also delineated as CTV3 (see Fig. 17.4).

In cases where the nodal disease has been surgically excised, the original nodal tumor bed with a 1- to 2-cm margin is outlined as CTV1, the remaining dissected neck is CTV2, and CTV3 is similar to the definitive setting (see Fig. 17.5). Only in the case of extensive ECE or node excision, a smaller volume may receive a slightly higher dose (see Fig. 17.6).

Dose

The dose to the initial target volume is 54 Gy in 30 fractions.

The boost volume dose is an additional 6 to 10 Gy in three to five fractions in the postoperative setting. The boost dose can be delivered as a concomitant boost as second daily fractions, with a minimal interval of 6 hours, during the last week of the basic treatment course. In cases of gross nodal disease, a dose of 16 Gy in eight fractions is delivered (smaller fractions size if boost is given concomitantly).

With IMRT, the preference is to deliver treatment in 30 fractions to all targets. With gross nodal disease, the prescribed doses are 66 Gy to CTV1, 60 Gy to CTV2, and 54 Gy to CTV3. An electron boost of 2 to 4 Gy in one or two fractions can be delivered to the gross nodal disease to bring the dose to 70 Gy. In the postoperative setting, the prescribed doses are 60 Gy to CTV1 (smaller higher-risk regions may receive 63 to 66 Gy), 57 Gy to CTV2, and 54 Gy to CTV3.

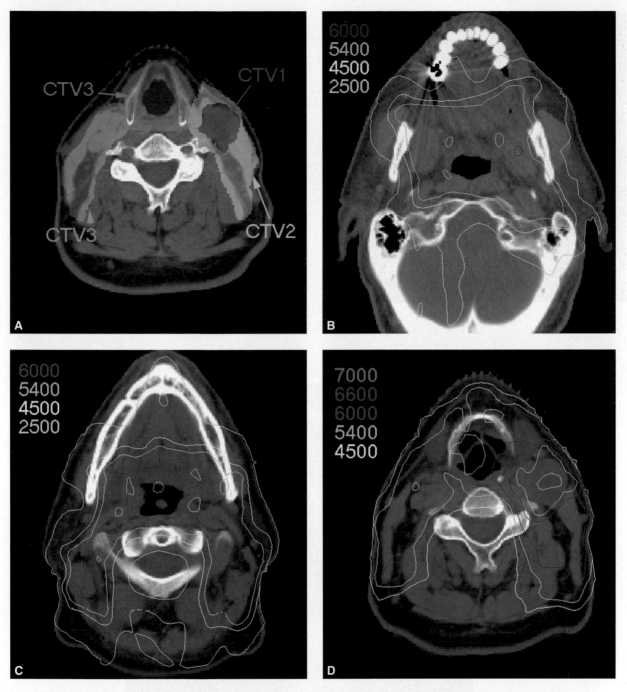

Figure 17.4 A 56-year-old man presented with T0 N2b squamous cell carcinoma of the left neck and received intensity-modulated radiation therapy (IMRT). The involved nodes and margin were identified as clinical target volume 1 (CTV 1) (69 Gy), the margin around CTV1 as CTV2 (60 Gy), and the pharyngeal axis, larynx, and remaining neck as CTV3 (54 Gy). **A:** Axial image at level III, demonstrating contour delineation. The larynx was outlined as a separate CTV3 to allow for the flexibility of planning to minimize hot spots in this structure. **B:** Axial image at the level of the inferior nasopharynx, with isodose distribution. The pharyngeal axis (including inferior nasopharynx, soft palate, and superior base of tongue), retropharyngeal nodes, and jugular fossae were identified as CTV3. The left (involved side) jugular fossa was included in the target, but not the right side, to allow more parotid sparing. **C:** Mid-oropharynx (including posterior wall, base of tongue, and bilateral tonsils) and bilateral neck and junction of oropharynx and hypopharynx (including vallecula and vestibules of the pyriform sinuses) **(D).** The mucosal sites and contralateral neck were in CTV3 (54 Gy); nodal level IB, IIA, and IIB were within CTV2 (60 Gy); and the gross node and margin were within CTV1 (69 Gy). The patient showed complete response and did not undergo neck dissection. He remains without disease for $3\frac{1}{2}$ years and has grade 1 xerostomia.

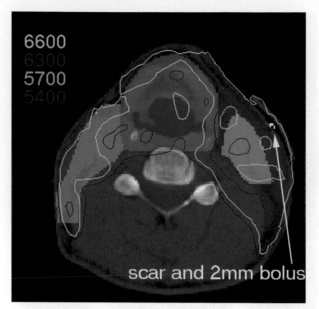

Figure 17.5 A 45-year-old man presented with a 4-cm left neck mass. It was thought to be a branchial cleft cyst and was excised, but histologic examination revealed squamous cell carcinoma. Complete workup showed no primary lesion and he was treated with intensity-modulated radiation therapy (IMRT). An axial CT image is shown with contours and isodose distribution. Clinical target volume 1 (CTV1) (*green*), delineated on the basis of imaging of the original nodal location, received a dose of 63 Gy. CTV2 (*purple*) represented margin around the original nodal bed that encompassed the nodal level at risk. The contour was drawn to just under the skin surface at the surgical scar (wired) and bolus was applied for treatment planning. CTV3 included the contralateral neck nodes (*maize*) and putative mucosal sites (*blue*) at the level shown. The doses delivered to CTV2 and CTV3 were 57 Gy and 54 Gy, respectively, in 30 fractions.

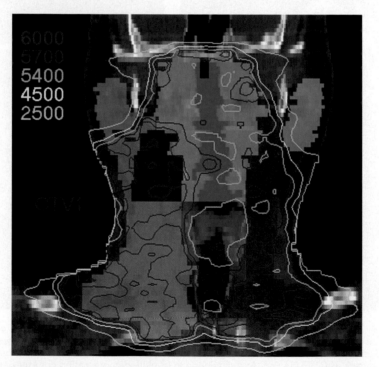

Figure 17.6 A 66-year-old man, former smoker, presented with right level II adenopathy. He underwent an examination under anesthesia with bilateral tonsillectomies, biopsies of the right and left nasopharynx and base of tongue and right pyriform sinus, and a right neck dissection. All the results of the mucosal biopsies (including the tonsil specimens) were negative, and the neck dissection revealed two level II nodes (largest 3 cm) positive for squamous cell carcinoma. He was treated with postoperative intensity-modulated radiation therapy (IMRT), which was delivered to the entire volume (including level 4 and supraclavicular nodes) in 30 fractions. Contours and isodose distribution are shown on a coronal image. Clinical target volume 1 (CTV 1), encompassing the right level IIA region with margin, receive a dose of 60 Gy (*blue* contour). An additional dose of 4 Gy in two fractions was delivered to level II nodal region, with 12-MeV electron beam. The remaining dissected right neck received a dose of 57 Gy (*yellow*). The left neck, pharyngeal axis, and larynx were defined as CTV3 and received a dose of 54 Gy. CTV3 was outlined as three separate structures for flexibility of planning. Notably, portions of the larynx received a slightly lower (within 5%) dose. He is without disease over 3 years from his treatment. He does have corrected chemical hypothyroidism and also has diminished taste and minimal xerostomia.

Dose Specification: See "General Principles"

Background Data

TABLE 17.1

THERAPY FAILURES BY NECK SURGERY AND IRRADIATION TECHNIQUE

Irradiation Site	Incisional Biopsy	Excisional Biopsy	Modified Neck Dissection	Radical Neck Dissection	Total
Neck only	0/2	2/4	1/6	4/8	7/20
Nasopharynx and oropharynx	1/11	0/3	1/6	2/6	4/26
Nasopharynx, oropharynx and hypopharynx	1/10	0/15	2/12	0/10	3/47
Total	2/23	2/22	4/24	6/24	14/93

Note: The 14 patients who failed therapy are shown both by the type of surgical procedure performed and irradiation technique used. A greater proportion of patients failed after having received irradiation to the neck only (7/20), as compared to those treated to the naso-oropharynx (4/26) or naso-, oro-, and hypopharynx (3/47). No correlation is seen between the incidence of failure and type of surgery used.
From Carlson LS, Fletcher GH, Oswald MJ. Guidelines for radiotherapeutic techniques for cervical metastases from an unknown primary. *Int J Radiat Oncol Biol Phys* 1986;12:2101–2110, with permission.

TABLE 17.2

CERVICAL LYMPH NODE METASTASIS: UNKNOWN PRIMARY CANCER

Site	Surgery	Irradiation	Combined Treatment
Nasopharynx	2	—	—
Maxillary antrum	—	—	1
Tonsil or faucial arch	4	—	1
Base of tongue, valleculae	4	—	—
Oral cavity, salivary glands	2	2	—
Aryepiglottic fold, epiglottis	1	—	1
Hypopharynx	6	1	1
Cervical esophagus	1	—	—
Thyroid	1	—	—
Total head and neck	21/104	3/52	4/28
New primaries	(20%)	(6%)	(14%)
Primaries below clavicles	5	3	1

Note: Location of primary lesions appearing after various treatments: 37 patients. Three years to unlimited follow-up. Data from the M.D. Anderson Cancer Center.
From Fletcher GH, Jesse RH, Perez CA. Cervical lymph node metastasis: unknown primary cancer. In: Fletcher GH, ed. *Textbook of radiotherapy.* 3rd ed. Philadelphia, PA: Lea & Febiger, 1980, with permission.

TABLE 17.3

REGIONAL FAILURE AND MUCOSAL SITE OCCURRENCE: LITERATURE REVIEW

First Author (yr)	No. of Patients	Neck Treatment	Regional Failure (%)	Radiation Technique	Primary Site Occurrence (%)
Grau (2000)	250	X—224	X—50%	M—224	M—13%
		X + S—26	X + S—38% (5-yr a)	N—26	N—23%
Weir (1995)	144	X—144	X—49% (5-yr a)	M—59	M—2%
				N—85	N—7%
Colletier (1998)	136	X + S—136	X + S—9% (c)	M—120	8%
				N—16	
Erkal (2001)	126	X—56	A—22% (c)	M—119	M—10%
		X + S—70		N—7	N—14%
Maulard (1992)	113	X + S—113	X + S—14% (c)	M—113	10%
Marcial-Vega (1990)	72	X—41	X—54% (c)	M—53	M—25%
		X + S—31	X + S—58%	N—19	N—16%
Reddy (1997)	52	X—21	X—52% (c)	M—36	M—8%
		X + S—31	X + S—10%	N—16	N—44%

X, radiation alone (following biopsy); X + S, radiation and neck dissection; A, all patients; M, radiation to bilateral necks and mucosal sites; N, radiation to the involved neck only; 5-yr a, 5-year actuarial; c, crude rate. Data from the M.D. Anderson Cancer Center.

SUGGESTED READINGS

Barrie JR, Knapper WH, Strong EW. Cervical nodal metastases of unknown origin. *CA Cancer J Clin* 1971;21:112.

Bataini JP, Rodriguez J, Jaulerry C, et al. Treatment of metastatic neck nodes secondary to an occult epidermoid carcinoma of the head and neck. *Laryngoscope* 1987;97:1080.

Colletier PJ, Garden AS, Morrison WH, et al. Postoperative radiation for squamous cell carcinoma metastatic to cervical lymph nodes from an unknown primary site: outcomes and patterns of failure. *Head Neck* 1998;20:674–681.

Coster JR, Foote RL, Olsen KD, et al. Cervical node metastases of squamous cell carcinoma of unknown origin: indications for withholding radiation therapy. *Int J Radiat Oncol Biol Phys* 1992;23:743.

Davidson BJ, Spiro RH, Patel S, et al. Cervical metastases of occult origin: the impact of combined modality therapy. *Am J Surg* 1994;168:395–399.

Dickson R, Vargas DR. Occult primary of the head and neck. *J Otolaryngol* 1979;110:427.

Erkal HS, Mendenhall WM, Amdur RJ, et al. Squamous cell carcinomas metastatic to cervical lymph nodes from an unknown head-and-neck mucosal site treated with radiation therapy alone or in combination with neck dissection. *Int J Radiat Oncol Biol Phys* 2001;50:55.

Fletcher GH, Jesse RH, Perez CA. Cervical lymph node metastasis: unknown primary cancer. In: Fletcher GH, ed. *Textbook of radiotherapy*, 3rd ed. Philadelphia, PA: Lea & Febiger, 1980.

Friesland S, Lind MG, Lundgren J, et al. Outcome of ipsilateral treatment for patients with metastases to neck nodes of unknown origin. *Acta Oncol* 2001;40:24.

Grau C, Johansen L, Jakobsen J, et al. Cervical lymph node metastases from unknown primary tumours. Results from a national survey by the Danish Society for Head and Neck Oncology. *Radiother Oncol* 2000;55:121.

Jacobs CD, Pinto HA. Head and neck cancer with an occult primary tumor. *N Engl J Med* 1992;326:58.

MacComb WS. Diagnosis and treatment of metastatic cervical cancerous nodes from an unknown primary site. *Am J Surg* 1972;124:441.

Marcial-Vega VA, Cardenes H, Perez CA, et al. Cervical metastases from unknown primaries: radiotherapeutic management and appearance of subsequent primaries. *Int J Radiat Oncol Biol Phys* 1990;19:919.

Maulard C, Housset M, Brunel P, et al. Postoperative radiation therapy for cervical lymph node metastases from an occult squamous cell carcinoma. *Laryngoscope* 1992;102:884.

Mendenhall WM, Mancuso AA, Parsons JT, et al. Diagnostic evaluation of squamous cell carcinoma metastatic to cervical lymph nodes from an unknown head and neck primary site. *Head Neck* 1998;20:739.

Reddy SP, Marks JE. Metastatic carcinoma in the cervical lymph nodes from an unknown primary site: results of bilateral neck plus mucosal irradiation vs. ipsilateral neck irradiation. *Int J Radiat Oncol Biol Phys* 1997;37:797.

Rusthoven KE, Koshy M, Paulino AC. The role of fluorodeoxyglucose positron emission tomography in cervical lymph node metastases from an unknown primary tumor. *Cancer* 2004;101:2641.

Strasnick B, Moore DM, Abemayor E, et al. Occult primary tumors. The management of isolated submandibular lymph node metastases. *Arch Otolaryngol Head Neck Surg* 1990;116:173.

Wang R, Goepfert H, Barber AE, et al. Unknown primary squamous cell carcinoma metastatic to the neck. *Arch Otolaryngol Head Neck Surg* 1990;116:1388.

Weir L, Keane T, Cummings B, et al. Radiation treatment of cervical lymph node metastases from an unknown primary: an analysis of outcome by treatment volume and other prognostic factors. *Radiother Oncol* 1995;35:206.

Subject Index